# Her Healthy Heart

# Praise for Linda Ojeda's
## MENOPAUSE WITHOUT MEDICINE

D r. Linda Ojeda has written a book that should be read by any woman concerned with planning for the future.... *Menopause Without Medicine* could be described as a 'wellness bible.' It really gives women an overall picture of their bodies and how to keep [them] running to optimum proficiency. As menstruation is the beginning of a woman's reproductive cycle, menopause should be seen as the culmination, not the bitter ending. **—Whole Life Times**

M *enopause Without Medicine* is more than another overview of symptoms: it probes the underlying beliefs and concepts about aging which can prove self-defeating, and presents suggestions and programs designed to combat and minimalize the depression and stress associated with menopause. **—The Midwest Book Review**

E xemplifying recent, more enlightened attitudes toward menopause, Ojeda regards her subject as a part of the natural evolution of a woman's body, not as a condition to treat or mask. She believes further that menopause is not the death of womanhood but the birth of a new life stage. Hence, she focuses on wellness, recommending natural ways—including dietary modifications, vitamins, exercise, and attitudinal adaptation—to cope with the body's changes during menopause.... She also packs the book with appendixes, charts, recipes, and suggested resources. These, combined with the accessible, reassuring, and female tone of her writing, make this a very useful resource. **—Booklist**

A n excellent book.... It is often easy to find books that tell us how wonderful estrogen is for menopausal women. It is not so easy to find a book that talks about alternatives. Linda Ojeda has written such a book. **—Miriam Diamond,**
**Elizabeth Blackwell Health Center for Women**

## DEDICATION

*To my family, who fills my heart with laughter and love:*
*Roland and Joseph Ojeda*
*Jillian and Erik Peterson*

# HER HEALTHY HEART

## A Woman's Guide to Preventing and Reversing Heart Disease *Naturally*

Linda Ojeda, Ph.D.

Hunter House PUBLISHERS

Hunter House Inc., Publishers
P.O. Box 2914
Alameda CA 94501-0914

**Library of Congress Cataloging-in-Publication Data**
Ojeda, Linda.
Her healthy heart : a woman's guide to preventing and reversing heart disease naturally / Linda Ojeda. — 1st ed.
p. cm.
Includes bibliographical references and index.
ISBN 0-89793-226-9 (cloth). — ISBN 0-89793-225-0 (pbk.)
1. Heart—Diseases. 2. Women—Diseases. 3. Heart—Diseases—Prevention.
4. Women—Health and hygiene. 5. Heart—Diseases—Alternative treatment.
I. Title.
RC669.O37 1998
616.1'2'0082—dc21 98-35412
CIP

**Project Credits**
Cover Design: Knockout Design, Cameron Park, CA
Production Coordinator: Wendy Low    Editorial Coordinator: Kiran Rana
Production Intern: Jennifer Gall    Editorial Intern: Jennifer Huffaker
Copyeditor: Rosana Francescato    Proofreader: Lee Rappold
Indexing: Kathy Talley-Jones
Marketing: Corrine M. Sahli, Susan Markey
Publicity: Marisa Spatafore
Customer Support: Christina Arciniega, Joel R. Irons
Order Fulfillment: A & A Quality Shipping
Publisher: Kiran S. Rana

Printed and Bound by Publishers Press, Salt Lake City, UT
Manufactured in the United States of America

9  8  7  6  5  4  3  2  1      First Edition

# Contents

## PART ONE: All Women Are at Risk

PART FOUR: Designing Your Program for Heart Health

# Acknowledgments

I owe a debt of gratitude to the many scientists, researchers, doctors, and allied health professionals who have contributed to the vast research on heart disease. Without their dedication, a book like this could not have been written.

Thank you to all the women in both northern and southern California who helped me distribute and who participated in a questionnaire asking women about their diets and knowledge about heart disease. Special acknowledgment to my neighbor Ursula Deuster, to Marilyn Grant and the women in her exercise classes in Hacienda Heights and Whittier, to Jillian Peterson and her co-workers at Rose Drive Friends Church in Yorba Linda, to the women in my exercise classes at Nautilus of Marin, to my friends at the Sausalito Woman's Club, and to the women at Hillside Church of Marin.

I am also grateful to

— my family and circle of close friends, who offered encouraging words and allowed me solitude when I needed it;

— my small group who prayed for me during the span from my initial proposal to the completion of the manuscript, thanks: Leta Altom, Jackie Sue, Denise Bowman Wylie, Leigh Schlichting, and Linda Nordling;

— my editors, Lisa Bach and Rosana Francescato, thank you for your insightful suggestions, valuable input, and painstaking work;

— the staff at Hunter House who were involved in the production process: Wendy Low, Jennifer Huffaker, Jennifer Gall;

— and to my publisher and friend, Kiran Rana; thank you for seeing the potential of this information and taking yet another chance.

# Part One

# ALL WOMEN
# ARE AT RISK

# Introduction

Above all else, guard your heart for it is the wellspring of life.

PROVERBS 4:23

T he reason for telling the story about women and heart disease is simple. It's killing us in record numbers, and much heart disease can be prevented and reversed if only we make minor changes in our diets, lifestyles, and attitudes. We can all recite the prescription for maintaining a healthy heart: a low-fat, low-cholesterol, low-salt diet, with regular exercise and minimum stress. But if this is all we're doing for our hearts, it's not enough. Not only is this commonly quoted formula inadequate for women—parts of it may not even apply. There is so much about heart health that has yet to be told, so much that has been omitted in the general information that is recycled in medical pamphlets and monthly magazines.

I have always been a little ahead of my time when it comes to presenting health information to women. When I study the scientific literature concerning nutritional remedies and see how little of this information filters down to women who need it, I feel an obligation to spread the word. My first book, *Exclusively Female*, was a pioneer endeavor that examined the nutritional treatment of a variety of menstrual problems. Many of you may not even remember a time when such studies were unavailable, but until recently, women did not know that they could change the way they feel before, during, and after their periods by altering their diet and lifestyle. My next book, *Menopause Without Medicine*, also stood alone on bookstore shelves for a long time before the now overwhelming deluge of menopause books arrived. My little weight-loss book for adolescents, *Safe Dieting for Teens*, still remains one-of-a-kind, since it is intended specifically for teens to read rather than for their parents.

Women and heart disease is an issue that has been overlooked and underplayed by the scientific community of researchers and doctors. Much is known, especially regarding diet and specific nutrients, and a lack of access to this information can severely lower the quality of your life. Much of the information in *Her Healthy Heart* will be new to you, but if you continue to watch the news and pay attention to reports on heart disease, you will see continued confirmation of this information.

What you don't know *can* kill you. The idea that women are immune to heart disease has been exposed as a myth, yet women remain unaware that this disease is shortening our lives in record numbers. The American Heart Association reported in the fall of 1997 that only 8 percent of American women think they are in danger of heart disease and stroke, a condition closely related to heart disease, despite the fact that those diseases kill twice as many women as what is perceived as the biggest threat—cancer.

Despite its prevalence and seriousness, we know far less about heart disease in women than we do about heart disease in men. Health and medical research has virtually ignored the female population, disregarding our obvious anatomical and hormonal differences. Most of the available data is based on research conducted on men and then extrapolated to women. Only recently have scientists admitted that women and men may not be the same when it comes to diagnosis, treatment, and prevention of heart disease. The scattered studies that have been done using women suggest that discrepancies do in fact exist.

When it comes to heart disease, women's and men's experiences do not compare. For years we have been told our hormones offer protection from the disease. Not true; women are not exempt. And this is just the tip of the iceberg when it comes to the facts concerning women's hearts. While women tend to be stricken later in life than men, their chance for recovery is dimmer. Because women's early warning signs for an impending attack are not always the same as those for men, both women and their doctors frequently ignore crucial signals. Diagnostic methods are less accurate for women; even after being diagnosed, women are unlikely to be treated as aggressively as men, and they appear to be less receptive to the wonders of surgery and drugs.

Risk factors for heart disease such as smoking and weight gain pose a greater threat to women. And the low-fat diet that is heralded as the foundation of heart health for men may not provide similar benefits to women. In addition, let's not overlook the complications that go with pregnancy, menopause, and hormone therapy.

What about hormone therapy after menopause? Does it lower the risk of heart disease? Some researchers quickly respond "yes" and others cautiously say, "I'm not so sure." Long-term studies have only just begun to evaluate how our hormones alter the picture of heart disease; it will be decades before we have definitive answers. Those of us who are over fifty are not in a position to wait and must base our decisions on the information that is available right now.

The issue of hormones is not clear-cut at this time. Studies do show that women taking hormones have 50 percent less heart disease. What is not so obvious is why. These same women are also better educated, are financially advantaged, and take better care of their health than those who do not take or cannot afford hormones. Until we have a study that accounts for all these factors, we won't know for sure whether hormones protect women from heart disease or whether women who take hormones tend to be healthier to begin with.

I want to be clear that I am *not* against the use of hormones for some women; women who are at risk for osteoporosis and heart disease or who have unbearable menopausal symptoms may require exogenous hormones. I do find unconscionable the indiscriminate prescribing of hormones for women who may not need them, in spite of the risks associated with taking hormones.

Heart disease in women is rampant not because of lowered female hormones but because of long-term assaults on the body, mind, and soul. Overwhelming evidence indicates that heart disease is multifactorial in causation and that diet, lifestyle behaviors, and attitudes each play costarring roles. This reality is no longer in question. Countless well-documented studies prove that a diet rich in specific nutrients, an active lifestyle, the ability to reduce or manage stress, and the ability to enjoy life and other people participate equally in slowing down the progression of heart disease, lowering blood pressure, reducing fatty blockages, and minimizing clotting in the blood.

Scientists have identified specific risk factors that increase an individual's probability of developing heart disease. I am sure you know what the main ones are: elevated cholesterol, high blood pressure, diabetes, and lack of exercise. What is not generally known is that one-third of all heart attacks occur in people who don't show any of these well-established risk factors. What is going on? Obviously, there is more to heart disease than what we have been told.

Some things we know with relative certainty. Our diet, for example, can either harm us or protect us. Few researchers question the fact that the all-American diet clogs arteries. The food we eat on a regular basis can set in motion a destructive process that causes cholesterol to creep into and close the arteries leading to the heart. There is a strong body of evidence that ties the beginning of the current epidemic of heart disease to the widespread use of hydrogenated fats and refined sugars, plus the omission of fresh antioxidant nutrients, over the last seventy years. Sadly, we are infecting other countries with our destructive dietary habits. The World Health Organization (WHO) predicts that heart disease will soar worldwide over the next twenty-five years, in part because of lethal habits spreading from the United States. We are exporting an unhealthy diet in the form of fast foods and packaged products. According to a WHO spokesperson, "Developing nations are overcoming malnutrition and infection only to fall prey to chronic diseases like heart disease and cancer."

Food can also exert curative powers. Good food contains restorative and healing properties. A nutritious diet can shield us with a chemical armor from the artery destroyers and even go one step further to reverse damage already inflicted. Certain foods can reduce cholesterol, thin the blood, dissolve clots, lower blood pressure, and keep blood sugar under control. Studies around the world show that people who follow certain dietary practices enjoy a life free from the fear of heart disease.

In terms of dietary recommendations for protection against coronary heart disease, people have been told simply to eat a very low fat, no-cholesterol diet. Evolving research shows that this paradigm is limited, to say the least. The diet-heart relationship is much more complex. Other important nutrients, such as vitamins A, B, C, and E, minerals such as calcium and magnesium, essential fats, and plant nutrients called phytochemicals also affect the heart. Without them, the heart is compromised; when they are added to the diet either in food or as supplements, the heart thrives.

A great deal of information about diseases of the heart and circulatory system is not widely published. Tucked away in a slew of studies in medical journals is extensive research concerning specific vitamins and minerals that has not been made available to the general public with the same enthusiasm as has, say, information about hormone therapy. Many researchers and doctors who have made important experimental findings on the heart benefits of specific nutrients hold back from endorsing supplementing the diet with vitamins and minerals while they wait for additional studies. I am not against further verification of research, but it is interesting to note that the same standards do not appear to apply when it comes to drugs that can turn a profit. The blanket endorsement of hormones for women over fifty is a prime example. The medical community freely and without hesitation encourages women to take hormones for their hearts, bones, and menopausal symptoms, even though the increased risk of cancer associated with taking those hormones hovers over their heads like a dark cloud. Yet, doctors and scientists remain cautious about recommending a harmless multivitamin tablet or antioxidant, when it could dramatically affect women's future health. It scares me that women feel protected from heart disease by popping a hormone pill but neglect the more important lifestyle and behavioral changes that could affect their lives in a positive way.

Whether or not to take supplements has been the subject of endless debates since I entered the field of nutrition some thirty years ago. Dietitians and nutritionists agree that the ideal place to get important nutrients is from food. The plain truth is that few women are eating the requisite number of foods on a daily basis. With advancing age the challenge is even greater, since nutrients are not as well absorbed. Hard as I try, I find it a major struggle to eat three servings of fruits and five of vegetables a day. Unless you work harder at it than I do, you will probably need to find additional ways to get these nutrients also. Not getting enough of them sets you up for deficiency and the repercussions that inevitably follow. The research is overwhelming that specific vitamins can prevent heart disease even more effectively than a low-fat diet. Once you read the information presented in *Her Healthy Heart*, I think you will agree. If you are still unsure about what to do, remember Pascal's wager from Philosophy 101? This French philosopher opted to believe in God, on the grounds that he had everything to gain if he was right and nothing to lose if he was wrong. If he didn't believe, he lost everything. You, too, have nothing to lose and much to gain.

Women, like men, need more than food to function as completely healthy beings. As crucial as the physical body is to life, we cannot overlook our emotions and our spiritual nature. To ignore these areas is to deny several possible factors that may be damaging our hearts. There is growing evidence that depression, hostility, isolation, and loss are risk factors for heart disease. Recognizing destructive behavioral patterns that continue to manifest in our lives and erode our health may dramatically contribute to the healing process. Even tapping into one's spiritual nature has been scientifically proven to exert discernable chemical changes in the body that alter its health. Could it be that science is finally recognizing the ancient truth that a whole and healthy person is one who learns to balance and integrate the body, mind, and soul?

*Her Healthy Heart* documents the expanding evidence about the multiple factors that contribute to a troubled heart as well as those that contribute to a healthy heart. The primary focus of this book, however, is on the prevention of heart disease through diet and supplemental nutrients. This is not a medical book, therefore I will not address the diagnosis and treatment of heart disease. You will find several wonderful books on the market that speak to the medical aspects of various heart problems, and I have listed my favorites in the reference section. If you have suffered from heart disease, the dietary information still applies, but make sure you discuss your program with your cardiologist or physician.

Heart disease can end your life in an instant, but it develops over years. The sooner we understand that what we eat, what we do, and how we behave strongly shifts the balance between a healthy heart and a troubled heart, the closer we are not just to strengthening our heart but to enriching our entire life. My primary goal is to share the data that is currently available and to provide practical suggestions that you can easily integrate into your daily routine.

Even small changes in your diet and lifestyle have the potential of adding years to your life.

I will provide the principles you need for designing your own plan. What I will not give you are structured menus to follow. This is not a rulebook but a guide. It is my experience that preplanned menus work only for a short time, and then are abandoned because they are too foreign to our tastes and are not convenient in the real world. In addition, people have individual dietary needs. It is not difficult to structure a healthy diet that satisfies your palate and that you can adjust to your schedule and lifestyle. But you will have to spend time evaluating what you are eating and what needs revamping. Only you can do this: this is not *my* program, it's *yours*.

Now it's up to you to determine how important your health is to you and what you want to do about it. Don't jump in too quickly or try to change your life overnight. Read the material, think about it, and start with one area at a time. There may be many areas that need attention. You may start by altering your diet or decide to add supplements. You may read something that touches your heart emotionally and choose to take a path that leads you to work on inappropriate or unhealthy behaviors. You may feel drawn to investigate your spiritual nature. There are many roads leading to heart health. Are you ready to start your journey?

# 1

# HEART DISEASE
# KILLS WOMEN TOO

Have patience with all that is unresolved in your heart
and try to love the questions themselves.

—RAINER MARIA RILKE

## THE HARD FACTS

W omen do not escape diseases of the heart. The fact is
that 2.5 million American women are hospitalized
annually for cardiovascular disease, and approximately
five hundred thousand women die of it each year. One in nine
women between the ages of forty-five and sixty-four shows some sign
of heart disease or blood vessel weakness, and the ratio escalates to
one in three by the time a woman reaches sixty-five, then levels off.
Women fear breast cancer more than any other single disease, yet
their risk of succumbing to heart disease is six times greater than
their risk of dying of the dreaded cancer. Nearly twice as many
women die of heart disease and stroke than of all forms of cancer
combined. (See figure 1.)

## GENDER DIFFERENCES

What we know about women and heart disease is a little sketchy.
The research on the subject has concentrated almost exclusively on
men, and women have remained in the shadows of science and public interest. Twenty-five times as many men as women have been

**Figure 1.** Leading Causes of Death in American Women

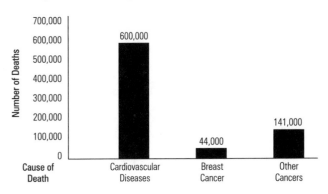

studied in major studies exploring the causes, risk factors, diagnosis, and treatment of heart disease, and the effects of dietary and lifestyle measures in preventing and reversing heart disease. In the past, researchers did not include women in their studies because they felt that menstruating women complicated test results with their erratic monthly hormonal fluctuations. What these researchers failed to acknowledge was that these same bothersome hormones that potentially skewed the data actually might influence and alter the way heart disease manifests in women. Researchers simply didn't think women were worth investigating.

I don't mean to suggest that women are totally unrepresented in the literature. A handful of studies, some on a major scale, provide clues that establish our uniqueness when it comes to heart health. But this is just the beginning. Major long-term studies that include women are currently under way, and this ongoing research will take into consideration the female anatomy, hormonal factors, and other gender-specific variables that relate to the prevention and treatment of this killer disease. Our day is coming, but until we have definitive answers, we must utilize the information at hand. Preliminary findings suggest that some of what we know about men and heart disease is applicable to women, and, as you might guess, some is not.

## SYMPTOMS

Let's face it: even if we have memorized the symptoms of a heart attack, the reality is not etched in our minds. Maybe we would take notice if we doubled over from chest pain, but our symptoms mask themselves more than men's. Women are likely to mistake the muddied signs of heart disease for acute indigestion, extreme fatigue, a panic attack, or the ever-popular diagnosis of stress—and passively wait for the discomfort to go away.

What's even scarier is that doctors don't necessarily catch on to a woman's symptoms any better than we do. Chest pain, the classic wake-up call for heart victims, actually signals a heart attack more frequently in women than in men, yet fewer women are referred for further diagnostic testing after complaining to their doctors of chest pain.

Without a doubt, there is evidence to support sex bias in the diagnosis and treatment of heart disease. In a large study conducted in Massachusetts and Maryland, complaints of eighty-five thousand women were reviewed. Women admitted to the hospital diagnosed with myocardial infarction (heart attack), unstable or stable angina (discomfort caused by reduced blood to the heart), chronic ischemic heart disease (reduced blood flow to the heart), and chest pain were less likely than men to undergo coronary angiography, coronary angioplasty, or coronary surgery. Another study published in the same journal determined that women had chest pain before a heart attack as frequently as and with more debilitating effects than men did, yet women underwent cardiac catheterization only half as often. Both studies controlled for age, race, economic status, and coexisting diseases.

Once women suffer a heart attack, they are then provided the same treatment as men. According to Bernadine Healy, M.D., former director of the National Institutes of Health, these findings demonstrate the workings of the "Yentl Syndrome." In other words, after a woman shows that she is like a man by having a heart attack or severe coronary disease, then she is treated like a man. In case you didn't see the movie *Yentl*, Barbra Streisand portrayed a young heroine who was allowed to attend school and study the Talmud only after she disguised herself as a man. Dr. Healy feels this film depicts the frustration women have experienced for decades trying to prove themselves equal to (or the same as) men before they get proper attention and respect.

## SURVIVAL RATE

*Question:* Do you know the first symptom of a heart attack? *Answer:* Sudden death. The prognosis for survival is less encouraging for women than for men. Tragically, their first symptom may also be their last. Depending on the study, it is estimated that 30 to 45 percent of women between the ages of thirty-five and sixty-four who have heart attacks die immediately or within one year of the heart attack, as opposed to 10 to 16 percent of the men in the same age bracket.

Experts aren't quite sure why women fare worse than men after experiencing a heart attack, but several theories seem plausible. As already mentioned, the diagnosis may be postponed because neither the woman nor the doctor suspects heart disease when a woman experiences chest pain or indigestion. In addition, women's coronary arteries are smaller and narrower than men's are, so it takes less plaque to accumulate and build up on the wall of the artery to create a life-threatening problem. Another problem is that women are generally older than men are when they succumb to their first heart attack and thus often have other confounding diseases, which lessens their chance of recovery and complicates treatment.

Women do not bounce back and resume normal activities as easily or quickly as men. Whether the causes are physical or emotional is up for grabs. Because women are typically older than men are when they have their attack, complications may prolong recovery. Women are also more likely to suffer from anxiety and depression following a heart attack or surgery. The reason why isn't clear: Are they more distraught because they take longer to recuperate, or do they take longer to recuperate because they are more distraught? Men usually rely on their wives to care for them after a heart attack, but who is available to provide TLC for women?

## DIAGNOSIS AND TREATMENT

Diagnostic methods, stress tests, and electrocardiograms are all used with a great degree of reliability for men, yet when it comes to women, their accuracy is questionable. Sometimes test abnormalities in women are difficult to interpret because, once again, the established standards have been based solely on the male body.

For reasons yet to be explained, interventional procedures like coronary bypass surgery and balloon angioplasty used to treat coronary artery disease remain riskier for women than for men. Medications and medical procedures found to elicit a positive response in men are not as successful in women. For example, clot-busting drugs that dissolve dangerous blood clots have far more serious side effects in women than in men. It is not even known if the same medications used for men, such as aspirin, beta-blockers, and calcium-channel blockers, work similarly for women. Cholesterol-lowering drugs like Mevacor and Lopid have not been sufficiently studied in women either.

## WHAT CAN GO WRONG

Any discussion of heart disease requires using some important medical terms. I realize that many people are intimidated by scientific jargon, so I will limit the terms to a few basic ones. If you have a general idea of what is going on and understand some of the basic vocabulary, it is much easier to make sense of books or articles that describe the process in greater scientific detail. Even a simple explanation provides a good foundation and can help you to discuss your individual concerns intelligently with your doctor.

Heart disease, also called *coronary artery disease (CAD)*, is a general heading that encompasses a variety of disorders involving the entire circulatory system, specifically the arteries that supply blood and oxygen to the heart. This circulatory system is extremely complex, but we don't need to understand the intricacies of everything that goes into and out of the heart to grasp what usually goes awry.

The heart is a muscular pump that moves blood throughout the body via a connected set of tubes called arteries and veins in order to supply each organ and cell with nourishment and oxygen. Starting from the right side of the heart, blood is pumped into the lungs, where it picks up oxygen, which it delivers to the left side of the heart and eventually to each and every cell in the body. After delivering its precious cargo, the blood, now depleted of oxygen, moves on to the liver and kidneys, where it removes unnecessary carbon dioxide and other waste materials, and it finally ends its trek by returning to the heart to start the cycle again. (See figure 2.)

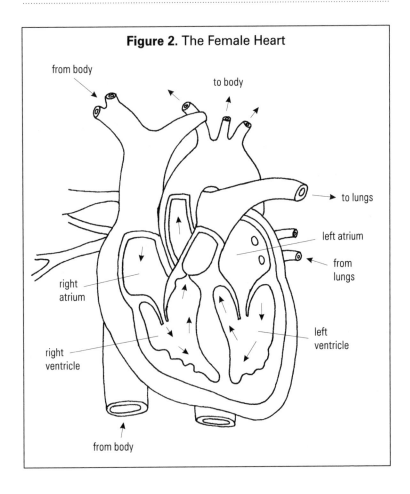

**Figure 2.** The Female Heart

When there is any obstruction to the blood as it moves through the body and returns to the heart, your body will let you know—maybe not at first, but certainly as the obstruction gets more serious. If the heart muscle doesn't get enough lifesaving oxygen and nutrients, the body may scream at you with chest pain or, as your doctor calls it, *angina pectoris*. Sometimes this crushing feeling precedes a heart attack or, in medicalese, *myocardial infarction (MI)* or *coronary thrombosis*. Blockage of the blood supply can affect other areas of the body besides the heart. For example, when the brain doesn't get enough blood through an artery *(ischemia)*, the result is a "brain attack" or stroke.

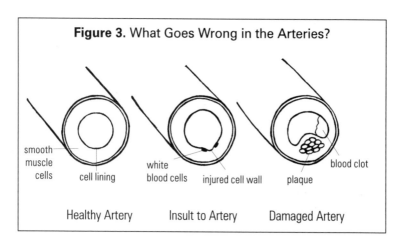

**Figure 3.** What Goes Wrong in the Arteries?

smooth muscle cells    cell lining    white blood cells    injured cell wall    plaque    blood clot

Healthy Artery          Insult to Artery          Damaged Artery

There are many reasons why blood may not flow smoothly to the heart. One common reason is that the walls of the arteries somehow get damaged, and a sludgelike material accumulates there, cutting off the access route. Researchers believed for years that circulating cholesterol was the primary culprit, clogging these vital arteries. Our present knowledge suggests cholesterol doesn't just collect in the artery without reason; something happens to attract it to a particular site. An "insult" or damage to the artery occurs first, which sets in motion a series of protective reactions by the immune system. White blood cells swarm to the cell wall, attempting to patch up the wound. But damage control gets out of hand and cholesterol, fat, waste products, and scar tissue collect at the weakened spot, creating what is called *plaque*. This waxy collection builds up, eventually narrowing the artery wall and leading to the most common type of coronary artery disease, *atherosclerosis*. (See figure 3.)

What is it that initially attacks the artery, leaving it vulnerable? As you might expect, the theories are all over the map. The condition could simply be caused by normal wear and tear in a genetically predisposed individual, or it might be brought on by high blood pressure, high blood homocysteine levels, high insulin, environmental insults, smoking, lack of nutrition, toxic emotions, or any combination of these. Whatever factors are involved, the process can be reversed and ameliorated with proper nutrition, regular exercise, practiced relaxation, and, for some, a change in attitude.

Cardiologists are only beginning to understand the various mechanisms that cause blocking of the arteries. It appears that the final straw in most heart attacks is not what you might think—more atherosclerotic plaque—but the breaking loose of a piece of plaque that forms a blood clot or thrombus and, once unleashed into the circulatory system, gets lodged in a narrowed artery and cuts off the blood supply. Furthermore, blood cells can get sticky and clump together, a condition called *platelet aggregation,* which also results in dangerous clotting and plugged arteries.

Some individuals are more prone to developing blood clots and therefore find themselves at greater risk for heart disease. Their doctors generally recommend an aspirin a day, because it thins the blood, making clumping less likely. Men are often advised to take one aspirin a day, but women's studies show that if we are susceptible, one-half that amount is adequate. I suggest that you not take any drug haphazardly as a preventive measure. Check with your doctor first to see if it might benefit you. Sometimes we forget that, as innocuous as aspirin appears, it is a drug with severe potential side effects (especially gastric ones) and therefore should be taken only if needed.

Obviously, I have not presented a full profile of cardiovascular disease or its diagnosis and treatment. That is beyond the scope of this book. I am dealing specifically with the aspects of heart disease that have been shown to respond to diet and lifestyle alterations. Unless the heart is damaged from a genetic weakness or other physical irregularity, the possibility of nondrug treatment is very good. Diet and nutrition have been shown to reduce fatty blockages and dissolve mineral deposits quite effectively.

## SIGNS OF A HEART ATTACK

The signs of a heart attack in women are not always obvious; in fact, they can be so subtle that you may not recognize them. In 40 percent of patients, there are no apparent clues, and when you examine the list in the next section, you may spot several symptoms that you have experienced that did not put you in the hospital. A bout of indigestion may be poor food combining; fatigue may be the result of overwork or inappropriate coping skills; heart palpitations frequently accompany hot flashes or too much alcohol or coffee; light-headedness can occur after several hours without food; and chest pain may accompany bronchitis, anxiety, depression, or gallbladder problems. How, then, can we determine how real our symptoms are? We can't. But if you have one or more of the following, please consult your doctor.

## Possible Symptoms of a Heart Attack

+ Chest pain—extreme pressure, a crushing or squeezing feeling (may or may not radiate to the arm and back). If it lasts longer than twenty minutes, seek emergency care.

+ Severe pain in your jaw, neck, shoulder, or arm.

+ Arrhythmia or abnormal heart rhythm.

+ Heart palpitations, irregular heartbeats, skipping of beats.

+ Fainting or feeling of light-headedness, blackouts.

+ Shortness of breath or difficulty breathing.

+ Extreme fatigue or exhaustion.

+ Bodily swelling or excessive sweating.

+ Intense indigestion (not relieved by antacids).

+ Feelings of impending doom.

Your life depends on getting attention as quickly as possible following your first symptom. From 50 to 80 percent of deaths occur within four hours after the onset of symptoms. Many women deny they could be experiencing a heart attack or fear they are and would rather not know. Get over it and get to the hospital.

# 2

# RISK FACTORS
# AND PHYSICAL TRAITS

Your biography becomes your biology.
—CAROLYN MYSS, PH.D.

A risk factor is an inherited trait, lifestyle activity, or behavior that can potentially increase your chances of developing a specific disease. It stands to reason that the longer your list of risk factors, the greater your probability of contracting the problem. I am certainly not suggesting that you are doomed to die of heart disease if you check off more than two or three of the risk factors described in the next few chapters. But you do need to be more conscientious about the factors that you can monitor in your life.

It is a good idea to evaluate where we stand in terms of our risk profile. Our genetic makeup and physical traits may predispose us to heart disease; unfortunately, some of these factors are nonnegotiable. For example, we do not really control our age, height, or sex. Women's risks differ from men's, but exactly how and to what degree the female hormones affect the heart remains in question. That annual physical exam that we frequently let slide can provide obvious medical clues such as high blood pressure and diabetes, and less well known clues such as elevated homocysteine levels. Your daily behavior and ways of dealing with people require the same attention and concern that you give your medical report. And of course, the diet/lifestyle connection to heart disease is well known.

To give you some appreciation of how much an individual risk factor can shorten your life, a new study, involving twenty-seven thousand Seventh-Day Adventists in California, has quantified how many years earlier, on the average, heart disease occurs in people with the following conditions:

| | |
|---|---|
| Diabetes | 8.3 years |
| Lack of regular exercise | 5.7 |
| High blood pressure | 4.9 |
| Smoking | 3.1 |
| Being overweight | 1.9 |

One risk factor in this list may not pose a fatal threat, but combine two or more and the risk increases exponentially. This is called *synergy*—when a second factor multiplies rather than simply adds to the effects of the first factor. The good news is that synergy can also work in your favor. When you improve your diet, drop extra fat, and engage regularly in physical activity, your body reaps synergistic benefits. You can lower your blood pressure, regulate your blood sugar, and improve your blood fat levels all at the same time. The cumulative action strengthens not only your heart but also all your glands, tissues, and cells.

## AGE

Age is one risk factor that we cannot control. The older we are, the greater our risk for heart disease. Women have a distinct age advantage over men by ten to fifteen years. Most women don't have to worry about dying from heart disease until they are over forty-five. Even then, the numbers are low. Consider the following:

+ Ages 35 to 44: 1 in 1,000 women show signs of CAD.

+ Ages 45 to 64: 1 in 7 show some form of heart disease or stroke-related problem.

+ Ages 65 and up: 1 in 4 succumb to heart disease; women reach parity with men.

The aging process itself partially explains the increased incidence of heart problems. We know the connective tissue in the

arteries becomes stiffer and less flexible with increasing years, causing a rise in blood pressure, which has been shown to contribute to
wear and tear on the arterial wall and also on the heart muscle itself.
Cholesterol levels climb with age in both sexes, as do those additional pounds. Adult-onset diabetes enters the medical profile of
many women in their midlife years, adding to the number of probable risk factors. After menopause, women also produce less estrogen,
the hormone that is thought to give us a protective edge during our
childbearing years.

Just because women do not die from heart problems until we
pass the half-century mark does not mean we should pretend heart
disease doesn't exist until we reach menopause. Heart disease
evolves slowly, starting long before the first symptom shows. In
studying a group of 364 women between the ages of fifteen and
thirty-four who had died from accidents, murder, or suicide,
researchers found that the fatty streaks and artery-clogging plaque
that predispose individuals to heart attacks appeared in the blood
vessels of even the youngest victims. We have had similar information regarding men for forty years. When autopsies were conducted
on young soldiers who had died in the Korean War, the men displayed fatty streaks and cholesterol lining their arteries. This is the
first study showing that the same destructive forces are at work in
women at an early age.

## RACE

The lack of research concerning women and heart disease is apparent, blatant, and frustrating. It becomes downright embarrassing
when it comes to ethnicity. While the reasons remain unclear, there
is evidence that African American women have more of the obvious
risk factors for heart disease than Caucasians—they are more likely
to be overweight, to smoke, and to have diabetes, high blood pressure, and high cholesterol. What confuses researchers is that, in
spite of their potential for multiple risk factors, black women are less
prone to CAD than white women. What's even more baffling and
seemingly contradictory is that the African American women who
do suffer heart attacks are 69 percent more likely to die from them

than their white counterparts. Economic disadvantage and inadequate health care may explain the poorer prognosis, but no one knows for sure.

## OBESITY

Obesity exacerbates many of the risk factors for heart disease, such as high blood pressure, diabetes, and elevated cholesterol. If you are just twenty pounds over your ideal weight, which is the classic definition of obesity, your risk of heart disease doubles. One of the latest reports from the famed Nurses' Health Study, an ongoing investigation that continues to follow more than 115,000 nurses, indicated that women who put on even modest amounts of weight after their teen years increased their risk of heart attack later in life. Compared with women who gained less than eleven pounds since age eighteen, the risk of having a heart attack increased as follows:

+ 25 percent higher in those who gained 11–17 pounds.

+ 64 percent higher in those who gained 18–23 pounds.

+ 92 percent higher in those who gained 24–43 pounds.

There were four times as many deaths from cardiovascular disease among those who gained more than forty-three pounds than among women of normal weight, and twice the number of cancer-related deaths—particularly from breast, colon, and uterine cancer. Those with the lowest risk of heart disease weighed less than the recommended government guidelines. Obviously, we need to rethink those trusty charts that decorate the examining room of our doctor's office.

The increasing prevalence of overweight individuals in many countries indicates that

### The Nurses' Health Study

Throughout this book I refer to the famed Nurses' Health Study. This is an ongoing observational study conducted by researchers at Brigham and Women's Hospital, Harvard Medical School, and Harvard School of Public Health. It began in 1976 and continues to use data provided by 120,000 women who were between the ages of 30 and 55 when they enrolled and now are 50 to 75 years of age. The women have been asked to fill out extensive questionaires every two years about their health, diet, and lifestyles. The more than one hundred reports compiled from this data have provided a foundation for additional research into women's health risks.

obesity may be considered pandemic. In the United States, government statistics as of June 1998 show that 97 million adults or 55 percent of the population are over their ideal weight or obese and thus at risk of contracting a host of chronic and potentially fatal diseases. Realizing that it was time to take action, the National Heart, Lung, and Blood Institute (NHLBI), in cooperation with the National Institute of Diabetes and Digestive and Kidney diseases, released the first federal guidelines to identify, evaluate, and treat overweight and obesity. A twenty-four-member expert panel reviewing the most up-to-date scientific evidence on excess fat and obesity determined that the assessment of overweight involves the evaluation of three key measures: body mass index (BMI), waist circumference, and patients' risk factors for diseases and conditions associated with obesity.

The number that pops up on the scale whenever we are bold enough to stand on it has been the sole criteria for judging one's weight status and risk profile. The current guidelines redefine overweight according to how much of our excess poundage is fat. This is regarded as a more accurate indicator of obesity as well as a measurement of general fitness. A confusing paradox exists when you evaluate your health status solely by how you look in the mirror. The fact is you can appear to be overweight and yet have a low percentage of body fat; correspondingly, you can look great in sleek jeans and still register high body fat.

There are several methods for determining your body fat. You can go to a hospital, gym, or health club and be tested by a health professional or, if you are anxious to know immediately, you can use the relatively simple calculation below to calculate something called your body mass index (BMI). The number you arrive at will give you some idea of whether your body fat is high enough to put you at risk for heart disease and other chronic conditions. It is applicable to women and men of all ages. Please also see appendix A for an easy-to-read BMI chart.

## Calculating Your Body Mass Index

1. Multiply your weight in pounds by 0.45 to get your weight in kilograms (for example, 130 pounds x 0.45 = 58.5 kilograms).

2. Multiply your height in inches by 0.025 to get your height in meters (5'5" or 65 inches x 0.025 = 1.625 meters).

3. Multiply your answer in step #2 by itself to get your adjusted height in meters squared (1.625 x 1.625 = 2.641).

4. Divide your weight in kilograms (step #1) by your adjusted height in meters squared (step #3) to get your Body Mass Index (58.5 / 2.641 = 22.15 BMI).

The federal guideline for overweight is a BMI reading of 25 to 29.9, and obesity is calculated as a BMI of 30 and above, which is consistent with the definition used in many other countries. According to the most recent analysis of the National Health and Nutrition Examination Survey (NHANES III), as BMI levels rise, average blood pressure and total cholesterol levels increase and average HDL levels decrease. Women in the highest obesity category have four times the risk of hypertension, high blood cholesterol, or both compared to women of normal weight.

Waist circumference is strongly associated with abdominal fat, an independent predictor of heart disease risk. A waist circumference of over 35 inches in women and 40 inches in men signifies a heightened risk, especially in those who have a BMI of 25 to 34.9.

Losing excess body fat, if you are appreciably over the acceptable range, relieves stress on the heart, lowers blood pressure and blood cholesterol, and keeps non-insulin-dependent diabetes under control, often without the use of drugs. Research is specific as to how effective weight loss can be in regulating the numbers:

*Cholesterol:* The combination of seventy studies on almost thirteen hundred overweight volunteers concluded that for every five pounds you lose, your total cholesterol level drops by 7 points, LDL (bad) cholesterol drops by 3 points, triglycerides (bad) drop by 14 points, and HDL (good) cholesterol rises by 1 point.

*Blood Pressure:* A great deal of research shows that blood pressure comes down when weight comes off. One study showed that 60 percent of people with hypertension were able to discontinue taking their medication after they lost just ten pounds.

*Blood Sugar:* Diabetics who shed at least fifteen pounds over a year lowered their blood sugar levels by 15 percent—without medication. Those who lost at least thirty pounds lowered their blood sugar by more than 40 percent, even though they remained over their ideal weight.

## WEIGHT FLUCTUATIONS

Debate continues as to whether weight fluctuations may contribute directly or indirectly to disease risk. Data from a Framingham study suggest that the risk is greater for women whose weight varies substantially over time than for women and men whose weight remains relatively stable. Additional support comes from the Harvard Alumni Health Study, which also indicated that alumni who maintained a stable weight had the lowest all-cause mortality. Observations of premenopausal women found an association between weight loss and weight gain and increased mortality from coronary heart disease. While other studies have failed to show a similar link, it is clear that there is something here that needs more scientific attention.

## BODY SHAPE

When you look at your body in the mirror, is the shape of you see that of an apple or a pear? The way fat is distributed on your body affects your susceptibility to conditions like heart disease, hypertension, and diabetes. The most unhealthy place to carry your excess weight is around the middle, like an apple, and the least harmful storage spaces are the hips and thighs, which give you a shape reminiscent of a pear. Stanford University researchers found that women with overdeveloped thighs have a lower risk of heart disease than women with midriff pouches. It appears that the fat cells in the thighs act primarily as storage bins for fat (awaiting that impending famine), whereas fat in the stomach is available and anxious to be converted into cholesterol. Did you ever think in your wildest dreams that you could be grateful for "thunder thighs"?

Experts have also developed a mathematical formula we can use to figure out if we are too round in the middle. It is based on your waist measurement divided by your hip size. Sure, you can go to the mirror and eyeball it, but that's hardly scientific—so go get your tape measure and calculator. The true location of your waist is at the navel, not below the belly, where some men fasten their belts. Don't cheat and hold in your stomach. We're going for accuracy. The widest point of your hips is where you want to put your tape. When you have your two numbers, punch them into your trusty calculator and divide. The magic number or the healthy ratio of waist-to-hip measurement should be

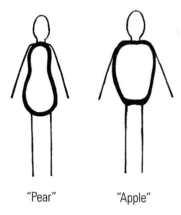

"Pear"            "Apple"

less than 0.8 for women. For example, if your waist measures 28 inches and your hips measure 36 inches, 28 divided by 36 gives 0.77, which is lower that 0.8, which is good.

## HEIGHT

Here's a new one. Those of us who are height-challenged share a greater risk for heart problems. Researchers at the Boston University School of Public Health found that women who are under 4'11" are at a 50 percent greater risk of heart attack than are women over 5'4". I fall right in the middle, which puts me where? It's really a moot point, since science hasn't come up with any wonder drugs or surgical procedures to give us that extra height boost.

## EARLOBE CREASE

The next time you find yourself at the mirror contemplating which fruit you resemble, zero in on your earlobe. If you should see a diagonal crease where your earring resides, it may indicate an inclination toward heart disease. Over thirty studies since the 1970s have shown this rather obscure correlation. The rationale for the significance of this hairlike line is that a decreased blood flow over a period of time may show up on the otherwise richly vascularized lobes. A crease alone is not predictive of heart disease, but some doctors pay attention to it as a secondary screening tool.

# 3

# MEDICAL PROFILE

*The universe will get your attention one way or another—*
*with a sip or a splash.*

—SARAH BAN BREATHNACH

## FAMILY HISTORY

Heart disease runs in families. But just because a relative in your gene pool died from heart disease doesn't mean your future is doomed. What counts is how close the relative was to you and at what age he or she had the heart attack. Your risk is greater if your father or brother experienced a heart attack before the age of fifty-five or your mother or sister suffered a heart attack prior to age sixty. Your genetic legacy also includes contributing factors for heart disease (or coronary artery disease, CAD), such as hypertension, high blood cholesterol, diabetes, and obesity. Furthermore, lifestyle traits also pass along the branches of the family tree. People who live together usually eat the same food, exercise together, or sit and watch TV as a unit. Children mimic their parents. When Mom and Dad inhale five doughnuts for breakfast or smoke a pack of cigarettes after dinner, guess who's watching and following suit. Whether a person succumbs to stress or has the ability to cope rubs off on family members, especially impressionable children.

There is new evidence that your genetic makeup may determine whether you will benefit from dietary changes that lower blood cholesterol. We are all born with specific molecules, called *apolipo-proteins*, which determine how cholesterol is transported in our blood. Some people who have a certain type of apolipoprotein, apoE4, appear to respond more favorably to dietary modification than those with other varieties. If you have been vigilant about your diet in the hope that it will bring down your cholesterol and after several months discover that the numbers didn't change, you may consider medical intervention. However, don't think that because your healthful diet did not improve your risk profile that it is not helping your body in other ways. Continue to pay attention to what goes in your body; the results will definitely show in other areas.

## CONGENITAL DEFECTS

More girl babies are born with defects than boy babies are. Some doctors speculate that because female fetuses are generally stronger than male fetuses, they are more likely to survive with a defect or abnormality. To be born with a congenital heart defect means you have a physical or structural malformation of the heart or surrounding arteries or veins leading to the heart. In some infants it is immediately apparent; other heart defects aren't detected until later in life. In my case, when I was a child the family doctor heard a murmur or a skipping sound during a routine examination. It wasn't until I was a teenager and underwent a heart catheterization that I learned the cause and nature of my specific abnormality. Like mine, many of these quirks are innocuous and don't interfere with life. Still, it's a good idea to have them rechecked as an adult in case they change.

## DIABETES

Diabetes is an especially serious issue for women and their hearts. Diabetic women are at greater risk than diabetic men for heart disease, and their chance for survival after a heart attack is less promising. Women with diabetes are more likely to be overweight and to have high blood pressure and high cholesterol, and they are twice as likely to suffer a heart attack as nondiabetic women.

It is a well-established fact that diabetes wreaks havoc with your cholesterol levels. If you are diabetic, you can expect to see more of the dangerous LDL cholesterol, less protective HDL cholesterol, and higher levels of triglycerides. Gerald Reaven, M.D., an endocrinologist at the Stanford University School of Medicine, calls it "a whole cluster of abnormalities that heighten your risk for coronary heart disease."

Diabetes is a chronic metabolic disorder caused by either a deficiency of the hormone insulin or impairment in the action of the hormone. There are two types of diabetes: Type 1 or insulin-dependent diabetes, which usually shows up in childhood and requires daily insulin injections, and Type 2 or non-insulin-dependent diabetes, a condition diagnosed later in life that typically can be regulated with diet. The two are really very different conditions with different causes and treatments. When I use the term *diabetes* in this book, I will be referring to the Type 2 variety, also known as adult-onset diabetes.

Diabetics have a problem clearing sugar from their blood. In medical terminology this is called *hyperinsulinemia* (too much sugar in the blood). Sugars and starches, which come from the carbohydrate food group, are eventually broken down into simple sugar (glucose). After you eat a bagel or an orange, the pancreas sends insulin out to the cells to help open the gate, so to speak, so the small sugar molecules can enter the cell membrane and be used for energy or stored as fat. In diabetics, the cells are resistant to the nudging of insulin, and thus, the sugar remains outside, floating in the blood, where it insidiously attacks the eyes, nerves, kidney, limbs, and heart.

Minor complications from too much sugar in the blood appear in the form of wounds that don't heal readily and infections that reoccur. You may experience digestive problems, sexual dysfunction, loss of sensation in the feet, and cataracts or other visual problems. If left unchecked, diabetes can result in blindness, nerve damage, limb amputation, and kidney failure. It is not something to take lightly.

Half of the fifteen million Americans that have Type 2 diabetes don't know it. Half of those who do know they have it typically did not find out for seven or more years after it had already been chipping away at their body and overall health. This can happen because it is rare in the initial stages to notice any overt symptoms. Like heart disease, diabetes lurks silently in the tissues and organs, rarely leaving clues. It is critical to get tested periodically for diabetes, especially if any of the following conditions apply. Waiting can be deadly.

## Test for diabetes if ...

+ You are forty-five or older.

+ You are obese (more than twenty pounds over your ideal weight).

+ You have a parent or sibling with diabetes.

+ You are African American, Asian, Hispanic, or Native American.

+ You developed gestational diabetes during pregnancy.

+ You gave birth to a baby weighing more than nine pounds.

+ You have high blood pressure (140/90 or higher).

+ You have a HDL cholesterol level of 35 mg/dl (milligrams per deciliter) or below and/or blood triglyceride level of 250 mg/dl or higher.

+ You experience several of the following signs: weakness, headaches, unusual hunger or thirst, frequent urination, blurred vision, leg cramps, itching, and minor vaginal infections.

In an effort to encourage earlier diagnosis, the American Diabetes Association (ADA), backed by federal health authorities, recently called for routine screening of all adults age forty-five and older every three years. Moreover, these experts decided to reevaluate the present definition of diabetes, which means that blood glucose levels that had previously been considered normal are now classified as too high. Until this meeting, the threshold for diabetes was 140 milligrams of sugar per deciliter of blood after an overnight eight-hour fast. The new marker will be 126 ml/dl, which the American Diabetes Association (ADA) believes will lead to many more people being diagnosed before they suffer irreparable damage. Even if your blood glucose is between 110 and 126 mg/dl, you are considered in a danger zone and need to act quickly to reduce your risk.

The ADA suggests that a simple blood test can just as easily replace the more expensive and time-consuming oral glucose tolerance test. This makes testing much more convenient, since it can be performed on the same sample of blood drawn to check such things as cholesterol levels. Diabetes caught early is controllable by managing blood sugar levels with diet, exercise, weight loss, and specific nutrients. Much of the information in *Her Healthy Heart* applies to maintaining constant blood sugar levels; however, if you have been diagnosed with Type 2 diabetes, I suggest you make an appointment with a registered dietitian or qualified nutritionist.

## INSULIN RESISTANCE

The ADA reported at its annual meeting in 1996 that insulin resistance is known to contribute to as much as 60 percent of cardiovascular disease in women and 25 percent in men. Resistance to the effects of insulin may be a major determining factor in if not the precursor to diabetes, high blood pressure, elevated triglyceride levels, low HDL levels, obesity, and ultimately, heart disease. In an ongoing study in New Orleans in which patients have been followed from birth for twenty years, it has been found that the first measurable change in the blood chemistry of an adult before the onset of diabetes, hypertension, obesity, and symptomatic cardiovascular disease is an elevated insulin level.

Insulin resistance is a condition in which the cells of the body have become insensitive and unresponsive to normal levels of insulin. In most individuals a small burst of the hormone will bring down blood sugar levels, but in the insulin-resistant a larger dose is required to do the job, so the pancreas continues to pump it out to the cells. High blood insulin levels plus a cluster of other risk factors for heart disease (such as poor blood fats, obesity, and high blood pressure) are particularly dangerous to the heart. Some clinicians are recommending that insulin level tests be used more regularly to diagnose potential problems.

It was estimated in research quoted by the *New York Times* (February 8, 1995) that at least 25 percent of Americans are insulin resistant. So how do we identify the one-quarter of the population who are living with such a serious risk factor? Two obvious clues may tip you off: the size and shape of your body. If you are extremely overweight and if you carry your excess weight around the middle rather than on your hips and thighs, you may be insulin resistant. According to leading authority Jean-Pierre Despres, Ph.D., director of the lipid research center at Laval University Hospital in St. Foy, Quebec, a waistline over thirty-nine inches in both women and men is yet another sign.

A more scientific indicator may be the fasting glucose test that is used to detect diabetes. Most susceptible individuals will register increased levels of glucose over 100 mg/dl. It is even more of a red flag if this number is combined with high triglycerides and a ratio of total cholesterol to HDL cholesterol greater than five (this ratio is explained on page 73).

Individuals who have weak pancreatic cells are probably genetically predisposed to be insulin resistant; however, obesity, lack of exercise, smoking, aging, and diet can induce or exacerbate symptoms in susceptible individuals. A great deal can be done to reduce insulin levels with diet and exercise. Cutting down on consumption of simple sugars and carbohydrates, plus losing weight and exercising regularly, have been known to successfully reduce insulin resistance.

## HIGH BLOOD PRESSURE

High blood pressure is clearly the most well known alarm system notifying us that it is time to pay attention to our health. Even mild hypertension boosts the risk for premature death and any number of heart-related complications. High blood pressure can erode the walls of the arteries, starting the process that ends up as atherosclerosis. Even though the body fights to repair the damage, fatty deposits build up within the arteries, clogging them and narrowing the opening for the passage of oxygen and nutrients. The pressure builds over time until, on a routine visit to the doctor, we discover that our body defenses are down and we need to take action.

The pumping of blood through the circulatory system creates blood pressure. When your heart contracts, blood flows into and through the arteries; this is when the pressure is at its highest. Then, as the heart relaxes, blood flows through and from the veins back into the heart, and the pressure reaches its lowest point. The blood pressure measurement expresses both the highest point (systolic) and the lowest point (diastolic). What commonly happens when the regulatory system goes awry is that the small arteries stay constricted and the blood pressure gets stuck on high.

A normal blood pressure reading is around or below 130/85 (systolic/diastolic), and hypertension is usually considered to be around and above 140/90. There is a tremendous variability in blood pressure among women, and even a so-called normal reading may be abnormal in a particular woman. If a woman is consistently 110/65 and suddenly jumps to 130/80, her doctor may suspect a problem. Reasons for the hike in blood pressure could be as innocuous as stress associated with visiting the doctor, trying a new medication, or devouring a bag of salty chips the night before. Determining the cause of any irregularity is always a good idea. Even the high end of normal may be too high for some people who have additional risk factors.

## Risk Factors for High Blood Pressure

+ *Age:* The older you are, the greater your risk. Prior to menopause, women usually have lower readings than men of the same age do. Between ages fifty-five and sixty-five, women and men level off, and after age sixty-five, women take the lead and are more likely to experience elevated blood pressure.

+ *Family History:* If your parents have it, you may too.

+ *Ethnic Background:* No one really knows why, but African American women are twice as likely as Anglo women to suffer from high blood pressure, even in their younger years.

+ *Weight:* Women who exceed their ideal weight by more than 30 percent are two to three times more likely to develop high blood pressure than women who are within their normal

range. A host of studies show that losing weight can profoundly affect blood pressure readings. One study found that
in 60 percent of people with high blood pressure, a loss of just
ten pounds allowed them to discontinue medication.

+ *Diabetes:* High insulin levels characteristic of non-insulin-
dependent diabetes is thought to play a major role in the
development of hypertension; therefore, diabetics face a
greater risk.

+ *Pregnancy-Induced Hypertension:* If you tested high during pregnancy, the chances of your blood pressure shooting up again
are very good.

+ *Oral Contraceptives:* Five percent of women will be unable to
take the pill because of high blood pressure.

+ *Alcohol:* While moderate alcohol consumption may protect
against heart disease, consuming three or more drinks a day is
associated with an increased incidence of hypertension.

+ *Salt:* Not everyone who eats salt will experience a rise in blood
pressure. But one-third to one-half of the population is salt-
sensitive, meaning their blood pressure rises and falls with the
amount of sodium in their diets.

+ *Minerals:* Research strongly suggests that a deficiency of the
minerals calcium, magnesium, and potassium may also
increase your risk for high blood pressure. Potassium, either
from food or in pill form, causes a drop in blood pressure
almost as effective as that caused by drugs.

+ *Lead:* Lead has been linked to high blood pressure, heart disease, cancer, and kidney disease. Avoid calcium supplements
made from oyster shell, dolomite, or bone meal. They are
known to contain lead.

+ *Stress:* Countless studies link chronic stress with hypertension.
More important than the amount of stress in one's life is the
way one handles it.

In many cases, high blood pressure can be treated with diet, special nutrients, and lifestyle changes. Daily menus that are relatively low in fat and plentiful in fruits and vegetables can substantially lower blood pressure. If you can't lower your blood pressure by eating healthy food, taking supplemental nutrients and herbs, and exercising, your doctor can prescribe medication.

## CHOLESTEROL COUNTS

Men are frequently concerned about their total cholesterol levels—with good reason. High blood cholesterol levels do in fact increase men's risk for heart disease, but for women the data are not so clear. The American Heart Association informs us that 200 is the magic number over which no one should go, yet studies that focus on women seem to suggest this may not be the right number for us. Consider the famous Framingham Heart Study, which showed that women under the age of seventy-five with cholesterol counts over 295 had the same or lower risk of heart disease as men whose cholesterol hovered around 200. A study from Scotland informed us that women between the ages of forty-five and sixty-four who had cholesterol levels over 278 had a lower risk of coronary heart disease than men with cholesterol levels below 193. Then, close to my home, researchers at the University of California at San Francisco analyzed data from nine different studies and noticed that healthy women whose high cholesterol level wasn't treated with diet or drugs were no more likely to end up with heart disease than those who were treated.

We need to rethink everything about women and cholesterol and heart disease, because the bulk of research has been conducted with men. After reviewing the handful of studies that included women, it is clear that research needs to be redesigned specifically to address women.

The most potent predictor of heart disease for women is a combination of low HDL (*high-density lipoprotein* or "good" cholesterol) levels with high *triglycerides,* a damaging form of fat. Even a small drop in HDLs is correlated with a substantial jump in risk of heart disease in women, whereas a rise in HDLs of only 1 mg/dl is associated with a 3.2 percent decrease in risk. Triglyceride levels can also signal danger to women, and unfortunately, it is a number we tend to overlook. The good news is that both HDLs and triglycerides are amenable to diet and lifestyle changes. Read chapter 7 for specifics.

One point stands out clearly: just knowing our total cholesterol level isn't enough for women, especially if there are other risk factors involved. It is especially critical for us to find out the values of the individual components, the HDL (*high-density lipoprotein* or "good" cholesterol) level as well as the LDL (*low-density lipoprotein* or "bad" cholesterol) level and the level of triglycerides. Ask your doctor to order a full lipid profile that measures all the various blood fats.

## HEALTHY GUMS

Few of you have probably heard that unhealthy gums may translate to a heightened risk of heart disease. Suggestions of such a link sprinkle the literature; however, until fairly recently the studies have not factored out the effects of smoking, which frequently contributes to gum disease. A recent study of more than thirteen hundred Pima Indians in Arizona, a group in which smoking is uncommon, showed that the ones who suffered from periodontal disease were 2.7 times more likely to have a heart attack than those with healthy gums. The researchers concluded that in this group, gum disease showed a stronger connection to the risk for developing heart disease than high blood pressure. The actual connection is as yet undetermined.

## MEDICAL TESTS THAT PROVIDE CLUES

A routine trip to the doctor may provide clues of a heart at risk. A blood test can indicate many things, though a thorough battery of tests is not typically included as part of a heart-healthy physical because added tests are costly and most insurance carriers won't pay for them. Let's hope that the future will bring more diagnostic tools to keep us informed of changes that may affect our health.

### Uric Acid Test

High blood levels of uric acid (hyperuricemia) have been linked to coronary artery disease and some of its other risk factors, such as high blood pressure, high blood lipid levels, diabetes, and obesity.

Uric acid is the end product of nucleic acids, the genetic building blocks that make up DNA and RNA. High uric acid levels in the blood are not harmful in and of themselves. However, some people with consistently elevated levels develop kidney stones, gout arthritis, hypertension, and heart disease. Normal blood levels of uric acid for women fall between 2.6 and 6.0 mg/100ml.

If you have made an appointment for your regular physical or are concerned about your uric acid levels, it's important to take a few precautions prior to being tested. For accurate results, a few days prior to your blood test you should limit your intake of foods high in the amino acid purine. These would include organ meats, scallops, sardines, anchovies, asparagus, mushrooms, and spinach.

## Fibrinogen Levels

An elevated fibrinogen level is an independent risk factor for heart disease and stroke, at least for men. *Fibrinogen* is a substance produced in the body to ensure proper clotting of the blood, especially when injury occurs. Levels are typically higher in women and in smokers. Diabetes and high blood pressure are also linked to boosted levels. Exercise reduces blood levels of fibrinogen, which may be one reason why regular physical activity protects against heart disease.

## Hematocrit Level

A simple blood test can determine the percentage of the total blood volume of red blood cells, or the *hematocrit level*. A higher than normal reading may indicate early signs of oxygen deprivation or narrowing of the arteries, which is associated with coronary artery disease. Normal values for women are between 37 and 47 ml/100ml.

## Blood Homocysteine Levels

Another red flag for heart disease is having too much homocysteine in the blood. While the mechanism by which it works is not known, it is thought to reduce the production of nitric oxide on the blood vessel wall, possibly causing the blood vessel to constrict. It may also interfere with the activation of a natural anticoagulant, protein C, and thus help to encourage the development of blood clots.

A fasting blood test is normally used to determine homocysteine levels. Sometimes a blood test is not sufficient to show a defect in the conversion of homocysteine to another amino acid, methionine, and an oral challenge test of 3 grams of L-methionine is better.

Regulation of this obscure amino acid depends in part on three B vitamins: B-6, B-12, and folic acid. Women are characteristically deficient in all of these and should consider taking a daily multiple vitamin tablet.

## Lipoprotein(a)—LP(a)

*Lipoprotein(a)* is a particle in the blood composed of protein, cholesterol, and other lipids or fats. It is abundant in the blood of many people whose vulnerability to coronary heart disease cannot be attributed to other obvious causes. LP(a) increases in diabetics with uncontrolled blood sugar levels and in menopausal women. It appears that when estrogen winds down after menopause, there is a rise in LP(a). Because estrogen or hormone therapy helps to bring it back down, replacement therapy may be indicated in women at high risk. Drugs and diet have no effect on LP(a) levels.

# OTHER MEDICAL TESTS

## Exercise Stress Test

The stress test, also called *exercise electrocardiography,* is used to evaluate the availability of blood to the heart during exercise. It provides a clue as to how well the heart functions under physical stress and can also determine your level of physical fitness, muscle strength, and endurance. Electrodes are secured onto the arms, legs, and chest, and a machine measures the heart's electrical activity while you walk or jog in place. The operator can check for heart arrhythmias, narrowing of the coronary arteries, and reduced blood flow to the heart muscle.

There is some doubt about whether the stress test is valid for women, because it has a high rate of false readings. Some women taking the test show signs of CAD when they have perfectly normal arteries, while others test negative and turn out to have blocked arteries. Exercise stress testing was developed for and refined on men; perhaps it will soon be used with the same reliability on women.

## Electrocardiogram

The *electrocardiogram*, commonly called the *EKG*, is used to monitor or verify any undesirable changes in the electrical activity of the heart. The electrocardiogram can tell you if you have already had a heart attack, if your heart is enlarged, if you have abnormal heart rhythms, or if a blockage exists in one or more of the coronary arteries. But it cannot always detect damage to the heart and may, in fact, register normal for half of all patients who complain of angina, even though they may have CAD.

The EKG is a noninvasive, painless test that is performed while the patient lies prone on a table in the doctor's office. Electrodes are attached to the chest, arms, and legs, either with an adhesive or suction cups. Wires attached to the electrodes feed into the EKG machine, and the heart's electrical activity is recorded on paper for the doctor to read. If a patient has a normal EKG and has not experienced symptoms, she will probably not require further testing.

## Echocardiogram

An *echocardiogram* uses sound waves to provide a picture of the structure of the heart, and is often used as a follow-up test to confirm heart disease. It can tell the doctor how efficiently your heart and its valves are working, the size of the cardiac chambers, and the direction in which blood is flowing. The test is relatively reliable in women, although if a woman has large breasts, the image may be fuzzy and hard to interpret, because the fat and muscle insulates the heart from the sound waves.

To undergo an echocardiogram, you lie on your side on the examining table while a technician moves a sound probe, called a transducer, touching various points on your chest. The probe emits small pulses of ultrasound, which reflect off your heart and are amplified and visually displayed on a monitor. If you had a sonogram when you were pregnant, this is basically the same procedure.

A newer type of ultrasound called *exercise echocardiography* seems to be particularly useful in detecting a common form of CAD in women—blockage from a single blood vessel. It can be used with exercise or in combination with specific medications that stress the heart in a way similar to physical exercise.

## Cardiac Catheterization

*Cardiac catheterization* is considered the "gold standard" of diagnostic testing for CAD. Not only does it show conclusively whether or not the coronary arteries are diseased, it also provides information that cannot be obtained using other methods. It can detect where the blockage is located, as well as which arteries are narrowed and by how much. It can tell if the flow of blood has been rerouted to collateral blood vessels—blood vessels that are formed when the heart muscle is starved of oxygen. With all this information, the cardiologist can determine with relative certainty the patient's probability of having a serious heart attack.

Cardiac catheterization is highly accurate, but it is an invasive procedure and does come with an element of risk. The procedure is performed in a hospital under local anesthesia. A plastic tube is inserted in either the arm or the thigh and passed through a blood vessel into the heart. A dye is injected into the catheter, and an X-ray follows the dye as it flows through the coronary arteries throughout the heart. It is a painless procedure except for a rush of heat when the dye is injected. Actually, if you are interested in medical procedures, it is quite fascinating to watch, as I did as a patient over thirty years ago.

There is a risk to this procedure: in one out of five hundred patients the procedure triggers a heart attack, stroke, or other serious complication. Therefore, doctors usually reserve it for potential candidates for angioplasty or bypass surgery.

# 4

# RISKS UNIQUE TO WOMEN

*If it's not one thing, it's another.*

—GILDA RADNER

In each of the chapters describing risks for heart disease, I have pointed out differences between women and men. However, none are as obvious as the ones relating to our female hormones. We women experience a monthly cycle, pregnancy, and menopause, all of which come with fluctuations in hormone levels. The hormones that course through our bodies touch each cell, tissue, and organ. It stands to reason that the hormones that we make naturally and the ones we take orally for contraception or replacement therapy will somehow affect the rest of our body, as will a lack of these hormones. The information on how they affect us is scant at this time, but studies are under way and answers will soon come.

## PREGNANCY

Pregnancy burdens even a healthy heart, but most women can endure the rigors of pregnancy and childbirth without any adverse effects on the cardiovascular system. For some women with preexisting diseases or undiagnosed heart conditions, getting pregnant may pose a serious risk. It all depends on the nature of the problem and the health of the individual. With the proper medical attention, women with heart problems such as congenital heart defects and damaged valves may be able to safely deliver a baby. Please consult your doctor if you have a known or suspected heart abnormality and are considering having children.

Female hormone levels change during pregnancy. Both estro-gen and progesterone levels increase dramatically to support the new life growing inside the uterus. This surge of hormones is respon-sible for the many physical and emotional changes women experi-ence during pregnancy, from morning sickness to swollen breasts, weight gain, increased urination, and insomnia.

Blood lipids, blood sugar, and insulin levels also shoot up dur-ing pregnancy (they return to prepregnancy norms once the baby is born), which make researchers question if pregnancy might affect a woman's long-term risk of developing heart disease. So far, the stud-ies are split: some say yes and as many say no. Two studies shed a lit-tle light on this issue. The Framingham Heart Study, which included data from over two thousand women over twenty-eight years, and the National Health and Nutrition Examination Survey, a govern-mental study that pooled data from more than twenty-five hundred women for twelve years, found that women who had been pregnant did have a slightly higher rate of coronary heart disease than those who had never been pregnant, but it was only statistically significant if a woman had been pregnant six or more times.

The heart works overtime during pregnancy, and a woman may be very aware of its activity. Blood volume increases by 40 to 50 percent, which is considerably more than the heart normally pumps. The heart also beats faster: ten to twenty times more per minute than prepregnancy, contracting more vigorously with each beat. A woman may notice palpitations and irregular beats even during quiet times. If she is stressed at all—and what woman isn't at some point during the nine months—her anxiety can further increase cardiac output and place an additional burden on the heart.

Hypertensive disorders that arise during pregnancy pose serious problems for both mother and baby. Any high-blood-pressure disorder is dangerous at this time, because the heart, forced to work harder, causes the blood vessels to constrict, which reduces the amount of blood and oxygen available to the unborn fetus. An estimated one-fourth of all women who give birth in the United States develop pregnancy-induced hypertension (PIH) by the end of their pregnan-cies. Women who are especially at risk are first-time mothers-to-be, expectant mothers over the age of thirty-five, overweight women, diabetics, and women who have a family history of PIH.

About 5 percent of women reach the most dangerous stage of hypertension, called *eclampsia.* Left untreated, it can result in seizures, coma, and possibly death to both mother and baby. Certainly, high-risk women need to be vigilant about having their blood pressure tested regularly during pregnancy. But really, all women need to be cautious, since anyone can get it. The good news is that if PIH is caught early, it can be controlled with rest and a good diet.

## ORAL CONTRACEPTIVES

Oral contraceptives have taken the lead as the birth control method of choice because they are convenient, simple, effective, and safe for most women. When I wrote about the birth control pill some fifteen years ago, grave concerns permeated the literature, many relating to heart disease and stroke. Since then, with the reformulation of a lower dose tablet, both the amount of estrogen and the risks have been greatly reduced. The question still lingering in women's minds is, Will the lower doses be found to be safer after decades of use? No one knows for sure, because there are not yet enough women who have taken them for that long.

There is a group of women who *must not* take the pill; I hope every woman of childbearing age knows this. If you smoke, you should not take birth control pills. The combination is deadly. Combining the two makes it easier for your blood to clot, thereby increasing your risk of heart attack and stroke. The likelihood that you will suffer a heart attack skyrockets to 30 to 40 percent with this dangerous combination.

It may be a good idea to have your blood pressure checked periodically after you have been on the pill. Roughly 5 percent of women using the pill will develop high blood pressure within five years. Only half of these elevated blood pressures will return to normal once the women stop taking the pill.

No medication is right for every individual. Women who may want to rethink oral contraception include those who have had a stroke or already have heart disease, and those with high blood fats, circulatory or clotting disorders, high blood pressure, or diabetes. You should also review your options with your doctor if you have or have had breast or uterine cancer, severe liver disease, abnormal vaginal bleeding, migraine headaches, depression, or sickle cell anemia.

## PREMATURE MENOPAUSE

Women who stop menstruating prematurely because they have undergone a complete hysterectomy (also called a radical hysterectomy, in which both ovaries are removed along with the uterus), have a threefold increased risk for coronary artery disease. Having the ovaries surgically removed before the mid- to late forties plunges women into instant menopause. An abrupt drop in estrogen during the reproductive years, when estrogen is naturally present, upsets the hormonal balance in the body and may pose future health risks to the heart and bones. The younger the woman is when her ovaries are removed, the greater the probability of developing these problems.

Premenopausal women who have a hysterectomy in which the uterus is removed but the ovaries remain intact do not enter menopause, because the ovaries continue to produce estrogen and progesterone until the time of natural menopause, which is usually around ages forty-eight to fifty-two. Some studies, such as the Framingham Heart Study, still find that the risk for heart disease is higher even when one or both ovaries remain. Researchers suggest that the ovaries do not function as well once the uterus is gone because of impaired blood flow, and therefore don't produce as much estrogen as they did prior to surgery. Moreover, and this may be the reason for the increased risk of heart disease, up to one-third of women who have a partial hysterectomy experience early menopause.

If both your ovaries have been removed long before your menopausal years, you are at a higher risk for heart disease and will want to consider hormone replacement therapy. If you have had a hysterectomy but still retain your ovaries, you can have a blood test for *follicle-stimulating hormone (FSH)*, and then your doctor can determine how much estrogen is being produced. This will tell you whether or not you are approaching menopause, so you can take steps to reduce your risks through diet and lifestyle methods and possibly hormone replacement therapy, depending on your age.

It makes sense to me that women who are not producing their own female hormones naturally in the amounts their bodies require prior to menopause should supplement with replacement hormones. It is important to mimic the cyclic phase as closely as possible until we reach menopause. To deny our bodies sufficient estrogen and progesterone before they are ready to wind down puts us at risk for heart disease and osteoporosis. The female hormones play many roles throughout the body that are not solely related to the menstrual cycle, sex, and producing children. When they are not present in their proper ratios, our health suffers.

## NORMAL MENOPAUSE

Women are said to lose their gender-edge for heart disease one year after menstruation ceases, at which time they are considered almost twice as likely to experience heart disease as premenopausal women. Furthermore, several studies indicate that postmenopausal women who take estrogen can expect a 30 to 50 percent reduction in the risk of coronary disease. But why? Is it as simple as one female hormone, estrogen? Is it the combination of lowered amounts of estrogen and progesterone? Women still make estrogen after menopause, albeit in much smaller quantities, but we don't produce any progesterone. Could progesterone play a larger role than we think?

I truly believe that women's risk of heart problems increases not with menopause but with age. Research supporting this issue centers around female hormones, specifically estrogen, but my sense is that a host of other factors are also involved that have yet to be quantified. It has not been established that heart disease is caused by a deficiency of estrogen, and to assert that estrogen therapy is a panacea for menopausal women is blatantly irresponsible. Is it a factor that women need to consider along with all the others? Yes, but let's not promote the idea that heart disease is a symptom of menopause.

## HORMONE REPLACEMENT THERAPY

The prevailing wisdom is that the female sex hormones protect women from heart disease. We know that women prior to menopause are at a relatively low risk for heart disease, and after the change of life, when the female hormones diminish, the risk of heart disease increases. Many experts therefore suggest that, since a drop in estrogen seems to increase the risk of heart disease, all postmenopausal women should routinely supplement with estrogen as a preventive measure. While the research is interesting, I have a few philosophical problems with this approach.

I oppose isolating one risk factor (in this case, lowered estrogen levels) out of a constellation of possibilities and focusing on it to the exclusion of all others. I do not believe in mandating that all women take estrogen without regard for potential harm, especially when there are so many less invasive methods for tempering risk factors. Some top experts agree that we need to be prudent about randomly prescribing hormones. Lynn Rosenberg, M.D., an epidemiologist who specializes in cardiovascular research, testified before a congressional committee in January 1993, expressing concern that estrogen replacement (ERT) and the combination estrogen/progesterone therapy (HRT) are being prescribed without adequate assessment of the risks, benefits, and alternatives. Elizabeth Barrett-Connor, M.D., another epidemiologist who has written several papers on hormone therapy, shared her apprehension in a 1993 journal article. She wrote, "No other prescription drug has been given on such a large scale to prevent disease in healthy women without proof of efficacy by a randomized clinical trial."

All the major risk factors need careful attention if coronary disease is to be markedly reduced. It is my opinion that thousands of women are taking their little maroon pills with false confidence that they are doing their part to control heart disease. Diet, good nutrition, exercise, weight loss, and stress reduction are relegated to a lesser role in favor of the wonder drug, miracle cure, and quick fix. Until daily habits are changed, we will not see a decline in heart disease in women, no matter how many drugs we swallow.

ERT and HRT may be the best bet for some women; however, many women cannot take these hormones because of preexisting conditions such as cancer of the breast or uterus, liver disease, gallbladder disease, uterine fibroid tumors, endometriosis, diabetes, and migraines. Others cannot tolerate estrogen because they experience side effects such as withdrawal bleeding, fluid retention and weight gain, lower abdominal bloating, headaches, nausea, anxiety, mood swings, and vaginal discharge.

While hormone therapy is appropriate for some women who are at risk for osteoporosis and heart disease, and it successfully manages very uncomfortable symptoms of menopause like hot flashes, there are lifestyle measures for all these conditions that are as effective in many women. For the management of menopausal complaints and osteoporosis without using hormones, read my book *Menopause Without Medicine*. I do not reject the research on hormones, but I would like to suggest that heart disease is more than a deficiency of estrogen; it develops after a lifetime of inadequate nutrition and poor habits. Yes, hormone replacement is an option for some, but lifestyle improvements should be required for all.

What are the long-term effects of extended hormone use? With women opting not to have children or postponing pregnancy until later in life, many will be taking hormones for decades. Tack on to the continuous years of contraceptive hormones another twenty years of postmenopausal replacement therapy, and we are talking possibly fifty years of additional synthetic drugs. What will that do to the body? We know it definitely increases the probability of developing breast cancer. But is that all? The research is insufficient at this time, and it will be at least twenty years before we have definitive answers. Tough dilemma for those of us who need to make educated choices today.

## Natural versus Synthetic Hormones

If you have decided to take hormones, I would suggest that you consider investigating natural hormones. A few studies have found that natural hormones have the same positive effects as the synthetic versions with few or none of the negative side effects. The largest hormone study to date, the Postmenopausal Estrogen/Progestin Intervention trial (PEPI), found that natural hormones were as effective as estrogen and progestin in decreasing LDL cholesterol and raising HDL cholesterol levels.

The term *natural* is confusing, because it means different things depending on how it is used. In the case of hormones, *natural* refers to the structure of the molecule. Natural hormones are believed to be biochemically similar to the hormone found in the female body. This is thought to be why women seem to tolerate them better than some of the synthetic versions.

We tend to think that natural means coming from nature. The hormones labeled "natural" are in fact derived from the wild yam and modified soy estrogen; however, so are many of the synthetic hormones on the market. But the drug companies that make these synthetic hormones change the molecular configuration and add other ingredients to make their product patentable, which means more profitable.

Natural estrogen and progesterone come in pill form just like synthetic hormones. You still need a prescription, so you must go through a physician or medical clinic. The research is relatively new on the natural varieties, so it is quite possible your doctor may not be well informed about them.

If you want to know whether you are taking the right hormones or would like to find out about your various options, contact a pharmacy that specializes in natural hormones. They will be happy to send you and your doctor studies and information on the benefits and uses of natural estrogen and progesterone. I have provided phone numbers of places to call in the reference section. Another great resource is Dr. Christiane Northrup's monthly newsletter *Health Wisdom for Women*.

Women have been trained not to contradict or question their doctors. But it's our lives we are talking about, so we should be able to use our own research and ask questions about our treatment. We have choices, and each of us should make the decision about whether or not we want to take hormones and, if we do, whether they will be natural or synthetic.

Should you go on hormone therapy? Only you can decide. Consider both sides and keep up with new information. It may be different tomorrow. Listen to your doctor's advice, read all you can about women and hormones, and then make up your own mind.

# 5

# RISKY BEHAVIORS

*It's not the tragedies that kill us, it's the messes.*
—DOROTHY PARKER

## ACTIVE AND PASSIVE SMOKE

Does anyone not know that smoking is bad for one's health? And it's even worse for women than for men. A fifty-five-year-old woman smoker is in more danger of having a heart attack than her fifty-five-year-old male counterpart. Smoking cigarettes heightens women's risk of heart disease in several ways: women smokers start menopause two to three years earlier than nonsmokers; smoking lowers women's levels of good HDL cholesterol and raises levels of bad LDLs; and smoking increases a woman's chance of developing severe hypertension.

A rather disturbing study in the January 14, 1998, issue of JAMA linked both active and passive smoking to hardened arteries. It stated that the arteries of smokers, ex-smokers, and those exposed to secondhand smoke harden much faster than those of nonsmokers. According to Dr. George Howard, one of the study's researchers at Wake Forrest University, "When you smoke, you are accumulating damage to your arteries, and when you quit, the rate of damage is proportional to the amount of smoking you've done." It appears that the speed at which the arteries harden has more to do with how many cigarettes were smoked rather than the length of time since one quit.

Those of you who think this doesn't apply to you because you smoke only a few cigarettes a day should be aware that even one to four cigarettes a day can increase your risk by two to three times. Of course, heavy smoking is worse, but even a few cigarettes a day can damage the walls of your coronary arteries, making it easier for plaque to attach to them. Smoking also activates your body's blood-clotting system, promoting clots that can lead to heart attack. Smoking is possibly the strongest factor involved in *peripheral vascular disease*, a narrowing of the blood vessels that carry blood to the legs, brain, and kidneys. This condition often precedes a heart attack.

Smoking has harmful effects on the bones, lungs, and other body parts. Women smokers have twice the incidence of pelvic inflammatory disease as women nonsmokers, have an increased risk for cataracts, and are more likely to experience restless sleep, snore, and have nightmares.

Secondhand smoke can wreak havoc in the heart as well. In a latter-day look at the Nurses' Study, scientists found that being exposed regularly to other people's smoke appears to almost double the risk of heart disease in women who don't smoke. The Harvard author is quoted as saying this is higher than previously noted and is "startling in terms of the strength of the association."

You may not be able to completely avoid secondhand smoke, but you do have control over your own smoking habit. And once you quit, your risk is greatly diminished. When you stop smoking, your body starts to reverse some of the damage that has been inflicted. Within a mere twenty-four hours, your chance of a heart attack starts to decrease. Within one year, your risk of coronary heart disease is half that of a smoker. Don't wait until it is too late. Make the decision to stop smoking today. I highly recommend a helpful book called *How Women Can Finally Stop Smoking* by Robert C. Klesges, Ph.D., and Margaret DeBon, M.S. (listed in the references section at the end of this book). If you can't find it at your local bookstore, call the publisher at 1-800-266-5592. Order it this week.

## AIR QUALITY

Outdoor pollution is getting worse in many cities, and we may not realize that it is unhealthy for the heart as well as the lungs. According to a study conducted at London's St. George's Hospital Medical School, air pollution may trigger one out of fifty heart attacks. Measuring daily pollutant levels between 1987 and 1994 revealed that elevated levels of the various chemicals in smog were linked to an increased risk of heart attack. Carbon monoxide seems to be particularly dangerous because it reduces oxygen levels in the blood, thereby putting an undue strain on the heart during physical activity. If you live in a city, I recommend not exercising heavily on days when air quality is poor.

## ALCOHOL: A DOUBLE-EDGED SWORD

A glass of wine with dinner seems to benefit women's hearts, as it does men's. Part of the ongoing Harvard Nurses' Health Study showed that women over fifty who drank up to twenty drinks per week (not all at once) had a lower risk of heart disease than non-drinkers. The rewards were greatest for those who were at risk for heart disease, meaning they had a collection of obvious risk factors. One must keep in mind when interpreting such research that other lifestyle factors or combinations of factors may have been responsible for the lowered incidence of heart disease, not just the alcohol.

Research shows that alcohol appears to protect against coronary artery disease in several ways: by raising the levels of HDL cholesterol, decreasing the "stickiness" of blood platelets, and lowering the level of fibrinogen, a blood coagulant and known risk factor for heart disease. We also know that red wine contains a variety of antioxidants that help prevent the oxidation of LDL cholesterol, another important contributing factor discussed further below.

### Red Wine: Protective Antioxidants

It is not clear whether all forms of alcohol have the same benefits in terms of heart health. To date it appears that wine confers the greatest benefits. Several studies contrasting the health benefits of white versus red wine show that the latter has more advantages. We know that red wine has more antioxidants than white, because the red skin and seeds from the grapes, the source of important antioxidants, are left in the barrel during fermentation. Red wine contains a large number of phenolic compounds, plant chemicals that have been found to be beneficial in numerous therapeutic applications. Phenols include antioxidant flavonoids such as quercetin, rutin, and catechins—each of which has been isolated and studied independently for its health-enhancing qualities.

One specific flavonoid, quercetin, has been tagged as one of the primary nutrients responsible for the "French Paradox," the fact that the French eat liberal amounts of fat and still have low rates of heart disease. Is it possible that the red wine compensates for rich sauces, liver pates, and whole cheese? A recent Dutch study lends weight (no pun intended) to this theory. A group of elderly men who regularly ate foods high in quercetin enjoyed a reduced risk of sudden heart attacks. The more quercetin, the lower the risk. For those of you who don't care to drink wine, grape juice, apples, onions, and green tea contain quercetin and may be just as protective.

## When Alcohol Is Not So Healthy

A little alcohol protects the body, but an excess poisons it. During the last few years, several studies have found lower death rates among moderate drinkers, meaning those who have one to two drinks per day. These findings suggest that risk rates follow a "U-shaped curve": the risk is lowest in the middle, for moderate drinkers, and highest on each end, where we find nondrinkers and heavy drinkers.

There is a special downside to heavy drinking for women. We do not metabolize alcohol in the same way as men do. Women do not produce as much of a special enzyme called *alcohol dehydrogenase,* which is needed to break down the alcohol molecule. Therefore, alcohol circulates in our bodies longer, making us more susceptible to liver disease and breast cancer. Even moderate alcohol use can raise blood triglyceride levels, a major risk factor for heart disease in women. Just a few drinks with dinner the night before a blood test can triple the level of triglycerides in your blood. Heavy drinking, in excess of two to three drinks a day, will cause a rise in blood pressure and add many unnecessary calories to the diet (a 3.5-ounce glass of wine has one hundred calories), and alcohol, when abused, may actually poison heart cells as well as liver cells. A recent study now raises another caution about the long-term health consequences of drinking alcohol; this one relates specifically to women taking estrogen. A Boston study found that when postmenopausal women who were on hormone replacement therapy drank the equivalent of just half a glass of wine, the levels of estradiol—one of the most potent forms of estrogen—in their blood nearly doubled. After they drank the equivalent of three glasses of wine, estrogen blood levels skyrocketed more than 300 percent. Researchers feel these findings could have significant implications, but what they are is still being studied.

High levels of circulating estrogen combined with moderate amounts of alcohol have been linked to breast cancer. Does this mean that drinking and taking hormones at the same time may escalate the risk of cancer? No one has been willing to make that connection yet. Elizabeth Ginsburg, M.D., a leading investigator in the Boston study, says she personally doesn't take a hard line on alcohol. She simply tells her patients that there is an association and then lets them make their own decisions. Dr. Ginsburg adds, "Association doesn't mean causation; it doesn't mean that if you drink you're going to get breast cancer. It just means that your risk is higher."

More than three drinks a day of any kind of alcohol—hard liquor or wine—can result in long-term nutritional deficiencies, a host of medical problems, premature aging, and death. Even in the presence of a fairly good diet, alcohol abuse inhibits the absorption of specific nutrients (vitamins C, E, D, B-1, and B-12, folic acid, and the mineral calcium) and increases urinary excretion of others (vitamin K, potassium, magnesium, and zinc). Alcohol provides little nutrition in relation to the calories it adds. It requires additional vitamins in order to detoxify in the liver (B vitamins: B-1, B-6, niacin, and biotin). It requires greater amounts of antioxidants (vitamin C, E, B-6, and B-12) to repair damaged tissues and rebuild new cells.

Alcohol in large quantities can be a nutritional nightmare. Certainly, popping a good multivitamin/mineral supplement will counteract some of these deficiencies and imbalances; however, it cannot protect the body from all of the toxic effects of alcohol or prevent fatty infiltration of the liver. Alcohol has the potential for raising blood pressure and drinking to excess increases your chances of stroke, stomach cancer, breast cancer, osteoporosis, accidents, and suicide. Women who drink heavily also seem to have higher rates of anxiety, depression, insomnia, menstrual cramps, abnormal vaginal bleeding, premenstrual syndrome, amenorrhea, infertility, and sexual dysfunction. And, of course, there's the potential for abuse.

Alcohol dependence is a very real concern for women: an estimated 4.6 million American women are alcoholics.

Not all women benefit from drinking even moderate amounts of alcohol. The list below identifies women who should absolutely *not* drink at all, or at least not during specific periods in their lives.

## Do *Not* Drink Alcohol If . . .

✦ You are pregnant or trying to conceive. Alcohol is known to induce miscarriage, birth defects, and Fetal Alcohol Syndrome.

✦ You are taking medications.

✦ You have a medical condition in which it may be contraindicated.

✦ You are a recovering alcoholic.

## Tips for Women Who Choose to Drink

✦ Stop at two drinks (one or less if you are at risk for breast cancer).

✦ Don't drink on an empty stomach. Soak up the alcohol with food.

✦ Never mix, never worry. Combining different alcoholic beverages can result in higher blood alcohol concentrations than if you stay with the same drink, even if the total amount of alcohol consumed is the same.

✦ If you have a family history of alcoholism, pay attention to how much and how often you drink.

✦ Drink purple grape juice as an alternative. It contains many of the same antioxidants as red wine, though in smaller amounts.

## SEDENTARY LIFESTYLE

Inactivity is just as potent a risk factor for heart disease as obesity, high blood pressure, and high blood cholesterol. Firsthand data now confirms that the cardioprotective benefits of exercise apply to women as well as men. In a very large study of women ages forty to sixty-five, it was found that the women who exercised were up to 44 percent less likely to suffer a heart attack than their more sedentary sisters.

## STRESS

Your deepest feelings and innermost thoughts touch your heart physically, just as they move you emotionally. The way you respond to life's major and minor irritations may send your blood pressure and cholesterol levels soaring into dangerous territory. Noted stress expert Dr. Hans Selye discovered years ago that repeated or unrelenting stress in one's life can thwart the body's natural built-in coping mechanism. Without a chance to recharge between major stresses, the entire body, mind, and soul suffer exhaustion, which can eventually turn into illness if left untreated. We need to rest and regroup as we struggle with death, divorce, job loss, moving, sickness, and such. One isolated event or several bad days won't send us to a coronary-care unit. It's constant and excessive stress over time that will wear our bodies down, leading to dysfunction and disease.

Your personality and actions, and the way you treat yourself and others, have been included among the factors that can either harm or benefit your health and your heart. Once again, most of the observational studies relating to life stress and the coronary-prone personality have focused on men, but what information is available for women does suggest similar conclusions.

A report by the U.S. Department of Labor announced that women who work outside the home rank stress as the most difficult problem in their lives. Complaints primarily came from women in their forties who had professional jobs and from single moms who said their worst nightmare is balancing work and family. At any age, whether you are single or married, an at-home-mom or an executive, life can be overloaded with frustrations and anxieties that, when internalized, can lead to ill health. You may be juggling two jobs, going to school and raising a family, staying at home feeling unfulfilled, struggling with guilt about leaving your children, tending to ailing parents, reparenting adult children, trying to find your niche in life, changing careers, surviving breast cancer, or living apart from your mate. No one is immune from life stress.

The term *stress* is highly subjective and obviously means different things to different people. Generally, we think of a stress as a negative reaction to an event or situation, but this isn't always the case. It could just as easily emerge from something long anticipated and very pleasant. I think, for example, of my daughter's wedding. The day went smoothly, with no disasters. A year of planning paid off, and we left that night with precious, treasured memories. So, why did it take me weeks to recover from that perfect celebration filled with beauty and love? As any mother or daughter out there knows, a wedding is more than a service and reception. Its significance extends far beyond the touching ceremony, fragrant flowers, and creative photography. A child's departure from home (even under the best circumstances) is loaded with feelings of loss, with nostalgia and memories, and future dreams for the entire family.

Many life events evoke unexpected emotions, which we ignore or overlook because they don't fit in with what we expect. Births, graduations, and holidays often stir up feelings that leave us unsettled, scared, frustrated, and sad. We're stressed and don't know why. I think it's a good idea to investigate disturbing feelings like these, especially when they appear repeatedly.

Long-term stress creates physiological changes in the body that place greater demands on the heart and can set the stage for a heart attack. We know that anxiety leads to elevations in blood pressure, which over time can damage vulnerable blood vessel walls. The inability to cope with stress also has the potential of triggering a rise in cholesterol levels far beyond the normal range.

One classic example is often cited in articles and books on stress to show how quickly people change their blood chemistry in a tense situation. Certified public accountants, during the height of tax season (between January and April 15) may show as much as a 100 mg/dl rise in blood fats as compared to their readings the rest of the year. And this is something that could happen to any of us: students taking tests, executives preparing proposals, actors performing on stage, women planning major events, parents concerned about sick children, people changing jobs or moving from one city to another, writers meeting deadlines. My sense is that we have all known situational stress, but we may not realize that it could be raising our blood pressure and blood cholesterol.

Women are said to be more adept at handling stress than men. We are better able to identify our feelings, share our frustrations with our friends, and cry more freely. We're more likely to try meditation, take a class in yoga, or go for a long walk when we need a break. All in all, I think women have better coping skills than men, which may be one of our best strategies for keeping our hearts healthy.

## DEPRESSION

Depression is a risk factor for heart disease that has been overlooked and underreported, but the numbers suggest that it deserves serious consideration. According to a Danish study, depressed and anxious women are 70 percent more likely to experience a heart attack than women who are not depressed. Since women report symptoms of depression twice as often as men, this is something we really need to "take to heart."

Many doctors speculate that depression is a severe form of stress. Depressed individuals show elevated levels of the stress hormones cortisol and norepinephrine, which are known to hike up the heart rate and blood pressure. Over time, depression causes the arteries to constrict and encourages platelets to clump together and form clots. Depressed people often turn to self-destructive habits for comfort, such as smoking or excessive eating and drinking, their nutrition is often poor, and they tend not to exercise—all of which contribute to poor health and premature death.

One particular problem with depression, much like heart disease and high blood pressure, is that it often goes unnoticed. Stephen Sinatra, M.D., cardiologist and psychiatrist, finds that many of his depressed patients are unaware of their problem. They don't consider themselves depressed, but when asked how they find pleasure in life, they are stumped for an answer. So, how do *you* find pleasure in life?

Mild depression, situational sadness, and bad days may yield to exercise, relaxation techniques, and meditation. But lingering mood disturbances require professional therapy. Look over the following list and see if any of these signs apply to you. If three or more do, consider talking to a therapist, counselor, minister, priest, or spiritual director.

## Signs of Depression

+ Fatigue or listlessness.

+ Feelings of sadness, hopelessness, or emptiness.

+ Feelings of guilt, worthlessness, or emptiness.

+ Loss of interest or pleasure in everyday living.

+ Sleeping too little or too much.

+ Loss of appetite, overeating, or overdrinking.

+ Difficulty concentrating or making decisions.

+ Irritability.

## THE ANGRY HEART

Of all the human emotions, chronic anger stands out in its ability to undermine the heart. Medical knowledge accumulated over two decades clearly points to unresolved anger and hostility as the most destructive emotions to our physical health. Most of the studies on the health consequences of anger grew out of the search to find a link between behavior and the risk of heart disease. Researchers were specifically interested in determining whether men with certain characteristics—namely, competitiveness, aggressiveness, impatience, and hostility—were especially susceptible to heart attacks. The data suggested there was indeed a link between this type of behavior, which researchers labeled Type A behavior, and heart disease.

The landmark book that came out of these studies, *Type A Behavior and Your Heart*, by cardiologists Meyer Friedman and Ray Rosenman, hit the bookstores in the mid-1970s. It sounded so plausible that soon everyone believed that someone who worked long hours and was driven to succeed would suffer repercussions later in life. Well, over two thousand papers and journals later, guess what?

The theory turns out to have a few bugs. Apparently, not all aspects of the Type A personality are equally detrimental; only those concerned with chronic anger and hostility are harmful. Being ambitious, competitive, and hardworking are no longer clumped together in the same group as the more toxic characteristics. Actually, the current data reveal that the Type A male heart attack victim actually fares better in recovery than his mellow counterpart.

In one study of over sixteen hundred women and men, episodes of anger seemed to trigger a heart attack in people with diagnosed or latent heart disease. In this study, Dr. Mittleman, the primary investigator, found that the risk of having a heart attack was 2.3 times greater than would otherwise be expected if the person had been angry two hours prior to the event. This is not to suggest that everyone who erupts into an occasional rage will experience symptoms or drop dead. If you are healthy, chances are slim that anything will happen. The unfortunate news is that many of the heart attack victims in Dr. Mittleman's study had no previous history of coronary artery disease, which indicates that these anger-prone individuals were probably unaware that their body was primed already, whether because of years of anger or because of an already weakened heart.

## Women and Anger

During the dark ages of the 1970s, it was unthinkable that a woman might pursue a career with the same passion and aggressiveness as a man. And, of course, women were not considered prospects for heart disease—so why study us? Well, as we now know, women can be high-powered executives, doctors, lawyers, senators, bankers, and business owners. And on top of that, many of us raise children, do laundry, and clean our own homes. We also struggle with emotions that make us candidates for heart disease.

According to a number of studies, women get angry as often as men do (about six or seven times a week), for pretty much the same reasons, and with the same degree of intensity. However, women's styles differ when it comes to expressing their anger. Unlike the hot-tempered male, women tend not to erupt on the spot when provoked but postpone their reaction until another time. It's not that women are less agitated—they just keep a lid on it, letting the heat pass unexpressed and unresolved. Anne Campbell, a psychologist at England's Durham University, explains that women might get angry at work but usually will wait until they are alone or with a friend or partner to vent.

Suffering in silence may seem noble, but it turns out not to be the best way to deal with anger. A Belgian study showed that squelching one's emotions can be as damaging as blowing up. Heart attack survivors who had a tendency to suppress emotional distress were 27 percent more likely to die within six to ten years than those who did not stifle their rage. It appears that neither swallowing your anger nor venting it on innocent bystanders are healthy approaches for controlling habitual anger. Learning what triggers it and practicing new responses can blunt the harmful biochemical reactions that are set in motion when anger takes over our emotional life.

Women have one advantage over men when they get angry: they allow themselves to cry. Crying was once labeled a sign of weakness, but now it is regarded as a healing tool. Science has confirmed that our tears stimulate hormones that strengthen the immune system. I have a theory: maybe it is our tears that protect us from heart disease rather than our hormones. Now there's a thought.

## Physical Response to Anger

Experiencing continual outbursts of anger is like taking a small dose of a slow-acting poison every day of your life—so believes Redford Williams, a professor of psychiatry at Duke University. According to him, chronic anger results in biochemical effects on the cardiovascular system that slowly destroy the body. The external signs of an anger attack are easy to spot. Along with the verbal explosion comes a raised, quivering voice, aggressive hand gestures, clenched fists, a tight jaw, or a reddened face. What's going on beneath the skin is not so obvious. Anger, like other stressors, signals the adrenal glands to pump large doses of both adrenaline and cortisol into the bloodstream. When the adrenaline reaches the heart, the heart starts to pump faster and harder, increasing blood pressure. The arteries that carry blood to the muscles open, or dilate, so that blood can flow more quickly. Arteries that carry blood to the skin, kidneys, and intestines, do the opposite—they close, or constrict. All systems pre-pare for fight or flight. The immune system shuts down, and your platelets get stickier so you are less likely to bleed if harmed. This is a wonderful mechanism if you need to fend off an attacker or save a child. Unfortunately, when we respond with this same intensity every time the car won't start or someone cuts us off on the road, we overload the system and it wears out.

So then, should we vow never to raise our voices in anger again? I don't think that would be either appropriate or possible. Even if we had such control, anger has a place in our lives. The world is not fair, and people do not always behave with the purest intentions. To express our righteous indignation and let others know when they have overstepped their bounds or wronged us is appropri-ate. It's when we overreact on a daily basis that we need to examine our behavior and see if it is detrimental to our health.

## Hostility Hurts

Of all the negative emotions, hostility is the one most damaging to the body. The word *hostility* probably conjures up different images in each of us. According to Dr. Redford Williams, certain traits that come under the broad heading of hostility are more likely than oth-ers to lead to serious illness. The cynical mistrust of others, the fre-quent experience of angry feelings, and the overt expression of this cynicism and anger through aggressive behavior all contribute to what is called the *hostility syndrome*. As a group, hostile people report common complaints:

+ Hostile individuals generally are unhappy, reporting more has-sles with others and negative daily life events and experiences.

+ They perceive less social support within their families and among their friends.

+ They are not good sources of support themselves; they are often considered physically, emotionally, and verbally abusive.

+ They report less marital satisfaction and more marital conflict.

+ They complain of less job satisfaction and more difficulty with work relationships.

◆ They are considered by friends and acquaintances to be frequently aggressive and abrasive in their interpersonal dealings.

◆ They often engage in self-destructive habits, such as over-eating, drinking excessively, and smoking.

If any of these ring true for you, think about making some behavioral adjustments. Many books are available that show how to diffuse unhealthy hostility and anger. I have listed the best ones in the reference section at the end of the book.

## SOCIAL ISOLATION

Are you content with your life, interested in people, active in a church or club, or involved in your community? If you are, you may be providing richer nourishment for your heart than if you ate oat-bran cereal and bought a treadmill. People who feel connected to other people, pets, and their environment experience fewer illnesses, are happier, and are better able to handle stress.

Researchers now consider the presence or absence of social support an independent risk factor for cardiovascular disease. The sense of belonging and connection to other people has the potential of lowering the incidence of heart disease as well as many other health problems. Furthermore, women who isolate themselves from others and confine themselves to their home, with little social contact, are creating an environment that is hostile to the heart.

Researchers from the University of Michigan tested over twenty-seven hundred adults between the ages of thirty-five to sixty-nine. They recorded the usual physical risk factors—blood pressure, cholesterol levels, and smoking. In addition, psychological interviews were conducted and evaluated in terms of the individuals' social relations. It was found that, independent of all the traditional risk factors, women with weak social ties had a death rate one and a half to two times higher than those with strong social connections.

A classic study from Alameda County in northern California correlated social isolation with a higher death rate from cardiovascular disease, cancer, and all other major causes of death, including suicide and accidents. Dr. George Kaplan and his colleagues tracked seven thousand healthy residents of Alameda County for several years to determine the various indicators of social connectedness. The number and intensity of all types of relationships were put under the microscope. They considered contacts with relatives and friends, marital status, church or club membership. Nine years later, the death rate of the group was assessed. For both sexes and all ages, mortality was greatest for those with the lowest number of social interactions. This correlation remained significant even when factors such as economic status, smoking, and other variables were removed.

Other scattered studies provide interesting facts about relationships and heart disease. Married people appear to have fewer heart attacks than single or widowed people. If one spouse dies, there is a greater risk for the remaining spouse. Doctors report many cases of sudden death after an individual learns about the loss of a loved one. Women appear to adapt better than men when faced with living alone, probably because they usually have more friends and social outlets. I remember my grandfather Henry died within one year of my grandmother Grace. I'm not sure what they gave as his cause of death, but no one questioned that Henry just didn't want to stick around without his Grace.

Contact with people and pets does wonders to keep us alive and happy. Studies have shown the value of owning and caring for an animal. Pets love you unconditionally, and they calm your nerves and lower your blood pressure. Clinical studies have shown that survivors of heart attacks who were greeted when they came home by loyal, nonjudgmental, loving animals had a higher survival rate than those who returned to an empty house. It is difficult to assess the exact mechanism at work, but we know that petting a dog or cat is soothing to the human psyche. Walking your dog provides not only exercise but social contact with fellow dog walkers. Even gazing at fish in an aquarium can take your mind off daily aggravations. The beneficial factor could be the love you receive from a pet, the love you give, a healthy distraction, or all of these.

## SELF-INVOLVEMENT

People who constantly talk about themselves have more coronary disease than those who are other-oriented. Over a decade ago, Larry

Scherwitz, a psychologist from the University of California at San Francisco, taped conversations with 150 people hospitalized for a heart attack or suspected of heart disease. During these structured interviews, he found that the patients with the more serious problems gave longer answers with more references to themselves. In other words, heart patients more often used the pronouns *I, me, my, mine* in responding to questions. Even when he took other facts into consideration, such as age, blood pressure, cholesterol, Type A behavior, and the illness itself, the results remained significant.

Redford Williams, M.D., believes that self-involvement may be tied to the hostile personality that has been shown to be particularly susceptible to heart disease. In his book *Anger Kills* he explains that a hostile person's distrust of others probably leads him or her to focus almost exclusively on his or her own thoughts and ideas. Recognizing this character trait in oneself and learning how to listen to others can help one to break out of this behavior pattern.

## WORKING WOMEN, STRESS, AND LOSS OF CONTROL

The more control you feel you have over your life, the healthier your heart. Women executives who hold positions of power were expected to exhibit greater stress because they were supposed to have that "male" cardiac-prone Type A personality. Wrong. High-powered executives, female or male, are not putting their lives on the line because they love their jobs and work long hours to succeed. Work itself is not the primary stressor we once thought; after all, it is often what gives our lives meaning. If you love your job and enjoy doing the work, but don't always fit in that vacation, you are not necessarily setting yourself up for a heart attack. Sometimes, taking time off work for a vacation just because it's scheduled may be a greater stressor. True, even people who love their jobs need a break; the trick is balancing work and rest, and knowing when to do each.

An interesting paradox exists concerning women who work outside the home. Even though they exhibit more obvious risk factors for heart disease than women who spend their time at home—in other words, they are more likely to smoke, drink more alcohol and coffee, and exercise less—when their blood is tested, it turns out they are healthier than their homebody sisters. We would expect the reverse.

A German study testing cholesterol levels in women employed outside the home found that employment may exert a beneficial influence on coronary risk in women because of their higher HDL levels. The study further concluded that when women quit their paying job to stay at home, their protective HDL levels took a dive. What does this tell us? Were these women happier and more fulfilled in an outside environment? Did they succumb to soaps and deny their creative expression at home? Were they overly tired and over-wrought taking care of young babies? Or did they feel they lost control over their schedules and lives? We aren't sure, but if there is a moral here, it's find what you love and do it.

Certain jobs appear to cause more stress for women than others. One study, conducted at Cornell Medical College by Peter Schnall, M.D., and his colleagues, identified types of work that created the most stress in an individual. Stressful jobs generally have two negatives in common: high emotional demands and low decision-making latitude. Jobs that force an employee to work hard and fast but allow little autonomy or control cause what researchers referred to as "job strain." Another study that adds credence to this theory comes from University College in London. This research tracked over seven thousand women and men in the British civil service from 1985 to 1993. The results matched the Cornell study, suggesting that a feeling of little or no control at work explains why the Dagwoods and Dilberts of the world have a greater risk of heart disease—50 percent higher—than those in the executive suite. This reverses everything we thought was true about who is most at risk in the workplace.

Many women work in situations that fit the description of high stress and no control—waitresses, secretaries, computer operators, retail clerks. So what do we do with this information? Quitting is not an option for most. Living without a paycheck while looking for the ideal working conditions just replaces one stressor with another. What you may consider is finding ways to feel more in control of your life and circumstances at home and during your leisure time.

# DISCRIMINATION

African Americans succumb to heart disease more often than any other group of Americans. Some researchers attribute this to genetics or personal habits such as eating a high-fat diet or smoking, while others believe that racial discrimination and poverty (with their accompanying problems, such as poor diet and lack of medical care) may be more significant factors. Three recent studies bring new possibilities to light.

A study from Harvard looked at four thousand black and white workers and found that when black workers experienced racial hostility in the workplace, their risk of hypertension increased significantly. Persistent emotional stress brought about by racial discrimination was more dangerous than smoking or dietary factors. This ties in with other research showing that hypertension risk is higher among workers with demanding jobs that offer little sense of control and limited job security. Black professionals who had more control over their circumstances were healthier.

The co-authors of the study, Drs. Nancy Krieger and Stephen Sidney, point out the obvious, that there is always damage inflicted by discrimination. The preliminary findings may be useful not only for addressing the problem of cardiovascular disease among African Americans but as confirmation of the health effects of inequalities between women and men.

# CHRONIC EMOTIONAL HEARTBREAK

The emotional wounds and scars we accumulate over time often initiate the process that eventually leads to fatal diseases. Sometimes, hurts that we think are long forgotten remain so deeply submerged that we fail to recognize them even when they ooze out into our lives in the form of obesity, alcoholism, hostility, or depression. In the book *Heartbreak and Heart Disease*, Dr. Stephen Sinatra, M.D., unveils another area for analysis: the heartbreaks of life. You probably never read or heard of heartbreak being a risk factor for coronary disease, yet more and more we are learning how emotional losses, disappointments, and painful childhood experiences can impact our emotional and physical adult lives.

Dr. Sinatra strongly believes that there is a connection between childhood heartbreak (defined as the loss of love and intimacy) and heart disease. A child who has been physically or emotionally abused or abandoned may partially close off her or his heart. To shut down the heart in order to survive, while at the same time being denied love, results in a behavior pattern that over the years gnaws away at the heart.

Denial protects the child from rejection and intense heartbreak. Since the loss of love can be so devastating, a child may feel that she could actually die and that the only way to survive is to forget and bury the emotions. Adults coming from these unfortunate homes rarely admit to it, even in therapy. They would much rather experience physical pain than tell a therapist or even their closest friend that they were not loved as children. While denial worked as a coping mechanism for the child, it isn't effective for an adult. Since the denial of feelings is an unconscious mechanism used to monitor our hurtful feelings, it actually blocks the perception of real impulses. All sorts of emotions get bottled up and eventually explode into anger and rage or implode as physical diseases. This denial of true feelings or of reality can contribute to behavior that puts you at risk for heart disease. A good therapist or spiritual advisor can help you through the heartbreak of early childhood and lead you into a healthy adulthood.

Scientific studies seem to favor research devoted to causes of sickness rather than causes of health. What are the behavioral traits that keep people healthy? Generally speaking (you can always find an exception), women and men who remain healthy and happy throughout their lives believe in the basic goodness of human nature. They treat people with respect, fairness, and consideration. They rarely exhibit resentfulness, irritability, anger, or hostility, and when they do, it is in a way that does not hurt others excessively, or linger. Modern science now agrees with the truths espoused over two thousand years by religious traditions around the world: A happy heart "is slow to anger" and "treats others as they would be treated."

# Part Two

# FOOD FOR THOUGHT

# 6

# CHOLESTEROL CONFUSION

Knowing the truth may mean stretching into untried, frightening,
difficult arenas .... Subsequent choices require we alter
our self-view and way of life, or let go of favored habits.

—MARSHA SINETAR

ost people are unclear about what cholesterol actually is,
what it does, and how it can escalate to unhealthy levels
in the blood. The food industry fuels the fire of confusion
with their misleading labeling practices. When we go to the grocery
store and attempt to search out healthful foods, we are drawn to
products labeled "low cholesterol" or "cholesterol-free," and if we go
by these labels we feel assured that the items dropped into our basket
are reasonably good for us and will not clog our arteries. Unfortunately, this is not always the case. Just because something is free of
cholesterol doesn't mean that it is low in fat or healthy in other
respects. The "cholesterol-free" label on an oil or bag of cookies
means only that the fat used in the product came from a plant and
not from an animal. Cholesterol is found *only* in the animal kingdom; plants do not manufacture cholesterol. So the label attached
to a vegetable oil or product cooked in vegetable oil is meaningless,
because of course it is free of cholesterol. What is obviously omitted
from the label is that the product may be just as or more destructive
to the arteries even though it is cholesterol-free.

# WHAT IS CHOLESTEROL, ANYWAY?

Cholesterol and fat are not synonymous. Cholesterol is a waxy, fat-like substance; it is classified as a *lipid*, which also means fat, but technically the two terms are not interchangeable. We get cholesterol from two sources: it comes into our bodies from food we eat, and we also make it ourselves naturally. It is a critical component of our cells and if we didn't ingest it, the liver would provide us with an ample supply. Although most people think that cholesterol does nothing but clog our arteries, it is actually a versatile and necessary compound, and we could not survive without it. It insulates the nerves and allows normal transmission of nerve impulses, it helps the liver to produce bile, and it is used to manufacture the steroid hormones, including our sex hormones. Now, doesn't that alter your opinion of cholesterol?

# WHAT'S SO BAD ABOUT CHOLESTEROL?

Excess cholesterol circulating through the body gravitates to the walls of the coronary arteries, eventually causing blockages, which inhibit the oxygen flow to the heart muscle. This can result in a heart attack. Cholesterol can also collect in other arteries, including those leading to the brain, which in time may result in a stroke.

Authorities agree that an elevated blood cholesterol level is associated with an increased risk of heart disease, and that the higher the level, the greater the risk. Furthermore, reducing total blood cholesterol holds great rewards. The Coronary Primary Prevention Trial, a landmark study by the National Heart, Lung, and Blood Institute, showed that each 1 percent reduction in blood cholesterol was associated with a 2 percent decrease in heart disease. If you cut your cholesterol by 25 percent, you reduce your risk of heart attack by nearly one-half.

Cholesterol levels climb out of control for a number of reasons. Your body may be genetically predisposed, or you may be eating too many foods rich in saturated or *trans* fats (unsaturated fatty acids found in margarine, fried foods, and packaged sweets) or not eating enough foods that contain critical nutrients. Finally, your general attitude about life and the way you deal with life's problems can contribute to elevating cholesterol levels.

## CHOLESTEROL TERMINOLOGY

There is no way of explaining the different types of cholesterol without introducing some basic definitions. Fortunately, technical terms have filtered into the daily news and most people who are interested in health issues are fairly familiar with them already. The root word for the different varieties of cholesterol is *lipoprotein,* so let's start there. Lipoproteins are molecules made up of fat and protein that transport cholesterol through the blood into individual cells. It takes a specialized molecule that is compatible with both the waterlike consistency of blood and the oily consistency of fat to carry cholesterol through the body.

Different lipoproteins are packaged differently in the blood and play quite different roles. Some are thought to promote heart disease and others to prevent it. The principal lipoproteins that transport cholesterol around the body are called *low-density lipoproteins* (LDLs) and *high-density lipoproteins* (HDLs). Because of their influences on the circulatory system, one has been branded "bad" (LDL) and the other good (HDL). The lousy LDLs do their dirty work by infiltrating blood vessel walls, where they latch onto the interior membrane and form a gummy, potentially deadly plaque. The healthy HDLs try to prevent the LDLs from attaching to the cell wall by extracting the harmful cholesterol from the blood and carrying it to the liver, where it is excreted. One of the fundamental steps for maintaining heart health is to lower the number of LDLs while augmenting HDLs. In this book I will offer a variety of ways to accomplish this.

*Triglycerides* are another group of fatty compounds that often travel in close contact with various kinds of cholesterol. They, too, can get out of hand and pose problems, especially for women. It is not clear what role they play in the development of heart disease, but triglycerides have been associated with premature narrowing of the arteries and the development of blood clots.

# TOTAL CHOLESTEROL

Most authorities recommend keeping total cholesterol levels below 200 mg/dl (milligrams per deciliter is how cholesterol is expressed in medical terms); others suggest that closer to 150 would be better, since men whose levels hover around this range rarely suffer from heart attacks. As mentioned in chapter 3, it is still open to discussion whether this is true for women. The studies so far seem to indicate that total cholesterol is not as critical in women as in men, but if you are a woman at high risk, I recommend monitoring your cholesterol level and following dietary and lifestyle practices to keep it under control.

The question that always arises when a benchmark is set is, If the desired number (200 in this case) is average or the standard, shouldn't I see if I can do better by going even lower? Not necessarily. In 1990 the National Heart, Lung, and Blood Institute met to discuss this very issue. Examining previous research, the researchers from the institute noticed a U-shaped association between blood cholesterol levels and subsequent mortality. It appears that the lowest incidence of mortality in men occurs when cholesterol levels fall between 160 and 200 mg/dl. Above 200, cardiac risk increases. Below 160, other problems arise: increased mortality rates related to cancer, respiratory and digestive problems, and miscellaneous factors, including injury. No explanation exists at this time for the association of very low cholesterol with higher risk of death, but it does make sense if you believe in the concept of "all things in moderation." When you exceed suggested ranges on either side of the spectrum, there are repercussions.

## Low-Density Lipoproteins: Aim Low

Low-density lipoprotein cholesterol clogs the arteries with fatty deposits and thus contributes to the development of heart disease. More than half of American women aged forty-five or older have LDLs higher than the desirable 130 mg/dl. Some researchers drop the healthy level down a few notches to 100 mg/dl. The good news is that LDL levels can be lowered by eating fewer saturated fats, choosing more fruits and vegetables, and losing weight if necessary.

## How Low Do We Go?

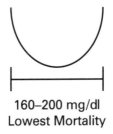

160–200 mg/dl
Lowest Mortality

*Below 160*
Increased risk of cancer
Respiratory problems
Digestive problems
Increase in violent deaths

*Above 200*
Cholesterol gravitates to artery wall
Oxygen flow is inhibited
Blockage is created
Possible heart attack

## High-Density Lipoproteins: Shoot High

High-density lipoprotein cholesterol helps pull the LDL deposits out of the arteries; sort of like Liquid Plumber. The more you have working for you, the better. Generally speaking, women are fortunate, because our HDL levels are naturally higher than men's, and we also have higher levels of a subfamily called cholesterol HDL-2, a factor that is critical in lowering the risk of CAD. Combine the effects of both, and we can come up with another valid explanation for why women are somewhat protected from heart disease. Estrogen may not be the only reason women don't tend to have heart problems until later in life.

Researchers suggest that HDL levels are a more powerful predictor of heart disease in women than in men. Even when total cholesterol levels are below 200 mg/dl, decreased HDL levels increase your probability of a heart attack. To give you an appreciation for its weight as a risk factor, if you have less than 35 mg/dl of HDL in your blood, your risk is the same as that of someone who is a moderate to heavy smoker—and you are well aware that is not good. Even at or below 45 mg/dl, you will want to pay attention to your food choices, exercise levels, and emotions. Shoot relatively high in this category: 60 mg/dl is ideal.

## Triglycerides: Go Low

Triglycerides don't get as much attention as the other two fatty compounds, but they are increasingly being recognized as an important risk factor for women, regardless of HDL levels. Triglycerides are the main type of fats found in the foods we eat and also the main type of fats found in the body. Blood levels of triglycerides are determined partly by our genes, partly by the fatty foods we eat, and partly by the amount of refined carbohydrates in our diet. Being overweight can elevate triglyceride levels, as can age, adult diabetes, oral contraceptives, and hormone replacement therapy. Losing weight, exercising, and controlling saturated fats, carbohydrates, and alcohol in the diet are tried and true ways of bringing triglycerides down to a desirable level of 150 mg/dl.

## Ratio of Total Cholesterol to HDL

Cardiovascular risk is frequently assessed in terms of a ratio that takes into account both total cholesterol and HDL values. It better represents the risk for individuals who appear to have inconsistent numbers; for example, they may have a low total cholesterol (good) and a low HDL (bad), or a high LDL (bad) and a high HDL (good). To determine your own ratio, you will need to do a little math, but it's very simple. You will need the numbers from your cholesterol profile, so if you haven't had a physical in a year or so, make an appointment for a fasting blood test and come back to this section when you have your figures. The lab or your doctor may do the calculating for you, but for your information here's the formula. Divide your total cholesterol value by the HDL, and this will give you your risk ratio. Say your total is 215 and your HDL is 93; your ratio would be 2.3, which is very good. A ratio of 4.0 or lower is suggestive of a low-risk profile.

| CHOLESTEROL VALUES | DESIRABLE | INCREASED RISK |
|---|---|---|
| Total Cholesterol | below 200 mg/dl | above 240 mg/dl |
| LDL Levels | below 130 mg/dl | above 160 mg/dl |
| HDL Levels | above 60 mg/dl | below 35 mg/dl |
| Triglycerides | below 150 mg/dl | above 190 mg/dl |
| Ratio of Total Cholesterol to HDL | below 4.0 | above 4.5 |

## FREE RADICALS: THE TRUE VILLAINS

The primary cause of plaque buildup in the arteries is actually not cholesterol—it is *free radicals* and the damage they inflict. These villainous oxygen molecules attack individual cells, which in time weakens the lining of the artery, creating crevices and rough edges that attract fat and cholesterol. If the arterial wall remained smooth and sleek, cholesterol would easily slide on through, but once it is compromised, plaque can easily attach and proliferate.

The highly reactive chemical compounds called free radicals have an affinity for LDL cholesterol. When they meet in the bloodstream, the free radicals attack the fatty LDL particles and initiate the process of *oxidation*. The body fights back by sending protective cells called *macrophages* to the rescue. As the macrophages engulf the fat globule they all mesh into what are then called *foam cells*. Once this stage is reached, the cell membrane becomes vulnerable to cholesterol attaching itself.

According to the current understanding of atherosclerosis, if you can stop this series of cellular events from taking place, LDL cholesterol should remain inert and harmless. Therefore, it is not the LDLs themselves that are ultimately dangerous to the arteries, it is the fact that they are transformed into toxic substances by free radicals in the blood, thereby creating an environment that is ripe for plaque formation. Free radicals also work by blocking the production of important hormones called *prostaglandins*, potentially leading to the formation of blood clots.

Oxidation is a natural process that occurs whenever fats are exposed to oxygen. All kinds of fats and cholesterol are radicalized by oxygen into toxic lipid peroxides. You witness this process when you leave your food too long in the pantry or refrigerator and it turns rancid. (My son Joey collects an interesting array of specimens, in case you don't have any of your own.) You may have surprised yourself by finding oxidation in progress when you accidentally left your metal gardening tools outside in the moisture and they started to rust. Similarly, our cell linings are constantly turning rancid and rusting because they have been exposed to rampant free radicals. This is something that happens naturally, but we want to keep it from getting out of control.

So, how do we stop these renegades from terrorizing our cell membranes? We can do this in several ways. Taking in less total fat is a reasonable start. A high-fat diet is a sure way to build an army of free radicals in the body. Heat is a catalyst for oxidation; therefore, the less you heat food, the smaller the band of roving radicals. Fresh, uncooked fruits and vegetables provide an array of antioxidants that both guard a healthy cell and renew an ailing cell. Taking mixed antioxidants in supplement form is an alternate plan for protecting the cells. The more food is processed and altered from its natural state, the more toxic free radicals are created; therefore, packaged products should be kept to a minimum in your daily diet.

Many substances that we come into contact with every day act as catalysts for free radical production. Limiting your exposure to the following is helpful:

+ Aluminum: cans, foil, antacids, kitchen pans, deodorants.

+ Cadmium: cigarette smoke, coffee, gasoline.

+ Carbon Monoxide: car exhaust, cigarette smoke, smog.

+ Chlorine: some tap water, pools.

+ Copper: some tap water, plumbing pipes.

+ Electromagnetic radiation: TV, computer screen.

+ Lead: dyes, paint, gasoline, plumbing.

+ Mercury: amalgam fillings, fish, paint, some cosmetics.

+ Nitrates and nitrites: processed meats.

+ Pesticides.

+ Radiation: X-rays.

Avoiding fat, high heat, and the free radical catalysts mentioned in this list is a good offensive strategy. Another approach is to bolster up a defensive team that will hold the line against invasion. Since oxidation is natural to the body, we also have an elaborate system that protects us against free-radical attack. The team is collectively called *antioxidants* (appropriately named) and they are produced from the nutrients that we ingest. You have probably heard of many of the major antioxidants, such as vitamin A (beta-carotene), vitamin C, and vitamin E. Not as well known are the minerals selenium, copper, zinc, and manganese, and specific sulfur-containing amino acids such as L-cysteine. Antioxidant nutrients temper the production of free radicals, intercept the damaging chain reaction that ends in destruction, and neutralize the oxygen before it attacks the body.

As we discussed earlier, it has been suggested that the French have a relatively low heart disease rate despite their penchant for rich sauces because they enjoy red wine, which contains antioxidants that inhibit LDL oxidation. They also eat many fresh fruits and vegetables, which are loaded with heart-healthy antioxidants. Wine may not harm the body and even be good for it if taken in moderation, but it is fruits and vegetables that are our best bet for keeping free radicals in check.

## DOES DIETARY CHOLESTEROL INCREASE BLOOD CHOLESTEROL?

The most renowned scientists and clinicians in the world hold radically differing opinions on whether dietary cholesterol increases blood cholesterol. One faction of distinguished authorities feels that the amount of cholesterol you eat daily raises the level of cholesterol in your blood. The other side, equally opinionated, says no, it doesn't matter how much cholesterol you ingest; your blood cholesterol levels will not be markedly altered. Both sides agree that saturated and *trans* fats are the worst offenders in creating unnecessary cholesterol; however, there is disagreement as to whether the cholesterol in food itself elevates blood levels. In a study conducted at both Northwestern University of Medicine in Chicago and the University of Texas, over eighteen hundred middle-aged men were tracked for twenty-five years. The study indicated that dietary cholesterol intake *was* associated with increased risk of death from heart disease. A long-time researcher and professor emeritus at Northwestern, Dr. Jeremiah Stamler, concluded "Cholesterol-rich foods promote heart disease even in people with low blood cholesterol." If this is the case, then it would behoove us all to monitor our intake of high-cholesterol foods.

Researchers at Oxford University in England recently published a meta-analysis examining over two hundred well-designed studies and found that the cholesterol in a single egg yolk raises blood cholesterol by 5.4 points. When you consider that an omelet usually consists of three eggs, that is not a small number.

Equally qualified experts uphold the view from the other side of the table. Paul Hopkins, M.D., a cardiologist from the University of Utah, recently analyzed twenty-seven studies on the subject and determined that eating foods rich in cholesterol *doesn't* make that much of a difference in the blood profile of most people. In his estimation, many individuals easily process eggs and other foods that are considered to be dangerous repositories of cholesterol, with no harm to the body.

Supporting this line of thinking is Dr. Edward Ahrens, a supervisor of research at New York's Rockefeller University. He states that only certain people need to worry about high-cholesterol foods. One of the New York studies found that about 20 percent of the men who ate three eggs daily for three weeks experienced blood cholesterol increases of more than 10 percent; 14 percent excreted the extra cholesterol; and the remaining 66 percent maintained the same blood cholesterol level. Dr. Ahrens explains that individuals respond differently when high loads of dietary cholesterol are dumped into their bodies. Depending on the individual's unique metabolism, three things may happen: (1) the excess cholesterol is metabolized and excreted, leaving blood levels unaffected; (2) the liver compensates for the overload by monitoring its own cholesterol production; or (3) the liver cannot handle the excess cholesterol in the body and subsequently stores it in the blood vessels and coronary arteries. It is the last group of people who are adversely affected by dietary cholesterol and therefore must reduce their intake. How do you know if you fall into this high-risk category? The answer is not simple, but the test is. Eliminate cholesterol-rich foods like meat, dairy, and eggs from your diet for two to three months, then have your total cholesterol rechecked. If it goes down appreciably, then cholesterol in foods is a problem for you. If you go back to your pretest diet for a few months and witness a dramatic rise, there is no question that your body requires a cholesterol-restrictive diet.

What do we do with this conflicting information? Wait until everyone is in total agreement before we act? My personal thinking on this matter is that if you have had a heart attack or know your risks are significant, do it all. Cut the fat, cut the cholesterol, take the vitamins, exercise, and learn how to relax. Why play the odds? When the research comes up with a more definitive answer, you can always revamp your plan. If you are the picture of health and have an impressive blood profile, you can be a bit more relaxed about ordering that Saturday omelet or indulging in a pat of butter now and then.

## Cholesterol Content of Common Foods

+ *Very High:* Egg yolks, liver, lamb chops, shrimp.

+ *High:* Veal, chuck roast, ham, bacon, steak, beef bologna, lobster, turkey, chicken, whole milk, ricotta cheese, waffles, pound cake, ice cream, pizza.

+ *Moderate:* Tuna, whole milk, cheddar cheese, yogurt, chocolate cake, bran muffins.

+ *Low:* Milk (1%), low-fat yogurt and cottage cheese, pancakes.

+ *Very low or none:* Egg whites, nonfat milk and yogurt, fruits, vegetables, grains, pasta, bread.

## BOTTOM-LINE FOODS FOR LOWERING CHOLESTEROL LEVELS

Blood cholesterol can waver in *some* people depending on what they eat or don't eat. Certain foods are known to hike up cholesterol levels and others can lower them. As a rule, the people who respond best to altering cholesterol levels thorough diet are those with the highest readings. If your blood profile registers in the unhealthy ranges, consider the dietary choices below.

| FOODS THAT RAISE CHOLESTEROL | FOODS THAT LOWER CHOLESTEROL |
| --- | --- |

*HIGH-FAT MEATS*

- ribs
- bacon
- sausage
- luncheon meats

*HIGH-FAT DAIRY*

- cheese
- butter
- cream
- milk
- yogurt

TRANS *FATS*

- stick margarine
- bakery products
- deep-fried foods
- doughnuts
- crackers
- processed foods (hydrogenated)

*MONOUNSATURATED OILS*

- olive
- canola
- avocado
- nuts

*OMEGA-3 FATTY ACIDS*

- salmon
- mackerel
- tuna
- sardines
- flaxseed
- walnuts

*SOLUBLE FIBER*

- oatmeal and oat bran
- apples
- carrots
- beans
- prunes

*ANTIOXIDANTS*

- fruits and vegetables
- alcohol
- garlic and onions

# 7

# FAT: FRIEND OR FOE?

We are what we repeatedly do.
Excellence then, is not an act, but a habit.
—ARISTOTLE

The library shelves are lined with journal articles implicating fat as the offender responsible for most major chronic health problems. Excessive amounts of fat in the diet and on the body specifically harm the heart by raising blood cholesterol levels, clogging the arteries, elevating blood pressure, contributing to diabetes, and preventing weight loss. No controversy here—too much fat destroys the heart. Or does it? A handful of researchers suggest there is indeed another side to this issue. The *amount* of fat may not be as important as and is possibly less important than the *kind* of fat consumed regularly in the diet.

The reigning low-fat, high-fiber diet evolved from research that began decades ago. Nathan Pritikin, among other pioneer researchers, studied cultures in which heart problems were nonexistent, and noticed that the diets of these healthy, robust people included very little fat and considerably more carbohydrates than is common in the United States. Observational studies that included subcultures within the United States, like the Seventh-Day Adventists, led to the theory that the low-fat, vegetarian diet should be the prototype for a heart-healthy diet.

Fat, in all forms, has emerged as the primary troublemaker for anything that goes wrong with the body. Heart disease, cancer, and other diseases are caused by too much fat in the diet. We are a fat-obsessed nation. But is the subject really that clear-cut and that simple? In our attempt to find something to blame, have we overlooked other evidence? What about those societies from which we have tried to learn? What else do they do on a regular basis that may be beneficial to their health? These are more recent questions that have been raised and that bear equal consideration. The Chinese and rural Japanese, for instance, are also highly active, and they eat an abundance of fruits, vegetables, seafood, and tofu. So why have we focused on fat intake alone when there are other elements of their lifestyles that may contribute equally to a lower risk of heart disease?

When we examine other cultures, we uncover some outstanding paradoxes regarding the fat issue. Take the Greenland Eskimos, for example. They consume an enormous amount of fat in the form of whale blubber, yet they have strong, healthy hearts. If the amount of fat were the only criteria for determining heart health, these people would be listed among the extinct. There is clearly more to heart disease than just the amount of fat consumed. The issue is far more complex, and to focus on this single factor alone is naive and potentially dangerous. In borrowing the "best" of another culture's diet we selectively choose what is easily salable to the American public. Consider that we are all dousing our bread in olive oil and drinking more red wine, but we're not eating whale blubber sandwiches.

More recently, scientists have been studying the dietary habits of still other cultures that consume what we would consider a prodigious amount of fat (up to 40 percent), because they too are showing us up when it comes to a lower incidence of heart disease. The Greeks, Italians, and French who live in the Mediterranean climates thrive on olive oil and rich sauces, and their hearts apparently are *not* suffering. Such paradoxes are shaking up the low-fat/no-fat community, and people are being forced to rethink this whole fat issue.

The type and amount of the fat eaten is being reexamined, and many scientists are suggesting that maybe they have carried fat restriction too far in their quest for an easy answer. For women, I find this issue particularly crucial and timely. So many women are cutting their fats to super-low levels, thinking they are prudently following heart-healthy guidelines. Not only may this be unnecessary, for women it just might be harmful. The evidence shows that the low-fat diet that works so well to lower total cholesterol and LDL cholesterol comes with a downside—it drags down our protective HDL cholesterol, which for women may be a more damaging risk than the extra fat in the diet.

## IN DEFENSE OF A LOW-FAT DIET

One greasy meal eaten by someone who has severely clogged arteries may be the last. Researcher George Miller of the Medical College of St. Bartholomew's Hospital in London states that for hours after a fat-rich meal, an individual is at higher risk of a fatal heart attack than at other times. Too much fat in the blood raises the levels of a protein called *factor VII*, which is instrumental in forming blood clots. The more factor VII in your blood, the larger the clot that will be created. It is not just clogging the arteries with plaque that is a problem; a sudden blood clot can also trigger a heart attack. One factor that determines the propensity to form clots is the amount of fat circulating in the blood. People whose arteries are gummed up with fat definitely need to examine both the amount and the type of fat they are ingesting.

Clinical trials have provided us with evidence that a low-fat diet does help to reverse heart disease. The most impressive research to date comes from Dr. Dean Ornish's Lifestyle Heart Trial. Dr. Ornish took men and women who already had partially blocked arteries and put them on a very low fat vegetarian diet that provided only 8 percent of calories from fat and virtually no cholesterol. After only a year, the blood cholesterol levels of the patients on the diet dropped dramatically, with averages falling from 213 mg/dl to 157 mg/dl. Moreover, coronary angiography, a relatively recent tool that provides a picture of the artery, showed that atherosclerotic plaques regressed in eighteen of the twenty-two people who completed the program. It must be noted here that fat reduction was not the exclusive variable in this study; modest exercise and meditation for stress reduction were also utilized.

A low-fat diet can reduce high blood pressure, which in turn lowers your risk for coronary disease. The Dietary Approaches to

Stop Hypertension (DASH) Trial, presented to the American Heart Association in November 1996, found that a low-fat diet, defined as 27 percent of calories from fat, is as effective in lowering hypertension as some drugs. For eight weeks, 459 participants whose blood pressure was higher than 140/90 ate a balanced diet that included small amounts of lean meat, chicken, fish, low-fat dairy products, cereals, fruits, and vegetables. After just two weeks into the study, these people's blood pressure began to fall; after eight weeks the average drop was 11.4 for systolic and 5.5 for diastolic.

How low in fat do we need to go in order to protect our hearts? When discussing the difference between the Spartan 10 percent–fat diet Dr. Ornish advocates and the more liberal 30 percent advised by the American Heart Association, we should distinguish between a reversal diet and a prevention diet. If you have survived a heart attack and you know your arteries are thick with plaque, then shoot for the lower end of the fat scale until you have seen a major improvement in your arteries or blood work. Then you can gradually add healthy fats to your diet while incorporating lifesaving nutrients, exercise, and stress busters. A diet to reverse and heal heart disease will generally be more stringent than one that is designed to prevent it.

For those of us who are concerned about maintaining healthy hearts, 30 percent of the monounsaturated and omega-3 fats is a reasonable goal. And guess what? As a nation, we are getting close to that target. According to a 1995 survey, dietary fat has decreased to about 33 percent of the total diet from the 43 percent typical in the 1960s. We are to be congratulated for our efforts. Now it is time to change focus from the *amount* of fats to the *type*. If that 33 percent fat is saturated or *trans* fat, as I suspect it is, we still have alterations to make—but we have proven that we respond to dietary recommendations, so it shouldn't be too much of a problem.

## WOMEN AND THE VERY LOW FAT DIET

A diet that is too low in fat is not necessarily a great idea for women. The low-fat diet that reduces LDL cholesterol in men has one major drawback: it lowers the protective HDLs as well. This may be fine for men, because their circulatory system is strongly influenced by

LDL levels. Women's hearts, on the other hand, respond more favorably to the effects of high HDLs. What to do? One alternative is not to go too low. According to Margo Denke, M.D., a heart specialist and member of the American Heart Association's Nutrition Committee, it is only when you reduce total fat consumption to below 25 percent of total calories that HDL levels fall; when fat makes up between 25 and 30 percent of total calories consumed, HDL levels are maintained. For most of us, this is a healthy range to stay within throughout our lives. If you have had a heart attack and are under the care of a physician who has you on a very low fat diet plan (10–15 percent), you can bump up those HDLs with exercise, more fiber, omega-3 fatty acids found in fish oils and vegetables oils, and specific nutrients.

## QUESTIONING THE LOW-FAT DIET

Prevailing weight-loss wisdom maintains that all we need to do to drop those unsightly pounds is cut out fat and stock up on carbohydrates: bread, rice, pasta, and cereal. It sounds reasonable and isn't terribly restrictive, but unfortunately, it's not working for a lot of women.

Substituting carbohydrates for fat, popularly thought to be a healthy way to eat, has not been satisfactorily proven to have salutary effects on serum lipids or, surprisingly, on long-term weight management. Despite the plethora of fat-free foods on the market, Americans are not getting thinner. According to the USDA's Continuing Survey of Food Intakes by Individuals, the real truth is that while Americans' fat intake is edging down—from the high of 43 percent to 33 percent by 1994—we're still getting fatter by eleven pounds a person on average. According to the Centers for Disease Control and Prevention, the percentage of overweight Americans has increased from 25 percent of the population in 1980 to 55 percent of the population in 1998.

How could this be? We have been told that we can pig out on all the carbs we want as long as they are fat-free. While this may be true for a certain segment of the population, for another group high levels of carbohydrates, especially simple sugars and refined carbohydrates such as pasta, rice, and white breads, hike up weight and serum lipids, putting them at risk for cardiovascular disease.

This condition, known as *insulin resistance*, sometimes accompanies you from birth, or it can surface over time. Basically what occurs is that insulin stays in your bloodstream longer than it should. The chain of events goes like this: you overeat carbohydrates, which provokes a very high blood sugar level, which in turn leads to insulin overload. The body cannot utilize the sugar surplus, so it stores it as fat. If you have found that you are not losing weight on a high-carbohydrate diet, it may not be the diet for you.

Women are obsessed by fat to the point of damaging their hearts. Low-fat diets generally are not based on whole foods and thus are low in essential fatty acids (EFAs). Not only do women shun red meat and cream sauces, we exclude nuts, oils, and fatty fish from our menus. *We women need some fat in our diets.* Since we cannot manufacture EFAs, we absolutely must get them from food. Every cell membrane is partially made of fat. EFAs are precursors to prostaglandins, hormonelike substances that are involved in the relaxation and contraction of our blood vessels. EFAs keep our platelets from clumping together, keep inflammation down, and help with other body functions too numerous to mention.

Extremely low fat diets may also produce deficiencies in fat-soluble nutrients such as beta-carotene and vitamins D and E, leading to an increased incidence of atherosclerotic disease and a host of other health problems. Many women are literally starving themselves on pasta and bagels and not getting adequate protein and fat. Listen to your body. Do you have symptoms that may be sending you a message? Do you complain of low energy, an insatiable appetite, uncontrolled sugar binges, loss of hair, acne, bloating, food allergies, mental confusion, irritability, thin skin, brittle nails, and menstrual problems? If this sounds familiar, it's time to temper those carbs and add some fat and protein to your diet.

So how do you know if the very low fat, high-carbohydrate diet is for you? Harvard doctors Frank Sacks, M.D., and Walter Willett, M.D., write in a 1991 *New England Journal of Medicine* article that individual patients may respond differently to the same diet. In other words, one size does not fit all. Most of the diet gurus would have us believe that their program is the best and only way to treat a health problem, and that it works for the entire population—women, men, young, old, active, and sedentary. Studies from around the globe tell us differently. The perfect diet that lowers cholesterol and strips the fat off one group of people may not offer the same benefits to another. Remember the Eskimos.

## EXERCISE AND THE LOW-FAT DIET

Endurance athletes who eat a very low fat diet may be damaging rather than protecting their hearts. Twelve male and thirteen female long-distance runners who averaged thirty-five miles per week were put on diets of varying degrees of fat (16 percent, 30 percent, and 42 percent). After four weeks their blood lipids were measured and compared. HDL levels rose on all the diets, but the ratio of total cholesterol to HDL cholesterol correspondingly escalated on the very low fat 16-percent diet. Since the ratio is highly predictive of heart disease, the authors concluded that this super low fat diet negated much of the beneficial effects of exercise on blood lipids. It is only fair to point out that this was a small study, but I am sure we will be seeing more work in this area. Meanwhile, maybe you exercise fanatics should consider whether or not going too low in your daily fat intake is appropriate. It would also be prudent to have your blood levels tested just to make sure.

## THE MEDITERRANEAN DIET: ONE OPTION

An increasingly popular alternative to a very low fat diet is the Mediterranean diet, which comes from the southern European countries bordering the Mediterranean Sea. When we look at the Italian, Greek, French, and Spanish people of that area, we find that heart disease is relatively rare in spite of their higher fat intake. According to several researchers, the Mediterranean way of eating appears wonderfully healthful, while providing a wide choice of foods and a great deal of satisfaction in general. It is my experience that you are more likely to follow a food plan if it is enjoyable and convenient. Not many people stick to a very low fat diet forever. They may be motivated at the beginning, but the results are not always worth the severe restrictions and duller flavors.

While there are many aspects to the Mediterranean diet, the

most studied one is the choice of fat. The Italians and Greeks primarily use olive oil, a beneficial monounsaturated fat that lowers LDL cholesterol while preserving HDL cholesterol. Additionally, it has anticlotting factors. Furthermore, they eat heartily of the local fish and shellfish, which are rich in omega-3 fatty acids. Essential fats, like the omega-3s, have been shown to help in lowering blood cholesterol, triglycerides, and blood pressure.

So it appears at first glance that eating more fats of the right kind could help prevent heart disease. Again, though, we need to ask the question: Are Mediterraneans avoiding diseases of the heart because they use liberal amounts of olive oil, or because they are *not* eating the quantities of saturated fats or *trans* fats that fill up our American pantries? Another question: Could it be that their diet also contains large amounts of fresh fruits and vegetables, legumes, and whole wheat, which provide important antioxidants? What about the fact that they walk more than we do and linger over a glass of wine during lunch, without seeming obsessed about getting back to work or on to the next event?

We are too quick to jump on the latest idea that provides an easy answer to good health. Olive oil now sits on the table at most "in" restaurants in the United States, and we douse our bread and coat our pasta in it because it is supposedly the healthy thing to do. I can't help wondering if we are getting caught up again in yet another false promise, taking one factor associated with a healthy population and plugging it into the American diet, without accepting the other parts of that population's diet and lifestyle as well.

I am not alone in my skepticism. Marion Nestle, Ph.D., head of the nutrition department at New York University, stated her concerns in an interview for the *Women's Health Advocate Newsletter* in January 1995. She points out that in Greece, where fat intake approaches the 40 percent level, people are extremely active and eat plenty of fruits and vegetables. Under those circumstances, a high-fat diet might be fine, but it is not clear that it is a good idea for Americans. What about the sedentary office worker or the woman who hates to sweat? Is it okay for her to add olive oil to an already high-fat diet? I don't think that is the message we want to convey, especially without stressing the importance of integrating exercise into the daily routine.

## SATURATED FATS

Experts may not agree about the amount of total fat we should consume, but on one point, agreement is universal. Saturated fats (found in meats, dairy products, butter, and tropical oils) and *trans* fats (hiding in margarine, fried foods, and packaged bakery products) must be limited. As far as heart disease is concerned, these two categories of fats are the chief suspects. Nothing can be said in favor of saturated and *trans* fats. They offer no nutrition and create a host of health problems. Both work equally to create cholesterol, interfere with the removal of cholesterol from the blood, weaken cell membranes, allowing bacteria and viruses to sneak in, dampen the immune system, and increase the risk of various cancers—and they make you fat.

How much saturated fat should we eat to stay healthy? The National Cholesterol Education Program (NCEP) and American Heart Association (AHA) recommend less than 10 percent. Many researchers say that is really an upper level. When you look at populations with next to no heart disease, you will find that their diets contain closer to 3 percent saturated fat. So why don't the experts come out and advocate a lower target rate? Scott Grundy, chairman of the NCEP's Adult Treatment Panel, explains that they are afraid that people will not make the change if it is too drastic. But how can physicians and nutritionists advise people if they are working with spurious numbers? And what is the goal here—to heal people or cater to their weaknesses? Personally, I feel it is our right to have correct information and be allowed to decide for ourselves whether or not making the necessary changes is feasible.

It is not easy to determine if you are getting 5 to 10 percent saturated fat in your diet, so I have provided a sliding scale in grams to help you estimate how much you might be getting in a day. If you have some idea about how many calories you eat regularly, then it's easy. If not, guesstimate. Take a look at the following list to see how

### Saturated Fat Allowance

| TOTAL CALORIES IN GRAMS | SATURATED FAT IN GRAMS | |
|---|---|---|
| | 10% | 5% |
| 1,000 | 11 | 06 |
| 1,500 | 16 | 08 |
| 2,000 | 22 | 11 |
| 2,500 | 28 | 14 |

easy it is to rack up the saturated fat grams. The idea is to find a food that you eat often and see where you stand. If cheese pizza is your downfall, two slices come in around 14 grams, which nudges the top range for most women.

## Where to Find Saturated Fats

(Serving size for meat, poultry, and fish is 4 oz., cooked)

| DANGEROUSLY HIGH (10 GRAMS AND ABOVE) | SATURATED FAT |
| --- | --- |
| Burger King Double Whopper with cheese | 24 grams |
| Alfredo sauce (½ cup) with 1 cup pasta | 20 |
| Taco Bell Taco Salad with shell | 19 |
| Chocolate mousse (½ cup) | 19 |
| Coconut (2 oz. dried) | 19 |
| Haagen-Dazs ice cream (1 cup) | 16 |
| American cheese grilled sandwich (2 oz. cheese) | 15 |
| Pizza Hut Cheese Pizza, med. (2 slices) | 14 |
| Cheesecake (4.5 oz.) | 14 |
| Arrowhead Mills Granola (2 oz.) | 11 |
| BLT sandwich (2 oz. bacon) | 11 |
| Porterhouse steak | 10 |
| Hostess Iced Honey Bun | 10 |

| HIGH (4–9 GRAMS) | |
| --- | --- |
| Regular ice cream (1 cup) | 9 |
| Ground beef (73% lean) | 9 |
| Ground beef (80% lean) | 8 |
| Ground beef (83% lean) | 7 |
| Arby's regular Roast Beef | 7 |
| Beef, sirloin, untrimmed | 7 |
| Butter (1 tbsp.) | 7 |
| Milk chocolate (1.4 oz.) | 7 |
| Coconut (2 oz. raw, shredded) | 7 |
| American and Cheddar cheese (1 oz.) | 6 |
| Cream cheese (2 tbsp.) | 6 |
| Beef, eye of round, untrimmed | 6 |
| Chicken wing with skin | 6 |

| | |
|---|---|
| Beef hot dog, Oscar Meyer | 6 |
| McDonald's French fries (large) | 5 |
| Milk, whole (1 cup) | 5 |
| Ice milk (1 cup) | 4 |
| Kraft Macaroni and Cheese | 4 |
| Nature Valley Granola (1/3 cup) | 4 |
| Beef, sirloin | 4 |
| Pork loin, center rib | 4 |
| Turkey leg with skin | 4 |

### MEDIUM (2–3 GRAMS)

| | |
|---|---|
| Beef, top or bottom round | 3 |
| Chicken thigh | 3 |
| Mackerel | 3 |
| Turkey breast with skin | 3 |
| Peanut butter (2 tbsp.) | 3 |
| Milk, 2%, (1 cup) | 3 |
| Cream cheese, light (1 oz.) | 3 |
| Sour cream (2 tbsp.) | 3 |
| McDonald's Chicken Fajita | 2 |
| Tuna salad sandwich | 2 |
| Milk, 1% (1 cup) | 2 |
| Sherbet (1 cup) | 2 |
| Yogurt, low-fat (1 cup) | 2 |
| Pancakes (3) | 2 |
| Biscuit (1) | 2 |

### LOW SATURATED FAT (1/2 TO 1 GRAM)

Ground beef, Healthy Choice Extra Lean

Chicken breast

Healthy Choice hot dog

Salmon, Atlantic or pink

Rockfish, scallops, trout

Cottage cheese, 1% (1/2 cup)

McDonald's low-fat milk shake

Mayonnaise, light

Canola oil

Breads

Graham crackers

Quaker Chewy Honey & Oats Bar

**LESS THAN LOW (LESS THAN ½ GRAM)**

Cod, flounder, halibut, haddock, perch, sole, snapper, tuna

Shellfish

Turkey breast

Beans, split peas, lentils

All vegetables and fruits (except coconut)

Nonfat milk, yogurt, or cheese

Bagel or pita bread

Breakfast cereals (except granola)

Non-fat granola

Fig bars

French and Italian bread

All grains

Pasta

Popcorn, air-popped

Pretzels

Tortillas

# DAMAGED FATS

Did you switch to margarine several years back when the experts suggested a no-cholesterol spread was healthier for the heart? Well, it's time for an update. A group of Harvard researchers examining the health and eating habits of eighty-five thousand middle-aged nurses found that those who reported eating the most margarine—more than four pats a day—were 50 percent more likely to fall victim to heart disease that those who did not. As it turns out, margarines and bakery products are constructed by altering vegetable oil, which creates compounds that react like saturated fats in the bloodstream. This process, called *hydrogenation*, turns the chemical structure of a liquid oil into that of a hardened fat. The conversion of the natural, flexible "*cis*" molecular configuration to the unnatural, more rigid "*trans*" form makes these oils unavailable to the body.

Hydrogenated fats are popular with food manufacturers for several obvious reasons: they are inexpensive to use, extend a product's shelf life, and make margarine spreadable and baked goods tender and flaky. This would be all well and good except for one important fact: hydrogenated fats cannot be used in the body like essential fatty acids to regulate cellular functions. Furthermore, they interfere with essential fats and block them from being metabolized. Hydrogenation also removes nutrients that are essential for a healthy heart—vitamins E and B-6 and the minerals chromium and magnesium. In addition, they may negatively alter—increase—levels of lipoprotein(a), another risk factor for heart disease.

*Trans* fats raise total cholesterol and LDL levels and appear to lower HDL levels as well. The literature, which has been growing for many years, suggests that foods like margarine, shortening, cookies, pies, cakes, frostings, chips, crackers, and fast foods made with hydrogenated oils elevate cholesterol much in the same way as do saturated fats. In 1993, the USDA conducted a study that proved consistent with these findings. Researcher Joseph Judd reported that a diet averaging only 10 to 20 grams of *trans* fat a day raised cholesterol levels as much as—or slightly less than—a diet high in saturated fat. "Until we know more, we can assume that each gram of *trans* raises LDL cholesterol about as much as a gram of saturated fat," says Judd.

The Center for Science in the Public Interest (CSPI), a nonprofit consumer advocacy group, publishes a wonderful newsletter titled *Nutrition Action Health Letter*. In the September 1996 issue the writers expressed their concern that the unsuspecting public not get lulled into thinking that "McDonald's French fries are healthy just because they claim to be cooked in cholesterol-free, 100 percent vegetable oil." According to their tests, the fries at McDonald's, Arby's, and Hardee's have as much artery-clogging fat as if they were fried in lard. Burger King and Wendy's are even worse. If you check this out in the McDonald's nutrition brochure, you won't read a word about *trans* fat; it discusses only the total saturated fat. I agree this is misleading, but does anyone out there really think that French fries are a health food?

The CSPI *trans* test generally confirmed a list of foods that harm the heart, including burgers, chicken nuggets, chips, and Fettuccini Alfredo. I will admit to a few surprises. They found that frozen supermarket potatoes like Ore-Ida Tater Tots and Snackin' Fries were no different from commercial fries. I am appalled that I used to give these to my kids, thinking they were seminutritious. Here's another surprise: a Burger King chicken sandwich ran neck and neck with a corned beef sandwich plus a bag of potato chips. And chicken is supposed to be the safe choice when ordering fast food. One of the worst offenders was Red Lobster Admiral's Feast of fried fish, French fries, cole slaw, and two pieces of garlic cheese bread. The CSPI compared it to a 12-ounce steak, a baked potato with butter, green beans with butter, and a slice of apple pie topped with half a cup of Haagen-Dazs premium chocolate ice cream. You know a steak is coronary city, but some people think fish is good for the heart, no matter how it is served. Wrong.

At least when it comes to saturated fat, food labels tell you how much you're getting; with *trans* fats, it's guesswork. The CSPI has jumped to the rescue and has petitioned the FDA to require that *trans* fats be included in food labeling. It is a monumental job, since the amount of *trans* fat in a food can vary depending on how "partially hydrogenated" the fat is. To complicate matters, although the FDA makes it easy for us to tell how much saturated fat is included in most products, and limits the amount of saturated fats in foods that claim "no" or "low-cholesterol," there are no limits on *trans* fats. And it is next to impossible to determine the amount of *trans* fats you are getting when eating out, so I have provided the following clues to help.

## Transitioning from *Trans* Fats

+ Avoid labels that read "hydrogenated oil." Partially hydrogenated is better, but no vegetable shortening is best.

+ Stay away from deep-fried foods (French fries, onion rings, fried cheese, fried zucchini).

- Substitute olive or canola oil for butter when you can.

- If you use margarine, buy tubs rather than sticks. To cut down on fat, get "whipped," "low-fat," or "fat-free."

- Use raw, natural nut butters in place of commercial brands.

- Try oil-free baked chips.

- For baking, you can sometimes substitute applesauce for butter.

A *note on olestra:* Olestra is not a healthy food because it has no nutritional value, it depletes beta-carotene, and it causes gas and indigestion in many people. However, it doesn't contain *trans* fats, therefore it is possibly a better choice for some.

## FRIENDLY OILS

Now that the cholesterol-building, artery-clogging fats have been exposed, it is time to focus on fats that we *can* eat without compromising our healthy hearts. Generally speaking, oils stand out as the safest way to integrate fat into the diet. Before I get into the best choices, I need to mention one group that was once high on the list and has since fallen from grace. A few years back, polyunsaturated oils such as safflower, corn, and sunflower oils were favored because they were thought to lower LDL cholesterol levels. But it turned out there was a downside; they also lowered HDL cholesterol. Polyunsaturated oils are more easily oxidized in the blood than other oils, which makes them highly suspect for preventing heart disease.

### More Monounsaturated Oils

Monounsaturated oils such as olive oil hold the favored stamp of approval. Like the polyunsaturated fats, monounsaturates reduce LDL levels, but the good news is they don't lower the HDLs. People who consume more olive oil and other monounsaturated oils appear to have a better HDL/LDL ratio. Monounsaturated oils may be helpful in another way, too: they appear to have antioxidant properties that fend off artery damage.

I'd like to digress from the heart for one moment and say a few words about the breast. A new study from Sweden was written up in the January 1998 issue of the *Archives of Internal Medicine*. It involved more than sixty thousand women and adds to the growing evidence that eating monounsaturated fats may significantly reduce the risk of breast cancer. Another reason to go for the oils.

No doubt, olive oil and other monounsaturated oils (canola, avocado, sesame) score highest on the list and thus should be substituted for saturated and *trans* fats. The questions that remain are, How much is good, and is more better? To add oil to a diet already high in fat would not contribute to heart health. Each tablespoon of olive oil, or any oil for that matter, consists of 14 grams and 120 calories of pure fat. And any fat we eat, healthy or not, is stored very efficiently in the body. Excess body fat is already at epidemic proportions in our country, increasing our risk of high blood pressure, diabetes, and heart disease. Yes, olive oil is healthier than butter, *trans* fats, and polyunsaturated oils, but eating a high-fat diet without additional exercise to burn it off results in that fat ending up on our hips and stomachs. And that isn't good for our hearts.

Most oils are not strictly saturated or unsaturated, monounsaturated or polyunsaturated; they consist of a combination of fatty acids. It is best if you select the ones with the highest proportion of monounsaturated oil. The two top monounsaturated oils for cooking are olive and canola. Olive oil is very stable against the free-radical effects of heat, air, and light. Some people use it on salads, but I prefer the lighter taste of canola oil. Canola oil has a high smoking point, which makes it great for cooking as well as enjoyable on greens. When fats and oils are exposed to high temperatures, they form chemicals that attack and destroy blood vessel walls; therefore, hunt for cold-pressed, expeller-pressed, and organic oils. I buy the smallest container possible, because each time you unscrew the bottle and expose the oil to air, oxidation occurs. And you do refrigerate your oils, right?

## OMEGA-3 FATTY ACIDS

A special category of fats collectively called the *omega-3 fatty acids* is causing quite a stir in the health industry. Research shows that if we ate proportionally more of these fats than the ones that we usually

| OIL | PERCENTAGE OF MONOUNSATURATED FATS | PERCENTAGE OF POLYUNSATURATED FATS | PERCENTAGE OF SATURATED FATS |
|---|---|---|---|
| Olive | 82.0 | 8.0 | 10.0 |
| Avocado | 70.0 | 10.0 | 10.0 |
| Canola | 60.0 | 34.0 | 6.0 |
| Sesame | 46.0 | 41.0 | 13.0 |
| Sunflower | 26.0 | 66.0 | 8.0 |
| Flaxseed | 24.0 | 70.0 | 6.0 |
| Safflower | 13.0 | 79.0 | 8.0 |
| Coconut | 6.0 | 2.0 | 92.0 |

do, we would be a much healthier people. The omega-3 fats are primarily concentrated in marine life, although some can be found in a few plants. They show great promise for preventing most degenerative diseases, including arthritis, diabetes, and heart disease. They are known to improve immune function and suppress tumor growth. Getting them in healthy doses is a challenge, though, because the richest sources are cold-water fish and flaxseed; not everyone likes salmon and mackerel, and few people know about flax. For a further discussion of flaxseed, see page 100.

The American diet is dominated by the more popular omega-6 fats from vegetable oil, seeds, nuts, grains, and the fat we eat in meat. The omega-6s are also essential fats, but they are more biochemically active, meaning they are extremely unstable when exposed to light, heat, and oxygen—which exposure routinely occurs during processing and cooking. Omega-6 fats easily change into toxic substances, which ultimately produce inflammation and promote blood stickiness and blood vessel constriction.

The preponderance of unhealthy fats in our diets pushes our cells into major malfunctioning, precipitating many chronic diseases such as heart disease, cancer, diabetes, and arthritis. With the proliferation of processed vegetable oils, burgers and fries, and packaged goodies, our cells are overburdened with foreign fats and starved for essential fats. This message seems to move at a snail's pace in reaching the consumer, but increasingly, concerned scientists are raising their voices. Artemis Simopoulos, M.D., president of the Center of

Genetics, Nutrition, and Health in Washington, D.C., wrote in the May/June 1988 issue of *Nutrition Today* that although it is largely unappreciated, our overconsumption of omega-6 oils, prevalent in margarines, salad oils, cooking oils, and processed foods, is helping to create a health disaster.

Most foods contain not one or the other but a mixture of omega-3 and omega-6 oils, usually with a higher concentration of one. The fact is that most Western countries consume too many omega-6s and too few omega-3s. Dr. William Lands, fish oil expert and formerly professor of biochemistry at the University of Illinois at Chicago, points out that Americans eat at least ten to fifteen times more terrestrial omega-6s than marine omega-3s—a horrible proportion. Canadian health experts believe omega-3s are important enough to warrant governmental recommendations. Denmark, too, is educating its population to ensure that they are getting an adequate supply of healthy fat.

## Go Fish

Eating more fish is an easy way to integrate more omega-3 oils into your diet. Researchers all over the globe are uncovering more and more evidence that fish oils are good for your heart and health. A long list of population and clinical studies validate the cardioprotective effects of fish. Across cultures, people who consume fish on a regular basis, even if their diets vary in other respects, appear to experience fewer heart problems.

A landmark study involving six thousand American men found that eating a mere ounce of fish a day cut fatal heart attacks in half. The men who consumed one ounce of mackerel or three ounces of bass each day were 36 percent less likely to die of heart disease than men eating less or no fish. Another study that spanned thirty years utilized data on 1,822 men who were employed at Chicago Western Electric. The relationship between baseline fish consumption and death from coronary heart disease was investigated. After three decades, the study concluded that participants who ate seven or more ounces of fish a week (which translates into one normal meal) were less likely to have a fatal heart attack than men who didn't eat fish.

A little fatty fish confers significant benefits to both women and men. David Siscovick and his co-workers conducted a study with male heart patients and their spouses at the University of Washington and found that for both sexes, those who reported eating one serving of fatty fish a week experienced half the risk of heart attack of those who did not consume fish. Most of the fish studies have not included women, but there is every reason to believe that it is protective for us as well. Research has demonstrated that fish can lower triglycerides and raise HDLs, both of which are of particular concern to women.

There is a strong case for the *preventive* properties of fish, but what about people who have had a heart attack? A two-year groundbreaking study called the Diet and Reinfarction Trial (DART) found that you can slash your risk of a second heart attack by one-third by including fish in your diet. Michael Burr, M.D., from the Medical Research Council in Cardiff, Wales, studied over two thousand men who had already suffered heart attacks. He divided the group into four sections. One section ate oily fish such as salmon, mackerel, or sardines, or took three fish oil capsules, at least twice a week; a second group cut their fats to no more than 30 percent of calories; a third group upped their fiber to 18 grams a day; and the fourth had no special dietary program. Two years later when the results were tallied, the death rate had dropped 29 percent in the fish-eaters compared to the non-fish-eaters. I don't think we can deduce from this one study that a low-saturated-fat diet or a high-fiber diet is ineffective, because so many other studies indicate that both have heart-healthy benefits. But I do think this study suggests that we need to broaden our scope to include a greater variety of possibilities for maintaining a healthy heart.

Omega-3 fatty acids have been used therapeutically to keep the arteries open after angioplasty, a procedure in which a balloon is inserted into a blocked artery and then inflated to widen the space through which blood can flow. The problem with angioplasty is that reclogging occurs in up to 45 percent of patients within six months. When these patients were given therapeutic doses of omega-3 fatty acids starting three weeks before angioplasty and continuing for six months following, their blood vessels remained less obstructed than those of patients not taking the omega-3s. If you are anticipating this procedure, though, please don't experiment by yourself. Consult with your doctor, give him or her this information if they are not already aware of it, and work together for your best treatment.

The fattiest fish provide the most omega-3 fatty acids: mackerel, anchovies, herring, salmon, and sardines. If you are like me and turn up your nose at the above-mentioned list, not to worry: you have other options. Although the fatty fish are undoubtedly superior for heart protection, it's not much use if you are not going to eat them. Check the following list for fish that suits your tastebuds and see how the omega-3s compare. Adding any seafood to your diet helps to readjust your fatty acid balance.

## Sources of Omega-3 Fatty Acids

| FISH (FRESH OR FROZEN) | MILLIGRAMS PER 3.5 OUNCES |
|---|---|
| Mackerel, Atlantic | 2,299 |
| Herring, Pacific | 1,658 |
| Salmon, Chinook | 1,355 |
| Whitefish, mixed species | 1,258 |
| Tuna, bluefin | 1,173 |
| Salmon, pink | 1,005 |
| Turbot, Greenland | 919 |
| Shark, mixed species | 843 |
| Bass, striped | 754 |
| Oysters, Pacific | 688 |
| Swordfish | 639 |
| Sea bass, mixed species | 595 |
| Trout, rainbow | 568 |
| Shrimp, mixed species | 480 |
| Halibut | 363 |
| Lobster | 373 |
| Snapper | 311 |
| Cod, Pacific | 215 |
| Clam | 142 |

| CANNED FISH | MILLIGRAMS PER 3.5 OUNCES |
|---|---|
| Anchovies, drained | 2,055 |
| Herring, Atlantic, pickled | 1,389 |
| Sardines, Pacific, drained | 1,604 |
| Tuna, albacore in water | 706 |
| Tuna, light in soybean oil | 126 |

If you absolutely hate the taste of fish, can you get the same benefits from supplements? At this time, the studies remain conflicting. Some research indicates that fish oil supplements reduced triglyceride levels an average of 25 percent after treatment. The downside is that you have to take eight to twelve capsules each day for the desired results. There is also evidence that fish oil taken in capsules can raise LDL cholesterol in some individuals, which is not the reaction we want.

Dr. Sheldon Hendler, author of *The Doctors' Vitamin and Mineral Encyclopedia,* does not recommend fish oil supplements for everyone but thinks they are appropriate for those with hypertension or any condition that predisposes the blood to clot. Dr. Hendler suggests a daily dose of 2 to 4 grams from either fish or supplements. If you take supplements, the best ones to choose are those combined with vitamin E. Fish oils easily turn rancid, and the antioxidant vitamin E protects against it. Diabetics and anyone known to bleed easily should *not* take fish oil supplements. Check with your doctor if you are considering supplemental fish oil.

## Flaxseed

Flaxseed and its oil is the primary source of omega-3 fatty acids in the plant kingdom. It is not as potent as fish oil, but it can provide an alternative for getting those essential fats if fish is not a part of your diet. Flaxseed also offers a unique set of benefits to the heart that we don't find in fish. It is a fair source of insoluble and soluble fiber, which is associated with cholesterol lowering. One-eighth of a cup (25 grams) of flaxseed offers 10 grams of fiber. Jack Carter, Ph.D., a professor emeritus at North Dakota State University and president of the Flax Institute, notes that adding flaxseed to the diet can beneficially alter lipid levels. Researchers have found cholesterol reductions on the order of 5 percent to 15 percent, primarily attributable to a decline in LDLs.

*Alpha-linolenic acid,* an essential fatty acid found in flaxseed, may protect against stroke. Alpha-linolenic acid, which is also found in some fruits and vegetables, has the ability to reduce platelet stickiness and blood viscosity. The Multiple Risk Factor Interventions Trial reported their results in the May 1995 issue of *Stroke.* It was found that participants with high blood levels of alpha-linolenic acid had a 37 percent lower risk of stroke.

Other components in flaxseed, specifically the lignan precursors, make them especially beneficial for women. During digestion, these compounds are converted by bacteria into phytoestrogens, hormonelike substances that may protect women against a number of hormone-mediated conditions like breast and ovarian cancer, hot flashes, and fibroid tumors. Phytoestrogens, found in many foods, spices, and herbs, have the versatility to function as either estrogens or antiestrogens, depending on their chemical structure and whether a woman is pre- or postmenopausal. Research on these phytonutrients will be filling the news more and more. Watch for it.

You can find flaxseed in both seed and oil form. The seeds are tiny, golden or brown, with a rich, nutty flavor, and they can be ground and sprinkled on cereal, salads, and soups, mixed in drinks, or added to breads, muffins, and cookies. To grind the seeds, use a high-quality coffee grinder or blender. Flaxseed oil is available at most health food stores. It is expensive and must be kept in the refrigerator in its original dark bottle because it spoils more rapidly than most oils. You may cook with it over low heat, but it is best cold, like in salad dressings.

When buying flaxseeds, whether as whole seeds or in granule form, freshness is essential. Store them in a cool, dry place. Once the seeds are ground, they should be eaten immediately or kept in the freezer. Commercial ground flaxseed flour maintains its freshness for several days or weeks at room temperature and several months in the freezer. You probably will have to find a health food store to purchase these products. I haven't seen them in regular markets yet, but I am sure that day will come.

Flaxseed is an excellent essential fat to add to the diet, espe-cially if you are one of those people who shun fat in other forms. You really do need some fat for basic body functions. If you are adding flax to an already moderately high fat diet, be sure to take the fat grams into account—10 fat grams per ¼ cup of seeds and 14 fat grams per tablespoon of oil. Even if it is healthy, too much of any fat is not good for the heart.

# NUTS

High-calorie, high-fat nuts just might be good for us. Can you believe that? In 1992, Joan Sabate and her colleagues at California's Loma Linda University observed the lifestyles of 31,208 women and men for six years, to determine why they had lower rates of heart dis-ease and cancer than other Americans. The results were intriguing, to say the least. Individuals who ate nuts more than four times a week were 38 percent less likely to die from heart disease than those who avoided nuts. These numbers held up even after age, body weight, smoking, blood pressure, blood cholesterol, and physical activity were considered.

I think we must tread lightly when interpreting results like those of this retrospective study. To be fair, we need to mention that the participants in the program were Seventh-Day Adventists, a reli-gious group whose lifestyle is superior in many respects to the stan-dard American one. They do not smoke or drink coffee or alcohol, and many of them avoid meat, which is probably why their nut con-sumption was more generous than the norm. Because Adventists are considerably healthier than most Americans across the board, maybe we should embrace these other aspects of their lifestyle, not just one segment of it.

This is not the full extent of the research. Dr. Sabate contin-ued to experiment with nuts, this time to measure specifically the cholesterol-lowering effects of walnuts. (Walnuts were used because the walnut industry funded the study.) There were two groups of nine men each: one group ate 3 ounces of nuts and the other ate a similar serving of meat. The remainder of the diet was identical, and the total fat content measured in at 30 percent. The men on the control diet averaged a total cholesterol level of 182, and the men on the nut plan came in around 160. Conclusion: the walnuts *did* lower cholesterol. But this really should not surprise the experts; when an unsaturated fat is substituted for a saturated fat in the diet, the response typically will be positive.

I am always thrilled when I can provide studies that include women—and yes, I did find one that lends credence to these results. In 1993, the Iowa Women's Health Study evaluated 41,837 women over fifty-five years of age. Again, nut eaters suffered fewer heart attacks, even after considering other known risk factors.

When you look at the composition of nuts, it makes sense that they can be incorporated into a healthy diet. They are low in saturated fat, rich in healthy monounsaturated fats, high in fiber, and packed with antioxidants like vitamin E and selenium, which also protect the arteries from the ravages of excess cholesterol. Because nuts are a compact source of fat (170 calories per ounce) you should not "go nuts" with them. But as an alternative to meat, a condiment for salads and vegetables, to spice up muffins and breads, and for an on-the-run snack, consider nuts.

# 8

# Fabulous Fiber

Think wrongly, if you please, but in all cases think for yourself.
—DORIS LESSING

F iber plays an important dietary role in the prevention of coronary disease. According to the Harvard School of Public
Health, the omission of fiber in the diet ranks alongside cigarette smoking, high blood cholesterol, and high blood pressure as an
independent risk factor for heart disease. Important as dietary fiber
intake is, the USDA's Continuing Survey of Food Intakes reports
that in 1995, Americans remained below par, scoring about 15 grams
per day when our goal should be 25 to 35 grams of fiber per day.

The formal study of fiber began in the 1960s with two medical
missionaries in Uganda, Drs. Denis Burkitt and H. C. Trowell. The
doctors noticed that their African patients were remarkably healthy
and free from common Western disorders like high blood pressure,
heart disease, diabetes, obesity, constipation, hemorrhoids, and gallstones. They also observed that the people of Uganda had swifter
and more bulky bowel movements than their English patients at
home. The simple correlation between a high-fiber diet, swifter, larger
stools, and a lower incidence of intestinal, metabolic, and cardiovascular disorders engendered an explosion of research that changed
dietary recommendations dramatically throughout the world.

A recent report from the Nurses' Health Study emphasized the
importance of dietary fiber in connection to one of the major risk
factors of heart disease in women—adult-onset diabetes. Over a six-
year period, women whose diets were heavy in refined carbohydrates

from white bread, white rice, pasta, and potatoes had two and a half times the risk for Type 2 diabetes as those who regularly ate a high-fiber diet containing natural whole-grain breads and cereals. Even after taking into account family history, weight, and physical activity, the verdict remained the same. A high-carbohydrate, low-fiber diet is a recipe for diabetes.

## WHAT IS FIBER AND WHERE CAN I GET IT?

Fiber is the textured portion of fruits, vegetables, and grains that is not digested and therefore passes intact through the stomach, through the small intestine, and out of the body. It is not absorbed, has no caloric value, and doesn't provide the body with any crucial vitamins or minerals, yet dietary fiber is one of the most important elements in a heart-healthy diet plan.

We speak of fiber as a single entity, but there are any number of foods that supply different kinds. Fiber is divided into two main groups, soluble and insoluble. *Insoluble fiber*, as the name suggests, does not dissolve in water, nor is it broken down by stomach acid, so it quickly moves through the intestinal tract, promoting swift elimination of fecal material. Insoluble fiber, as found in whole-wheat products, wheat bran, fruits, and vegetables, is excellent for relieving constipation and preventing hemorrhoids and diverticuli (painful pouchlike sacs in the colon), and it works wonders in curbing colon cancer.

*Soluble fiber*, on the other hand, does dissolve in water, even though it remains intact in the body. It functions quite differently from insoluble fiber. In the intestines, soluble fiber forms a gellike mass that binds with bile and cholesterol, promoting their excretion from the body. Because of this action, it has a potent cholesterol-lowering effect, reducing both total cholesterol and LDLs. It also plays a role in modulating other important risk factors as well. It improves sugar metabolism, reducing blood insulin levels, and it delays the emptying of the stomach, which produces a feeling of fullness after eating—which makes it helpful as part of a weight-loss program. Soluble fiber is obtained from a wide variety of sources, including psyllium seed, beta-glucans, pectin, and guar gum. You may be more familiar with the following sources: grains, oats, beans, barley, soybeans, fruits, and vegetables.

# OAT BRAN

Dozens of studies conducted since the 1960s have proven that a specific fiber found in oats called *beta-glucan* is effective in causing a moderate reduction in blood cholesterol. So is there a magic muffin that can take the place of a low-saturated-fat diet and exercise? No. But along with adopting a good diet and other positive lifestyle measures, eating oat bran can promote changes that may lower your cholesterol.

As little as 2 ounces of oat bran a day has been shown to reduce cholesterol by 7 to 20 percent. To give you an example of how strongly government representatives feel about oat bran, the Food and Drug Administration (FDA) is allowing food manufacturers to claim nutritional benefit on the labels of breads or cereals that are made from oats. The FDA keeps a close reign on food manufacturers so they don't get carried away making spurious claims, so being allowed a statement such as this is quite of coup for food manufacturers. There is a caveat on the label as well, so the public won't think that a bowl of oatmeal can counteract a cheeseburger and fries. The manufacturers must also use wording on labels to the effect that "soluble fiber from foods such as oat bran may reduce the risk of heart disease when it is part of a diet low in saturated fat and cholesterol."

We know oat bran works, but we don't really understand how. Experimental studies confirm that soluble fiber slows the liver's production of cholesterol. It is thought that the soluble fiber beta-glucan binds with cholesterol-rich bile in the intestinal tract, preventing the body from reabsorbing cholesterol into the bloodstream. This seems a reasonable assumption, since this is the way two cholesterol-lowering medications, cholestyramine and colestipol, work. Since the action is similar, and the drugs are expensive and carry possible side effects, while a bowl of oat cereal is safe and costs next to nothing, which option sounds the more reasonable? While I am not suggesting that you stop your medication without your doctor's knowledge, I do want to make the point that food can be as effective as medication for some people.

Studies vary as to how much of a change you can expect and how long it might take. While estimates range from 3 to 20 percent, the latest recommendation suggests that on average, 3 grams of soluble fiber per day will lower cholesterol by about 5 to 15 percent. Cholesterol levels start dipping within a matter of a few weeks after your first bowl of oat bran cereal, but to see appreciable results, I would wait three to six months before retesting.

The following list gives you an idea of the amount of cereal it takes to give you 3 grams of beta-glucan fiber. The list is by no means comprehensive. You might check some of your favorite cereals to see how they add up.

Be careful when you buy some of the new oat bran products flooding the market. Many of the muffins, cookies, crackers, and chips contain enough fat to offset any cholesterol-lowering effects the oat bran may have. Check the label for the fat content or ask for low-fat products at your bakery.

Oat bran works better for some people than for others. It is most effective for people whose cholesterol tops 230 and for individuals who show high HDL levels. This is also true of other high–soluble fiber foods. If your cholesterol level is already below 200, the probability of it dropping further is minimal. Younger women rarely see the marked declines that older women do. Individual differences apply to all recommendations, whether we're talking about nutrition or medicine.

If oats aren't your favorite, there is a wide variety of soluble fibers from which you can choose. Read on.

## Adding up Your Oats

| CEREAL | AMOUNT NEEDED FOR 3 GRAMS BETA-GLUCAN FIBER |
|---|---|
| Quaker Oat Bran Hot Cereal | 1 cup, cooked |
| Quaker Oat Bran Cold Cereal | 1½ cups |
| Quaker Quick or Old Fashioned Oats | 1½ cups, cooked |
| Quaker Instant Oatmeal | 3 packets |
| Quaker Toasted Oatmeal | 3 cups |
| Quaker Oatmeal Squares | 3 cups |
| Quaker Quick'n Hearty Microwave Oatmeal | 3 packets |
| Kellogg's Common Sense Oat Bran | 2¼ cups |
| General Mills Cheerios (original only) | 3 cups |
| Health Valley Oat Bran Flakes | 1¼ cups |

## BEANS AND OTHER LEGUMES

Beans may be a worthy rival to oats when it comes to lowering cholesterol. The studies aren't as extensive yet, but at least fifteen investigations of various legumes consistently have indicated that the mighty bean lowers blood cholesterol levels both in people with high levels and in those with not-so-high or normal levels. On the average, $1/2$ cup of beans a day will reduce cholesterol by about 15 percent. All types of beans work—dried, fresh, or canned. Pick your favorite—pinto, kidney, black, navy, lentil, lima, chickpea, and soybean.

Beans are a healthy choice for a number of reasons. As well as being a rich source of fiber, beans offer a low-fat substitute for meat protein, and they are packed full of nutrients like B vitamins and calcium. Both beans and legumes can easily be integrated into soups, salads, and casseroles. They are handy as dips for company and late-night snacks. My husband and son love beans and tortillas any time of the day or night.

A side effect I am sure you are well aware of is gas. If you avoid beans because of personal discomfort or public embarrassment, I have a couple of suggestions. Try cutting back on the amount of beans you eat for a brief period, then slowly increase it by a tablespoon more each time till you are back at your usual level. This is also a good idea when you start adding greater quantities of fiber to your diet. Take it slowly, and let your body adjust to these new foods.

A shortcut to eliminating odor is to take Beano, an enzyme supplement that helps you digest the carbohydrate in beans. It is available at most grocery stores, and it works. As you eat beans more frequently, your body will adapt and you won't have the uncomfortable side effects. One more suggestion to eliminate gas: if you are cooking up dried beans from scratch, prepare them the night before. Place the beans in a pan and cover them with water, add a touch of baking soda, boil for ten minutes, and soak overnight. Then pour off the water, rinse, cover again with water, and cook three hours or as directed. This method doesn't work for everyone, because some people do not have adequtae enzymes to digest beans, but try it and see.

# APPLES

You know what they say about an apple a day. It just might be true. Apples contain a soluble fiber *pectin*, which has been shown to lower LDL cholesterol. French researchers instructed a group of healthy middle-aged women and men to add two to three apples each day to their regular diet. After a month, LDL levels dropped by more than 10 percent in 80 percent of the participants. It should also be noted that HDL levels went up as well. Something very interesting about the apple study: it had a more pronounced effect on women than on men. I certainly would like to see more studies on apples. It is one fruit that is plentiful year-round, convenient, and versatile. It is great thrown into green salads and fruit salads, mixed in casseroles, baked as a side dish, cut up as a snack, or in my all-time favorite, pie (but you shouldn't eat the crust, of course, which is usually high in saturated shortening).

# CARROTS

Carrots aren't just good for the eyes—they benefit the heart as well. Like apples, carrots are loaded with pectin and other anticholesterol soluble fibers. Studies from all over the world show that a few carrots a day can both raise good cholesterol and lower bad cholesterol. In one study, participants ate two medium raw carrots each morning for three weeks. This one simple dietary change resulted in an 11 percent reduction in cholesterol. Philip Pfeffer, Ph.D., and Peter Hoagland, Ph.D., scientists at the U.S. Department of Agriculture's Eastern Regional Research Center, calculated that eating a couple of carrots a day can potentially lower cholesterol by up to 20 percent. According to Dr. Pfeffer, it doesn't matter if the carrots are raw, cooked, frozen, canned, chopped, or pulverized. Always keep carrots peeled and sliced in your refrigerator to munch on when you're bored. Each carrot has only about 30 calories, and by eating one a day you can fulfill your daily quota of beta-carotene and get a good deal of your fiber as well.

## WHOLE GRAINS

Whole-grain breads and cereals combine both soluble and insoluble fibers and are among the newcomers to the literature on cholesterol-lowering foods. The most recent study on fiber was conducted at Harvard University and involved forty-three thousand male health professionals between the ages of forty and seventy-five. The men who reported eating an average of 29 grams of fiber per day had a 36 percent lower risk of developing heart disease than those who consumed fewer than 15 grams. Every 10 grams of fiber added to the diet—whether it was from bananas, bran, or baked potatoes—lowered the risk of heart attack by 19 percent. But the researchers noted that it was the fiber from grains, rather than from fruits and vegetables, that was "most strongly associated with a reduced risk." In the Iowa Women's Health Study, a lower risk of heart disease was recognized in women who consumed dark bread rather than white bread, even when the loaf wasn't specifically a whole-grain product. Apparently, small changes do make a difference. With all the wonderful, tasty grains available, we are still a predominantly white-bread society. An estimated 80 percent of us eat crunchy grains less than once a day. Maybe it's an old habit that's hard to break. We were so accustomed to our mom serving white bread, white rice, and sugarcoated cereals that it goes against tradition—or our comfort level—to change. It could be out of convenience that we neglect the natural grains. Or maybe it's because of the confusion in labeling. We might think we are buying grainy bread when what we're really getting is a brownish-looking, spongy carbohydrate that looks like bread but is devoid of all natural vitamins, minerals, and fiber.

It is worthwhile to experiment. Diversify your diet, and try tasting different varieties of stone-ground whole-grain breads and cereals—you know, the textured ones that force you to floss after eating. Not all brown breads on the shelves possess the heart-healthy traits of the whole grain. Read the labels carefully and make sure they live up to their claims. "Light" products are usually not just lighter in weight and color but also in nutrients, so reach beyond them to the 100 percent whole-grain breads.

When choosing cereals, hunt for ones that are both whole grain and high in fiber. If you like a particular brand of cereal and it doesn't seem to have as much fiber as you want but you are unwilling to give it up, combine it with another product that has higher fiber content. I mix and match several grains, just to cover my bases.

## Pasta

Pasta is a hit both in restaurants and at home. It is low in fat, providing you don't cover it in cream sauce, and it can be prepared as a hot or cold entrée, with vegetables, fish, or meat. Depending on how it is served, pasta can indeed be healthy. But guess what? It is not necessarily a high-fiber food. Most pasta is made from refined white flour, which means it does

| WHOLE GRAIN | MOSTLY REFINED GRAIN |
|---|---|
| **COLD CEREALS** | |
| Cheerios | Basic 4 |
| Granola or Muesli | Corn Flakes |
| Grape-Nuts | Frosted Flakes |
| Nutri-Grain | Just Right |
| Raisin Bran | Kix, Corn Pops |
| Shredded Wheat | Product 19 |
| Total | Puffed Wheat |
| Wheat Germ | Rice Krispies |
| Wheaties | Special K |
| **HOT CEREALS** | |
| Oat Bran | Cream of Wheat (Farina) |
| Oatmeal | Cream of Rice |
| Quaker Multigrain | Grits |
| Ralston High Fiber | |
| Roman Meal | |
| Wheatena | |

not have the healthy fiber you are looking for. If pasta is one of your favorites, you can get whole-grain versions. Just check a specialty store or your local health food market.

## SOLUBLE FIBER AS SUPPLEMENT

What if you avoid cereal, rarely munch on apples and carrots, and can't tolerate brown breads? Can you take a dietary supplement and expect the same results? Most nutritionists would not advise this as a first choice, but yes, fiber in pill form does work to lower cholesterol.

The fiber source that has been used for the majority of the research so far is *psyllium*, a natural grain from India and the Mediterranean. At least seventeen trials have evaluated psyllium supplements and concluded that they are as effective as oat bran in lowering cholesterol. On the average, about 10 grams of psyllium per day was shown to lower cholesterol levels by up to 15 percent within two to four months. It is widely available under many brand names, the most popular being Metamucil. If one is displeasing to you, there are many more you can experiment with. Should you choose this route, be sure to start slowly, even more slowly than the directions may advise. Start with a teaspoon before breakfast, continue for a few days, and then gradually build up to the same dose for each meal. If you feel discomfort, take it only before one or two meals a day.

In Jean Carper's wonderful new book *Miracle Cures*, she writes about a particular blend of pectin fiber that is obtained from the rinds and membranes of grapefruit and combined with another soluble fiber called guar gum. When tested clinically, almost everyone who took it had dramatic results, even when cholesterol-lowering drugs failed. One woman watched her total cholesterol plummet from 295 to 208; her LDL and her triglycerides followed a similar pattern. The unexpected side effects for her were a loss of fifteen pounds in three months, more energy, and the cessation of her former food cravings.

The unique grapefruit product that Ms. Carper writes about is called ProFibe. It was developed by medical professor James J. Cerda at the University of Florida College of Medicine. As exciting as the change in blood fats was, this solitary fiber pill also cleared clogged arteries in some people, and when tested on pigs, whose cardiovascular system is similar to that of humans, the results were equally encouraging. Double-blind tests continue with humans to further determine how effective grapefruit fiber is in opening up arteries and reversing atherosclerosis. But you don't have to wait. The standard dose used in clinical studies is 15 grams of fiber, which translates to roughly 1/3 cup a day, to be divided in three mealtime doses. Dr. Cerda states that many people see results from even 5 grams a day of his product.

## THE BOTTOM LINE ON FIBER

Soluble fiber reduces the risk for heart disease by lowering cholesterol and regulating blood sugar levels. Almost any form of soluble fiber will do if taken in sufficient amounts. Smaller studies have branched out and tested other sources of soluble fiber, such as barley, prunes, and sugar beets, and all passed with flying colors. Obviously, there are a number of foods that have this heart-healthy fiber. Even though not all have been subjected to scrutiny, we can assume most will deliver similar results when put under the microscope. It behooves us to include as many as we can in our daily food plan to maintain our cholesterol levels or to bring our numbers down.

How much soluble fiber does one need in the diet for optimum health? Let's start with total fiber first, because both kinds of fiber are required for an all-around healthy diet. Most authorities recommend an average of 25 to 40 grams per day total, about one-third of which should be from soluble fiber. About 12 grams of soluble fiber a day is the amount to aim for when planning your dietary strategy.

## Sources of Dietary Fiber

| FOOD | PORTION | TOTAL FIBER | SOLUBLE FIBER |
|------|---------|-------------|---------------|
| *CEREAL* | | | |
| Kellogg's Bran Buds | ⅓ cup | 8.0 | 3.0 |
| Kellogg's All Bran | ½ cup | 12.9 | 2.1 |
| Quick Quaker Oats | 1 cup | 3.0 | 2.0 |
| General Mills Fiber One | ½ cup | 11.9 | 0.8 |
| 40% Bran Flakes | ½ cup | 4.3 | 0.3 |
| Post Grapenuts | ½ cup | 5.6 | 1.6 |
| Kellogg's Heartwise | ½ cup | 2.8 | 1.4 |
| Raisin Bran | ¾ cup | 5.3 | 0.9 |
| *BREADS* | | | |
| Bagel, plain | 1 bagel | 1.4 | 0.6 |
| Pita bread | 1 pita | 1.0 | 0.4 |
| White bread | 1 slice | 0.6 | 0.3 |
| Whole-wheat bread | 1 slice | 1.5 | 0.3 |
| *LEGUMES* | | | |
| Chickpeas, cooked | ½ cup | 4.3 | 1.3 |
| Kidney beans, cooked | ½ cup | 6.9 | 2.8 |
| Lentils, cooked | ½ cup | 5.2 | 0.6 |
| Pinto Beans, cooked | ½ cup | 5.9 | 1.9 |
| Split peas, cooked | ½ cup | 3.1 | 1.1 |

| FOOD | PORTION | TOTAL FIBER | SOLUBLE FIBER |
|------|---------|-------------|---------------|
| **FRUITS** | | | |
| Apple | 1 med. | 2.8 | 1.8 |
| Grapefruit, fresh | 1/2 med. | 1.4 | 0.9 |
| Peaches, fresh | 1 med. | 2.0 | 1.0 |
| Plums, red, fresh | 2 med. | 2.4 | 1.2 |
| Prunes, dried | 3 med. | 1.7 | 1.0 |
| Strawberries | 1 1/4 cup | 1.8 | 0.6 |
| **VEGETABLES** | | | |
| Asparagus, cooked | 1/2 cup | 1.9 | 0.7 |
| Broccoli, cooked | 1/2 cup | 2.4 | 1.2 |
| Brussels sprouts, cooked | 1/2 cup | 3.8 | 2.0 |
| Cabbage, fresh | 1 cup | 1.5 | 0.6 |
| Carrots, fresh | 1 med. | 2.3 | 1.1 |
| Potatoes, cooked | 1/2 cup | 1.5 | 0.8 |
| Sweet potato, cooked | 1/3 cup | 2.7 | 1.2 |

Nutritionists all agree that it is best to get your fiber from foods, but if you have studied the list and decided these foods are never going to appear on your plate on a regular basis, you might consider the supplement route. You won't reap the same rewards from supplemental fiber pills that you do from fresh fruits or whole grains, because you will miss out on all the other known and unknown nutrients that are in the whole food. Still, it is better than doing nothing. And remember, if your diet is currently low in any fiber, add both fibrous foods and supplements slowly. Too much too soon may result in uncomfortable bloating, embarrassing gas, or diarrhea.

# 9

# PROTEIN:
# ANIMAL VERSUS PLANT

True life is lived when tiny changes occur.

—LEO TOLSTOY

R esearch to date favors plant protein over animal protein as the means of maintaining a healthy heart. But what if we crave a burger now and then? Are we putting our life on the line for a few moments of gustatory pleasure? In my opinion, no. When it comes to the fine points of dietary selection, there is a wide latitude of choices. Whether you are a strict vegetarian or prefer eating meat, you can still maintain excellent health.

The majority of doctors and authors who write health books dogmatically adhere to one side or the other of this debate, rarely admitting to the possibility that both can be right. At one extreme we have the high-carbohydrate, very low fat crowd; at the opposite pole is the bunch that contends a high-protein, higher-fat diet is the true path to optimum health. I believe each is partly right and partly wrong.

Fifty years ago, Roger Williams coined the term *biochemical individuality,* which refers to the fact that people differ as dramatically on the inside as they do on the outside. If this is true, and I believe it is, why do we think that only one meal plan will work for all people, whether we are talking about the heart, stomach, or pancreas? One of my pet peeves about diet and health books is that writers try to convince us that their program is the only path for *all* people. I have a difficult time swallowing this, whether they are referring to diet, exercise, relaxation techniques, or religious beliefs.

Proteins are ubiquitous in foods derived from both the plant and the animal kingdom, which is probably why protein deficiency is almost unheard of. The American diet is rarely deficient in protein, except when we get caught up in the diet scheme of the month, which sometimes leads to people winding up weak from lack of protein, fat, or important nutrients.

When we continuously fall below the normal range for any of the major food groups, we will suffer imbalance and, eventually, ill health. If our daily diet falls short of its protein needs for any length of time, we may experience a number of subtle clues: fatigue, mental confusion, irritability, loss of hair, thin skin, brittle nails, food cravings, menstrual irregularities, lack of sex drive, and susceptibility to colds and infections. On the other hand, if we are following a diet that is heavy in protein and too restrictive of carbohydrates, we may experience dehydration, headaches, light-headedness, mental fatigue, and bad breath. Without adequate carbohydrates to fuel the system, the body produces chemical waste products known as *ketone bodies*. These toxic compounds, which are generated from the breakdown of stored fats, result in both short-term symptoms and long-term disease. An overload of protein burdens the kidneys and liver, causing significant loss of calcium from the bones. Consuming too much meat protein has been linked not only to osteoporosis but also to kidney stones, arthritis, and several types of cancer. Protein needs vary depending on the individual. If you recognize some of the signs in either direction, or if you aren't feeling up to par, you may want to review your protein intake.

## VEGETARIAN DIETS AND HEART HEALTH

The fact that vegetarians have a lower risk for heart disease is well documented. The vegetarian diet has been shown to reduce blood pressure and maintain or achieve desirable blood cholesterol levels, which reduces the incidence of atherosclerosis. Furthermore, vegetarians have lower rates of cancer and a lower chance of developing Type 2 diabetes, gallstones, kidney stones, diverticular disease, osteoporosis, and arthritis. They tend to maintain a normal body weight and to have a strong immune system. All this makes a strong case for converting to a vegetarian way of life.

Eating a vegetarian diet to combat heart disease was first suggested to the public in the 1970s, when Nathan Pritikin showed the world that he and hundreds of heart attack survivors were able to throw away their medications and live vital, healthy lives long after suffering a heart attack. His impressive results were not scientifically verified at that time; however, they could not be ignored, and numerous medical universities and private research labs seriously undertook the cause of evaluating and experimenting with low-fat vegetarian diets to cure and control heart disease.

The current high-profile advocate of the high-carbohydrate, low-fat diet is Dr. Dean Ornish from Sausalito, California. Armed with a few decades of data and with modern technology, he is the first clinician to document that heart disease can be stopped and reversed by changing diet and lifestyle. Based on his internationally acclaimed scientific study, Dr. Ornish's program has catapulted the vegetarian lifestyle into mainstream medicine. While Mr. Pritikin gave us anecdotal evidence of positive results, Dr. Ornish gave us the scientific proof the medical world requires.

We also have population studies attesting that in countries where people thrive on little or no meat, heart disease is minimal or nonexistent. In certain parts of Asia and the Mediterranean region, where people eat diets rich in fresh fruits and vegetables, grains, and legumes, diseases that we have come to consider unavoidable in the United States are rarely seen. And the reason is not genetics, as you might think. Once the inhabitants of other countries abandon their ancestors' eating patterns and assimilate to our Western-type diets— and probably other lifestyle habits as well—heart disease, cancer, and other diseases slowly emerge. This phenomenon has been proven time and again.

Subpopulations of vegetarian communities have received considerable scientific attention. The Seventh-Day Adventists in particular have been repeatedly studied because of their low rates of heart disease. According to a study of over twenty-five thousand women and men Seventh-Day Adventists, individuals who did not eat meat had substantially fewer fatal heart attacks. In order to clarify here,

### Protein Content
### of Selected Foods

| | |
|---|---|
| Tofu | 34 percent |
| Beans | 26 percent |
| Oatmeal | 16 percent |
| Tomatoes | 16 percent |
| Almonds | 12 percent |
| Corn | 12 percent |
| Potatoes | 11 percent |
| Carrots | 10 percent |
| Rice | 8 percent |

the term *vegetarian* can have different meanings. Strict vegetarians (vegans) eat nothing that has been made from an animal product; others just avoid poultry and red meat. In this study, about half of the Adventists reported following the no-animal standard and half ate eggs and dairy foods. All rejected meat, poultry, and fish. Members of this religious community clearly impress us with their flourishing health records. But is it good science to conclude that their secret lies in the absence of meat alone, when we know that Adventists also avoid coffee, alcohol, and cigarettes and they eat more fruits, vegetables, and whole grains? A vegetarian diet may be one part of the equation, but let's not make it the only answer to heart disease and good health.

A well-planned vegetarian diet can be lifesaving for some and all-around healthy for others. Many of you may be wondering where you can get protein if you restrict your diet to fruits, vegetables, and starches. Not to worry—virtually all unrefined foods have some protein. Consider the following list:

You may think that the vegetarian diet is too time-consuming because you have to combine your foods in a certain way in order to make a complete protein. This is no longer considered necessary. The essential and nonessential amino acids seem to find each other in the stomach regardless of whether they arrived for breakfast, lunch, or dinner. As long as you select a variety of grains, vegetables, and beans, you shouldn't lack protein or nutrients. All of us would benefit from eating more vegetarian meals, even if we choose not to entirely give up meat.

If you have survived a heart attack or are considered at high risk, you may want to consider going vegetarian or partially vegetarian. How strictly you follow the plant-based lifestyle depends on your health situation and how amenable you are to living without meat.

A therapeutic diet that reverses heart disease obviously is going to be more structured and austere than one meant for protective maintenance. You may want to check out Dr. Dean Ornish's program, attend a group organized by one of your local hospitals, or consult a dietitian or health care professional.

## Vegetarian Diets Don't Work for Everyone

A vegetarian diet may not be feasible for you for the long term, or it may not agree with your internal chemistry. As impressive as the research is, we are not all the same, and some people are just not biologically suited for a high-carbohydrate diet. While some individuals claim they are energized when they eliminate meats from their menus, others report feeling lethargic and sluggish. Christiane Northrup, M.D., author of *Women's' Bodies, Women's Wisdom,* noticed that when she integrated animal foods into her otherwise vegetarian diet, her cravings for sweets decreased dramatically, she was less groggy in the morning, and the abdominal bloating that she used to feel after almost every pasta- or grain-based meal was gone. I have since noticed a similar response when I overdo carbs. Dr. Northrup also noticed she started slowly losing body fat. I'm still waiting.

In her monthly newsletter, *Health Wisdom for Women,* Dr. Northrup shares a few more concerns about the very high carbohydrate, low-fat diets that work so well for men. "Over the long haul, I have found they often lead to increased carbohydrate cravings and, according to some studies, may even lower your HDL 'good' cholesterol and raise artery-clogging LDL 'bad' cholesterol." In addition, because these diets are so low in fat and protein, they may result in decreased muscle mass, increased fat storage, and depression, and you may be left feeling hungry after you eat.

We have been conditioned to think we can eat all the low-fat and fat-free carbs we want and still lose weight, but it is just not true. People respond differently to carbohydrate loading. Research from Stanford University determined that about 25 percent of the population hyperreact to the overconsumption of starches. Nutritionist Ann Louise Gittleman thinks that for overweight people, the percentage is considerably higher, possibly as high as 75 percent.

You know what happens when we eat too much sugar? The same response is triggered in some individuals when they load up on bread and spaghetti or bagels and fruit. To refresh your memory, the blood sugar levels immediately escalate, with insulin following shortly thereafter. Excess insulin causes the remaining sugar in the blood to be quickly stored as fat—not the reaction we want if we are already overweight. Furthermore, insulin blunts the fat-burning hormone *glucagon* and prevents it from releasing the already stored body fat from the cells. That makes two strikes against women who are struggling to lose fat. The condition of *hyperinsulinemia* (too much insulin in the blood) or insulin resistance (blunted cell response to insulin) leads to weight gain, prevents weight loss, and is associated with a higher risk for Type 2 diabetes and heart disease. Clues to determine whether you fall into either category may be high triglyceride levels, low HDLs, over-normal body fat, and diabetes.

If a high-carbohydrate weight-loss diet isn't working for you, consider that you may need to balance your carbs with more protein, even if it means adding fat. Your body may actually require more protein and fat in order to lose weight. A large amount of carbohydrates eaten at a single meal may be inhibiting weight loss. If losing weight is an issue for you, experiment with smaller portions of carbohydrates and balancing your grains and starches with 3 ounces of meat, chicken, fish, or tofu.

## MEAT IS NOT A FOUR-LETTER WORD

Meat is having a tough time shaking its unwholesome reputation when it comes to heart disease. It is definitely high in saturated fat and cholesterol, and therefore it tends to be shunned by those who work hard at keeping healthy. But I think we have gone too far. People who have had a heart attack or are at high risk can enjoy small amounts of beef, lamb, and veal, and individuals who exude health can eat slightly larger portions of these meats without worrying about ending up in the cardiac ward.

When you look at cultures that have fantastic health records, you realize they are not all exclusively vegetarian. Small amounts of meat, poultry, and fish are found in the diets of a good number of the plant-based societies. We should concentrate on removing the saturated fats that come from packaged and fried foods before we totally eliminate meat protein from our diets.

Red meat contains valuable nutrients that are difficult to get elsewhere, especially on a strict vegetarian diet. These include iron, zinc, and vitamin B-12. To obtain these nutritional benefits, small portions (3½–4 ounces cooked) will suffice. Furthermore, trimming the fat will greatly cut down on the saturated fat we so badly want to eliminate. As for the cholesterol content of meat, there is roughly 20–25 mg of cholesterol per ounce, which is the same as for poultry. One or two servings a day still keeps us under the 300 mg of cholesterol that the American Heart Association recommends as the upper-limit allowance.

A study in 1990 reported in *Food Chemical News* showed that low-fat beef had the same salutary effects on blood cholesterol and lipid profiles as did fish and chicken. Beef's fat content varies widely, but lean cuts are as low in fat as skinless chicken and broiled fish. Trimming all visible fat before cooking and keeping the portions to the size of a cassette tape or deck of cards further limits the amount of saturated fat.

Fatty meats are heart destroyers and should be restricted, if not totally avoided. Several studies tell us that the real culprit is not the protein part of the meat but the fat that accompanies it. Researchers from Australia put this theory to test by placing ten healthy women and men on a high-beef diet, which came out to about a pound of beef a day for three weeks. The beef was thoroughly trimmed of fat, making it ultra-lean. When the participants' blood cholesterol levels were tested, rather than going up as you might expect, they had dropped an average of 20 percent. Taking this experiment one step further, the researchers added beef fat drippings during the fourth and fifth week, retested, and found that the cholesterol readings were elevated again. I would love to see more studies like this to help us avoid feeling guilty each time we order a piece of lean meat. We are often led to believe that something is all good or all bad, but a strong case can be made for small portions and moderation.

A number of nutrition advocates believe that the problem with red meat today is the way it is raised. Our health problems, they say, are due not to the meat itself but to the effects of tampering with the meat. Cattle used to graze in the countryside on acres of lush, green grass. But nowadays, cattle are fed on prepared grains and fattened up in feed lots after being injected with a healthy dose of a growth hormone called *stilbestrol*. This change in feeding practices is thought to alter the type of fat that is stored in the animals' muscles. When we eat the meat, we introduce hormones into our bodies that clearly are not meant to be there. Choosing free-range beef, which is devoid of hormones and antibiotics, is one way to ensure that the beef you are eating is as safe as possible.

As a conscientious consumer looking for low-fat cuts of meat, utilize the USDA grading system. Grading is a voluntary service established by the U.S. Department of Agriculture to evaluate meat according to the amount of marbling, the white streaks of fat that run through the flesh and give meat its flavor and juiciness. Ironically, the cuts with the most fatty marbling are given the highest grade—Prime—followed by Choice and Select.

On the average, a cut of Select-grade beef has 5 to 20 percent less fat than Choice, and 40 percent less fat than Prime. Since grading is optional to the meat packer, not all beef on the market is graded. A rule of thumb: if the meat is sold under the store brand, you can be sure it is either Choice or Select. Supermarkets rarely stock Prime meat. Those scrumptious fatty cuts go directly to your favorite restaurant, and that is why the beef you order there tastes better than the same cut you serve at home.

The following chart will help you evaluate how much total fat as well as saturated fat you are getting from the meat you eat. It is generally recommended that women not exceed 30 percent of fat in our total diet, and of that, no more than 10 percent should come from saturated fats. For most women, this translates into 40 to 60 grams of total fat per day and 4 to 6 grams of saturated fat.

## Comparing Beef Cuts

(3 1/2 ounces trimmed and cooked)

| CUT OF MEAT | CALORIES | TOTAL FAT (GM) | SATURATED FAT (GM) |
|---|---|---|---|
| Ground beef, regular | 289 | 21 | 8 |
| Ground beef, lean | 272 | 18 | 7 |

| | | | |
|---|---|---|---|
| Ground beef, extra lean | 256 | 16 | 6 |
| Blade roast, Prime | 318 | 21 | 8 |
| Blade roast, Choice | 265 | 15 | 6 |
| Blade roast, Select | 238 | 12 | 5 |
| Ribs, whole, Prime | 280 | 19 | 8 |
| Ribs, whole, Choice | 237 | 14 | 6 |
| Ribs, whole, Select | 206 | 10 | 4 |
| Bottom round, Prime | 249 | 13 | 5 |
| Bottom round, Choice | 193 | 8 | 3 |
| Bottom round, Select | 171 | 5 | 2 |
| Tenderloin, Prime | 232 | 12 | 5 |
| Tenderloin, Choice | 212 | 10 | 4 |
| Tenderloin, Select | 200 | 9 | 3 |
| Sirloin, Prime | 237 | 12 | 5 |
| Sirloin, Choice | 200 | 8 | 3 |
| Flank, Choice | 237 | 13 | 6 |
| Porterhouse, Choice | 218 | 11 | 4 |
| T-bone steak, Choice | 214 | 10 | 4 |
| Eye of round, Prime | 198 | 8 | 3 |
| Eye of round, Choice | 175 | 6 | 2 |
| Eye of round, Select | 155 | 4 | 1 |

## Comparing Other Red Meats

(4 ounces cooked)

| CUT OF MEAT | CALORIES | TOTAL FAT (GM) | SATURATED FAT (GM) |
|---|---|---|---|
| Pork ribs, untrimmed | 449 | 34 | 13 |
| Lamb loin, untrimmed | 357 | 26 | 11 |
| Duck, with skin | 381 | 32 | 11 |
| Pork rib roast | 294 | 18 | 7 |
| Ham, leg, untrimmed | 285 | 16 | 6 |
| Pork chop, loin untrimmed | 271 | 15 | 5 |
| Veal sirloin, untrimmed | 228 | 12 | 5 |
| Pork shoulder, arm | 258 | 14 | 5 |
| Lamb, shoulder blade | 236 | 13 | 5 |
| Duck, no skin | 227 | 13 | 5 |

| Pork rib roast | 244 | 11 | 4 |
| Lamb loin | 244 | 11 | 4 |
| Pork chop loin | 228 | 9 | 3 |
| Veal loin | 198 | 8 | 3 |
| Lamb shank | 203 | 8 | 3 |
| Veal leg, top round | 170 | 4 | 1 |

Purchasing the leanest meats and cooking them properly will keep saturated fats in your diet to a minimum. The best cooking methods are roasting, grilling, broiling, or baking. Don't fry or braise, and if you use meat in a soup or stew, skim off the fat before serving. If you have time, refrigerate it so you can see the hardened beads of fat more clearly. Bypass the fatty cuts of beef, pork, and lamb (spare ribs and organ meats) and especially processed meats like bacon, sausages, hot dogs, and cold cuts. If and when you do indulge, trim as much of the visible fat off as possible.

Cooking meat at a very high temperature, as in grilling, broiling, or barbecuing, is very tasty but can be hazardous to your body in a number of ways. When you brown meat and poultry, and to a lesser extent fish, toxic agents called *heterocyclic amines* (HCAs) are created. These powerful substances can stimulate the formation of cancer cells and free radicals, which are known to damage the blood vessels and heart.

I am sure you will not totally give up your summer barbecues (me neither!), so take a few precautions. To reduce the number of HCAs, trim the meat closely to keep fat from dripping onto the coals and flaring the flame. You can also precook the meat in the microwave for two minutes before grilling so that some of the fats will drip off and you can then discard them. According to nutritionist Jean Carper, tests in California showed that precooking a hamburger in the microwave for two minutes before putting it on the grill reduced the HCAs by 90 percent.

You can remove up to half the fat from ground beef that will be used for spaghetti sauce or chili, or for any recipe that calls for ground meat, by taking the following steps: (1) crumble the beef into a frying pan or bowl and cook it over the stove or microwave it on high for a couple of minutes; (2) using a fork, break up the meat some more and pour off the grease; (3) continue until the meat looks cooked; and (4) place the cooked meat in a strainer and press out more fat or place it on paper towels and blot out the fat.

Another tip from Jean Carper to cut down those hazardous HCAs in burgers is to mix in soy protein before cooking. Even a small amount of soy can block the formation of 95 percent of these cell-damaging mutagens. The soy also replaces some of those ugly saturated fats, which makes the meat even more healthy. The recipe from Carper's *Stop Aging Now* is $1/2$ cup textured vegetable protein (TVP) mixed with two tablespoons of cold water and combined with a pound of lean ground hamburger. Knead all the ingredients together and form into patties. The rest of the household will never know the difference.

## CHAMPION CHICKEN

Chicken is a hot item on any menu these days. Most health-conscious women have switched from beef to chicken and fish, with the emphasis on chicken. As people examine their choices and consciously decide to lower their daily fat content, transitioning to chicken and turkey seems to be one of the easiest and most convenient tactics.

Poultry is undoubtedly the most versatile of the meats. It can be roasted, broiled, grilled, sautéed, stir-fried, poached, or deep-fried. It lends itself to a variety of seasonings, sauces, and toppings. The variety chicken offers and the fact that it is economical, rather than its low fat content, is probably why it is a staple in practically every culture's cuisine.

Chicken is comparable to beef in quality of protein, and both supply approximately the same amounts of vitamins and minerals, except that beef has slightly more iron and zinc. Although the cholesterol content is similar to that of red beef, the fat in chicken is less saturated. When cooked, skinless light-meat chicken is 40 to 80 percent leaner than trimmed cooked beef. Chicken breast, the leanest part of the bird, has less than half the fat of a trimmed Choice-grade T-bone steak. The light meat of poultry has less fat than the dark meat, so by switching from dark to light, you can slash 5 grams of fat in a $3 1/2$-ounce serving. You cut even more fat by avoiding the skin;

chicken skin derives 80 percent of its calories from fat. Turkey is even lower in fat.

A misguided few are under the impression, though, that as long as it's chicken, it's healthy. Wrong. A low-fat bird can easily be turned into a high-fat entrée, depending on the way it is cooked. Fried chicken may be a popular American dish, but it is one of the most unhealthy ways to prepare chicken. The breading absorbs a good part of the oil, taking a nice, light piece of poultry from 6 grams of fat to a whopping 15 grams. Instead of frying your bird, opt for roasting, baking, grilling, sautéing, or stir-frying. I am sure you already know this, but as a reminder, you don't always have to use oil in your preparation. Substituting broth, wine, or a nonfat spray works just as well.

## Comparing Poultry Parts
### (3½ ounces cooked)

|  | CALORIES | TOTAL FAT (GM) | SATURATED FAT (GM) |
|---|---|---|---|
| **CHICKEN BROILER/FRYER** | | | |
| Breast, with skin | 197 | 8 | 2 |
| Breast, without skin | 165 | 4 | 1 |
| Dark meat, with skin | 253 | 16 | 4 |
| Dark meat, without skin | 205 | 10 | 3 |
| Drumstick, with skin | 216 | 11 | 3 |
| Drumstick, without skin | 172 | 6 | 1 |
| Wing, with skin | 290 | 20 | 5 |
| Wing, without skin | 203 | 8 | 2 |
| **CHICKEN STEWERS** | | | |
| Dark meat, without skin | 178 | 9 | 2 |
| Light meat, without skin | 203 | 8 | 2 |
| **TURKEY ROASTERS** | | | |
| Breast, with skin | 153 | 3 | 1 |
| Breast, without skin | 135 | 1 | 1 |
| Leg, with skin | 164 | 5 | 1 |
| Leg, without skin | 159 | 4 | 1 |
| Wing, with skin | 207 | 10 | 3 |
| Wing, without skin | 163 | 3 | 1 |

| | | | |
|---|---|---|---|
| *DUCK* | | | |
| No skin | 201 | 11 | 4 |
| *CAPON* | | | |
| Meat and skin | 229 | 12 | 3 |

Poultry may or may not be graded for quality by the USDA. As with beef, the processors must pay a fee for this service; therefore, you will often find ungraded chickens at the market. If the product is graded, it is likely to be Grade A; lesser-quality meat is often sold to food manufacturers for processed products. More and more, you may be noticing chickens labeled "free-range" and "hormone-free." Unlike most caged chickens, these birds are allowed to roam freely on the farm and are not injected with hormones. Besides not being pumped with hormones, free-range chickens are said to offer more essential fatty acids and less saturated fat. Shelton Farms, Foster Farms, and Harmony Farms advertise organically raised poultry.

Take-out chicken may not be as healthy as you think. Researchers from Tufts University found that consumers are not getting all the facts when it comes to foods they consider nutritious. Tufts researchers came up with some amazing findings. Roasted chicken, which we all assume to be superior to the artery-clogging fried version, isn't all that much leaner. KFC's new Colonel's Rotisserie Gold variety breast and wing has only one gram less of fat than a similar portion of the Original fried recipe, which totals 432 calories and 25 grams of fat. Of course, you can remove the outer skin from both dinners and cut down the fat, but when you smell the aroma and touch the crunchy texture, temptation often wins out.

A rotisserie-cooked half-chicken with skin from Boston Market is not what you would call diet fare, either. Even without the tasty side dishes of potatoes, stuffing, and cooked squash, it weighs in at over 650 calories and 39 grams of fat, about the same as a McDonald's Big Mac and large fries. And then there are the side dishes. If you choose mashed potatoes, stuffing, and squash, tack on an additional 524 calories and 17 grams of fat. A serving of coleslaw from Roy Rogers contains 295 calories and 25 grams of fat, and the corn bread from KFC contains 228 calories, 13 grams of fat, and 194 milligrams of sodium—more on all three counts than a small order of McDonald's fries.

Appetizers can sneak in and ruin an otherwise healthy meal. Take the ever-popular chicken wings. How harmful can a little bite be while you're waiting for the main course? Say you are going to share a ten-piece order with a friend. Half a plate of wings from Domino's Pizza racks up 170 calories and 10 grams of fat. If you plan to scarf down the whole order at KFC's because you get only six, before you even glimpse your entrée, you will have added 471 calories and 33 grams of fat to your meal—more than half your total daily allotment. Dunk those little morsels into blue cheese dressing like many people do, and the calories and fat grams skyrocket. Just one tablespoon of blue cheese dressing contains 75 calories and 8 grams of fat. It adds up quickly, doesn't it?

If I haven't burst the it-must-be-healthy-because-it's-chicken bubble yet, stay with me. A very popular light lunch choice among women is the Oriental chicken salad. Delicious, yes—light, no. This skinless chicken breast over a mound of lettuce sprinkled with a few rice noodles weighs in at 750 calories and 49 grams of fat, 12 of which are of the saturated variety. If this is one of your favorites, you don't have to give it up; just learn to tailor your salad by ordering a lower-fat dressing or asking for the dressing on the side and sprinkling on just enough to savor the flavor but cut the fat. The same thing applies to the chicken Caesar salad. Use the dressing sparingly.

It is possible to find low-fat meals in restaurants and fast-food establishments. Grilled chicken sandwiches are available almost anywhere, with a mere 8 grams of fat. Be careful though when you add the bacon, cheese, and mayo; as juicy as it is, you jump to a very high-fat sandwich, with 30 grams of fat. Other decent choices are available, including stir-fried chicken, chicken soups and stews, or chicken with rice, pasta, or vegetables. Because of the endless number of ways to prepare chicken, chefs create new recipes every day. If you are in doubt about the fat content of the sauce or dressing, just ask, or if you are not comfortable doing that, ask for the sauce on the side.

## UNSCRAMBLING EGGS

In the years since cholesterol first became a widespread concern, eggs, because of their high cholesterol content, have been banished from heart-healthy menus. Yet gradually, some researchers are suggesting that eliminating eggs may not be necessary. There is consensus that saturated fat has a greater effect on blood cholesterol than dietary cholesterol—and eggs are not a major source of saturated fat. A whole egg yolk contains about 5 grams of total fat, of which less than 2 grams are saturated.

A few more words in defense of the much-maligned egg. It is an inexpensive source of high-quality protein (about 6 grams in one large egg) and an important source of vitamins, minerals, and amino acids. Vitamin E and the B vitamins are critical to heart health, and they are richly supplied in eggs. Eggs are high in lecithin, which, surprisingly, serves as a cholesterol-lowering agent. An individual egg doesn't contain as much cholesterol as we once thought. With the use of better cholesterol testing measurements, a study conducted by the USDA found that one large egg contains about 210 mg of cholesterol, not the 275 mg that is still reported in many texts.

Eggs can be integrated into a low-fat diet. The much-loved omelet can continue as your weekend treat if you cut down on the number of whole eggs. Extend the volume by adding one or two egg whites to a single egg, and no one will know the difference. Some restaurants will do this for you if you ask. Italian frittatas are my favorite, especially when they are filled with fresh spinach, broccoli, and mushrooms. Many chefs add cheese to frittatas, but they are just as good without it or with only a hint for flavor. Egg-based dishes like quiches, soufflés, and *stratas* are traditionally prepared with cream, butter, and cheese, but they don't have to be. Experiment with substituting nonfat milk, cottage cheese, and reduced-fat cheeses if you like making them at home.

The question remains, Will cholesterol in eggs raise blood cholesterol and clog the arteries? Some studies suggest that it raises total cholesterol, while others show it does not. As I have recommended before, if you have dangerously elevated cholesterol levels, do everything you can to bring them down: watch both saturated fats and cholesterol, and add fiber and healing nutrients. To be on the safe side, those of us with benign cholesterol levels and low risk should follow the advice of the American Heart Association and eat no more than four egg yolks a week.

## HOW TO "DO" DAIRY

Americans are raised from the cradle to drink milk as insurance for healthy bones later in life. We grow accustomed to the taste of fresh whole milk and tantalizing dairy-derived products like butter, cheese, and ice cream. Milk is synonymous with Mom's apple pie and goes great with homemade cookies. But now we find out our wonderful comfort foods rank second to beef as the largest source of unhealthy saturated fat in our diets.

Heart disease isn't the only condition related to an excess of high-fat dairy foods. Others include chronic intestinal discomfort, arthritis, allergies, sinusitis, acne, benign breast conditions, fibroids, and breast and ovarian cancers. Gynecologist Christiane Northrup suggests that there might be some correlation between overstimulation of cows' mammary glands due to hormones used for fattening, and subsequent overstimulation of our own, resulting in benign breast conditions. If you have experienced abnormalities in your breast tissue, it may be wise to consider how much cheese and ice cream creep into your daily diet. An ice cream cone now and then, however, will not put you at risk.

Milk isn't for everyone, in spite of what the billboards claim. In fact, people in three-quarters of the world's cultures thrive without drinking any milk after weaning. The majority of adult Americans cannot biochemically tolerate dairy products, either because they were not genetically blessed or because they have stopped producing the enzyme *lactase*, which is needed to break down the sugar in milk, called *lactose*. Lactose intolerance causes the undigested milk sugar to move into the colon, where it ferments, resulting in bloating, gas, pain, and diarrhea. A large proportion of African American, Greek, Asian, and Jewish people suffer from lactose intolerance.

Lactose isn't the only reason some people cannot utilize milk products. *Casein*, a protein in milk and cheese, cannot be assimilated by many individuals and may accumulate undigested in the upper intestine. As it putrefies, it produces mucus and toxins that eventually lead to a weakening of the gastric, intestinal, pancreatic, and bile systems. A greater amount of oxygen is needed to carry hemoglobin to cells enveloped with mucus; therefore, individuals who struggle with digesting casein may find their thinking dulled and their reactions slowed.

Not many women I know drink whole milk anymore. Most of us are aware that the 3.5 percent fat does not mean that our inno-cent glass contains less than 5 percent fat. The reality is that whole milk derives a whopping 50 percent of its calories from fat. Even the so-called 2 percent is not a low-fat product as advertised. Once you subtract the weight of the water from the total, you are left with a product that derives 38 percent of its calories from fat. If you are not ready to go to nonfat, 1-percent milk is a good compromise. It gets 23 percent of its calories from fat.

There are nondairy substitutes that you might try in place of milk. My favorite is rice milk. It is a 1-percent-fat, nondairy beverage with vitamins A and D plus calcium. This particular product is called Rice Dream and is derived from certified organic brown rice with a small amount of expeller-pressed oleic safflower oil. An 8-ounce glass provides 120 calories and 20 calories from fat. I pour it on my high-fiber cereal and really like the slightly sweet taste. My editor Rosana shared that she has had good results substituting it for milk in recipes. Soy milk is likewise available to drink straight or to add to cereal. If milk has been upsetting your stomach or you just want to try alternatives, experiment with several brands before deciding which is for you. Some are tastier than others.

Many options are available for reducing the fat content of dairy products or for substituting something else with less saturated fat. The food industry has been most cooperative in offering low- and nonfat milks, cheeses, sour creams, cream cheeses, yogurts, frozen desserts, and nondairy creamers. But be careful in choosing nondairy products; they are sometimes loaded with hydrogenated fat, which is just as bad as saturated fat. Try low- and nonfat diary products in place of the called-for whole versions in your favorite recipes. Most of the time no one will guess you have switched. Even if you replace just a portion of the whole milk with nonfat milk, you are on your way to cutting down on saturated fats.

If you like to experiment, you can make your own sour cream by pureeing low-fat cottage cheese in a blender with a touch of lemon juice or buttermilk. Try it on a baked potato instead of butter.

At first you may wince because it isn't butter, but let your taste buds get used to these new flavors, and you may be surprised how quickly you learn to like them. This low-fat sour cream as well as nonfat yogurts can also be used as a base for dips. During one of my food demonstrations I experimented with several low- or nonfat dip recipes and tried them out on my unsuspecting friends. Regular sour cream was also available for comparison. The most flavorful, according to this group, was not the high-fat sour cream/mayo dill recipe, but the yogurt/low-fat mayo dip. I have tried it several times for parties, and no one has guessed that they were enjoying a low-fat recipe.

Cheese is the tough one. Who doesn't love the creamy taste and texture of cheese covering a plate of pasta, sliced on a cracker, piled on bread, sandwiched between two flour tortillas, dripping on eggs, covering pizza, or topping apple pie? Imitation cheeses fill the deli cases now, but they are not the same. If you find them bland, rubbery, and tasteless, try simply cutting down your cheese portions and eat it infrequently. When I do order something with cheese, I ask that they sprinkle on a small amount. If I forget, then I carefully remove as much as I can. You might be surprised to find that when you scrape most of it off, the food still carries much of the flavor. Substituting cottage cheese for ricotta in lasagna works well; if you don't want to do this, try the part-skim-milk ricotta or mozzarella, which has a little less fat. No way around it—we all need to go light on cheese.

Making informed decisions requires knowing the facts. To help you in this process, I have provided the following list of calories and fat content for some favorite dairy products. Certainly there will be times when we splurge and enjoy higher-fat dairy foods, but a daily diet of high-fat dairy is not conducive to heart health.

## Comparing Dairy Products
(1/2 ounce or 1/2 cup)

|  | CALORIES | TOTAL FAT (GM) | SATURATED FAT (GM) |
|---|---|---|---|
| *DAIRY PRODUCTS* | | | |
| Heavy cream | 345 | 37 | 23 |
| Light cream | 292 | 31 | 19 |

| | | | |
|---|---|---|---|
| Sour cream | 214 | 21 | 13 |
| Half and half | 130 | 12 | 7 |
| Evaporated, whole milk | 134 | 8 | 5 |
| Evaporated, skim | 78 | <1 | <1 |
| Whole milk, 3.7% | 64 | 4 | 2 |
| Low-fat milk, 2% | 50 | 2 | 1 |
| Low-fat milk, 1% | 42 | 1 | 1 |
| Buttermilk | 40 | 1 | <1 |
| Nonfat milk | 35 | <1 | <1 |
| Yogurt, whole | 61 | 3 | 2 |
| Yogurt, low-fat | 63 | 2 | 1 |
| Yogurt, nonfat | 56 | <1 | <1 |

## CHEESE

| | | | |
|---|---|---|---|
| Cream cheese | 349 | 35 | 22 |
| Cheddar | 403 | 33 | 21 |
| Colby | 394 | 32 | 20 |
| Fontina | 389 | 31 | 19 |
| Roquefort | 369 | 31 | 19 |
| Monterey Jack | 373 | 30 | 19 |
| Blue Cheese | 353 | 29 | 19 |
| Brie | 334 | 28 | 17 |
| Swiss | 376 | 28 | 18 |
| Parmesan | 392 | 26 | 16 |
| Mozzarella, whole milk | 318 | 25 | 16 |
| Mozzarella, part skim | 280 | 17 | 11 |
| Ricotta, whole milk | 174 | 13 | 8 |
| Ricotta, part skim | 138 | 8 | 5 |
| Cottage cheese, creamed | 103 | 5 | 3 |
| Cottage cheese, 2% | 90 | 2 | 1 |
| Cottage cheese, 1% | 72 | 1 | <1 |

# GO FISH

An ocean of evidence supports a strong association between eating fish once or twice a week and a reduced risk of cardiovascular disease.

Like meat and poultry, fish and shellfish offer an excellent source of protein; yet, unlike the animal foods, fish is relatively low in saturated fat and calories. Surprisingly, all seafood is not lower in cholesterol. Most fish or shellfish rank about the same as skinless chicken breast or lean beef. The exception is shrimp, with 195 milligrams of cholesterol per 3¹/₂-ounce serving, but it is so low in saturated fat that it is tough to criticize. Fish is also a good source of many vitamins and minerals, including vitamin B-12, iodine, phosphorus, selenium, zinc, and ubiquinol, or coenzyme Q10.

The best thing about fish, other than its low levels of artery-clogging saturated fat, is that it is oozing with the clot-busting, cholesterol-lowering omega-3 fatty acids. These ultra-healthy fats, touted for their cardiovascular protective effects, may also be helpful in combating inflammatory disorders such as arthritis, high blood pressure, psoriasis, kidney disease, and possibly some forms of cancer. Numerous research projects are feverishly under way to determine the extensiveness of the health benefits of the omega-3s.

Research suggests that the higher the fat content of the fish, the better the cardiovascular benefits. Here is one time you can eat something fatty and not feel guilty.

## Fat Content of Fish

|  | TOTAL FAT (GM) | SATURATED FAT (GM) |
| --- | --- | --- |
| Shad | 18 | 6 |
| Mackerel, Atlantic | 18 | 4 |
| Fresh and canned herring | 12 | 3 |
| Salmon, red | 11 | 2 |
| Tuna, bluefin | 6 | 6 |
| Orange roughie | 9 | 1 |
| Catfish | 6 | 1 |
| Swordfish | 5 | 1 |
| Trout, rainbow | 4 | 1 |
| Sea bass | 3 | 1 |
| Red snapper | 2 | 1 |
| Haddock | 1 | 1 |
| Tuna, yellowfin | 1 | 1 |

The healthiest of foods can be harmful to some. If you are taking anticoagulants or any blood-thinning drugs, keep your fatty fish consumption to a minimum. Very high amounts of oily fish or fish oil capsules tend to prolong bleeding time and thus are contraindicated in people with a tendency to hemorrhage or bleed easily. This effect is rare, according to Sheldon Hendler, M.D., but still something to keep in mind.

Seafood is sometimes contaminated with poisons, such as industrial chemicals, agricultural pesticides, fertilizers, and human waste. The Environment Protection Agency estimates that 10 percent of America's waterways contain potentially dangerous levels of toxic chemicals and heavy metals. All of these pollutants can be absorbed and stored in the intestinal organs and fat of fish and passed on to us when we ingest them.

The most dangerous poisons that are passed from industry to water to humans are the polychlorinated biphenyls (PCBs) and methyl mercury, which are known reproductive toxins. PCBs, dioxins, and chlorinated hydrocarbon pesticides are thought to contribute to cancer. Until the government sets standards that will protect the consumer from these toxins, it is imperative that we take the initiative to protect ourselves.

One precaution is to cook our fish. Even the freshest fish may carry some bacteria, viruses, and microorganisms, but cooking will kill most of them. Sushi is popular now, but the risk of illness is high, so eating sushi is a real gamble. Certain shellfish—clams, mussels, and oysters—retain bacteria and viruses along with everything else they absorb. Raw shellfish can thus be a source of hepatitis and can cause gastrointestinal problems and many other infectious diseases. Raw fish, as found in sushi bars, has been found to house parasites such as tapeworms and roundworms, as well as bacteria and viruses. I don't wish to be an alarmist, but know the dangers and be careful.

Nothing, neither careful preparation nor high heat, can totally protect you from chemical contamination from lead and mercury. The best you can do is minimize your risk. Variety has been a cornerstone of dietetics, and it certainly applies here. Don't eat the same fish from the same body of water on a regular basis. Choose different species, favoring saltwater fish over freshwater, and deep-water offshore fish to coastal species.

Some think that the best way to buy fish is from a fish farm. It depends. Water in fish farms can be contaminated with agricultural runoff, pesticides, or river water. The fish farmers may also add drugs (including growth-promoting hormones, antibiotics, and sulfa drugs). The FDA does inspect fish farms, but some critics believe the system is inadequate. The surest way of getting untainted seafood is to buy it from a reputable dealer, whether it is your local market or a fish farmer.

To get the maximum benefit from the good fats, bake or poach your fish. Frying and adding vegetable oils high in omega-6 fatty acids decreases the omega-3 potency. It is quite easy to turn a healthy food into an artery-clogging nightmare; how we prepare fish could be more threatening to us than what was done to it in the water. Smothering your beautiful filet in cream sauce or frying it to a crisp negates those wonderful, health-giving benefits. The fast-food fish fillet sandwich you thought a good choice has more fat grams than many burgers. A fried seafood combo or popular Captain's platter contains 74 grams of fat, 26 of which is saturated. If you throw in the side of fries, coleslaw, and biscuits with two pats of butter, that number skyrockets to 130 total fat grams. We are talking heart attack waiting to happen.

Instead of preparing or ordering fried fish, try your fish broiled, baked, blackened, poached, steamed, or grilled. Herbs, spices, and vegetables enhance the flavor as much as a rich cream sauce. If you get stuck ordering a fish with a rich sauce, scrape it off. It is not rude to be careful about your health. Also try not to eat the fish skin, as it is a prime depository of chemicals.

## SAVOR SOY

Keep your eyes and ears open: soy is emerging as one of the all-stars when it comes to heart health. More than eighty years of accumulated evidence indicates that eating soy protein as opposed to animal protein significantly affects blood cholesterol levels. Early researchers searching for meat substitutes that were healthy, yet palatable, inadvertently discovered that the subjects testing soy-based meat alternatives were experiencing an improvement in their cholesterol profiles. In the mid-1970s the first systematic tests measuring the effects of soy protein on blood cholesterol levels were conducted by Dr. C. R. Sirtori of the University of Milan. He and his colleagues found that in just two weeks on a soy protein diet, cholesterol was lowered by an average of 14 percent, and by the end of three weeks it had declined by 21 percent.

Continuing research confirms the merits of soy. In controlled clinical trials, soy consumption repeatedly lowered total cholesterol, LDL cholesterol, and triglycerides, and in some cases it even raised HDL levels. The changes in blood cholesterol in people experimenting with soy have been substantial. In an analysis of thirty-eight studies involving a total of 730 volunteers, the average reduction in total cholesterol was 23.2 mg/dl or 9.3 percent; LDL cholesterol lowered 21.7 mg/dl or 12.9 percent; and triglycerides dropped 13.3 mg/dl or 10.5 percent.

For women who have not experienced significant results with the regular low-fat diets and find themselves frustrated, a soy-based diet may be worth a try. In a 1995 study at the University of Illinois, sixty-six postmenopausal women who had high cholesterol levels (above 200 mg/dl) went on a six-month diet. Half the women ate a low-fat diet in which the protein provided was nonfat milk; the others were given soy as their protein alternative. Although all had a significant reduction in total cholesterol levels, only the women eating soy had a significant reduction in LDL cholesterol, as well as a substantial rise in HDL cholesterol. In most of the studies, soy protein was substituted for animal protein without adding or subtracting calories. Individuals who benefit most from a soy-based diet are those with moderately high cholesterol. It doesn't seem to affect the number for individuals who fall within the safe range.

There is good reason to believe that soy can effectively lower dangerously high cholesterol as well. Italian clinicians have been diligently studying individuals who have very high blood cholesterol because of an inherited disease called *familial hypercholesterolemia*. In most cases, a low-fat diet (defined as 25 percent total fat daily) has not been effective, and these unfortunate individuals have no recourse but to constantly take medication in order to keep their skyrocketing levels under control. Soy was substituted in place of animal protein, and surprisingly, it worked. The LDL cholesterol levels dropped by 26 percent. It has become a practice of the Italian government to freely provide textured vegetable protein (TVP) as a dietary treatment for this condition.

I am not suggesting that if an error of nature has handed you frighteningly high blood cholesterol levels and a doctor has been treating it with drugs, you should stop your medication and fill your shopping bag with tofu and soy shakes. Take this information to your doctor and see if you can work together at lowering your cholesterol levels with less medication.

## How Does Soy Work?

Exactly how soy lowers cholesterol and protects the heart is not known. There is some evidence that the principal phytoestrogen in soy, *genistein*, may work in the early stages of atherosclerosis by hindering the overgrowth of the epithelial cells lining the arteries, which promotes plaque buildup and clogged arteries. Furthermore, genistein appears to thwart the activity of an enzyme, *thrombin*, which promotes blood clotting, potentially leading to heart attacks and strokes. Genistein may possibly increase the flexibility of the blood vessels, helping to prevent spasms that can trigger a heart attack.

Genistein not only appears to be a potent antioxidant that protects the arteries—it also possesses wide-ranging anticancer activity. In the lab, it directly inhibits the growth of several types of cancer, including breast, colon, skin, lung, and prostate. For women, genistein has an antiestrogen effect similar to that of tamoxifen, which blocks the overproduction of estrogen, thus curbing the growth of breast cancer. And I can't move on without mentioning how useful soy is to menopausal women. It counters the effects of bothersome hot flashes and night sweats, and it helps to keep vaginal tissues moist and healthy. As a woman still enmeshed in the throes of the transition, I can personally attest to the wonders of soy. As a rule, I tend to cringe when reading that one food or nutrient appears to solve a multitude of problems, but it is difficult not to get excited about the research surrounding soy.

Another reason soy is good for the heart is that it has a modulating effect on blood sugar. The amino acids in soy, glycine and arginine, decrease the level of insulin in the blood, thus tempering blood sugar levels. High blood insulin participates both in raising blood cholesterol levels and aggravating adult-onset diabetes, a major risk factor for heart disease. Diabetics and insulin-sensitive individuals can benefit tremendously from adding a little soy to their diets.

An elevated homocysteine level in the blood is considered as significant as high cholesterol in contributing to the clogging of arteries and eventually to heart disease. It is generally accepted that keeping homocysteine under control depends on three primary B vitamins: folate and vitamins B-6 and B-12. Can you guess? Soy is rich not only in these three, but in many other vitamins as well.

Possibly it is the soluble fiber in soy, the same fiber that is found in oats, rice bran, fruits, and vegetables, that makes it heart-healthy. There could be any number of phytochemicals we are only beginning to investigate, such as saponins, phytosterols, isoflavones, or lecithin, which are responsible for its super status. In any case, soy provides many health benefits, so do you really care if it's the protein, the fiber, the B vitamin, or the phytoestrogen that strengthens your heart, protects you from cancer, and helps you glide through menopause?

## How Much Do I Need?

In thirty-eight studies involving over seven hundred subjects, the average amount of soy that provided the benefits mentioned was 47 grams of soy protein a day. My sense is that this is probably not feasible for most of us and maybe not be desirable even for a heart patient who is highly motivated. I don't want to speak for all women, but I think I'm not too far off when I say that if we had to eat this much tofu and drink this much soy milk every day, most of us would probably take our chances with heart disease. Let's face it—soy is a foreign food to most, and our penchant for sticking with the familiar is often overpowering. Just try to incorporate as much soy into your diet as possible.

Good news: As studies continue to come in, a more doable dose of soy is advised. Several reports are telling us that only 20 to

25 grams of soy are needed to effect a change in blood cholesterol. A Japanese study found that when 20 grams of soy was added to the present diet of their participants, cholesterol levels dropped. The American Heart Association meeting in November 1997 agrees with this number, indicating that 20 grams of soy protein is adequate to lower cholesterol, reduce blood pressure, and ease hot flashes.

When a group of perimenopausal women from North Carolina were given two tablespoons of soy protein powder daily, which they either added to juice or milk or sprinkled over cereal, they reduced their LDL cholesterol by an average of 11 percent. Additionally, their diastolic pressure (the lower number) went down six points. The benefits occurred within a six-week period, and as a bonus these middle-aged women experienced fewer severe hot flashes and night sweats. A heaping spoonful of soy powder concealed in your morning cereal is a painless way to improve your heart.

## Soy Nutrition

Soy contains all of the major macronutrients we need for human nutrition—protein, carbohydrates, and fat. Soybeans provide a complete protein—in fact they are the only vegetable food that qualifies as complete, meaning they are essentially equivalent in quality of protein to meat, milk, and eggs. About 30 percent of the fiber in soy is of the soluble type, which lowers cholesterol. Soy products are low in saturated fat, highest in a polyunsaturated fat called linoleic acid, and contain up to 8 percent linolenic acid, an omega-3 fatty acid found primarily in fish oils and credited with lowering the risk of heart disease.

If you have heard that soy is high in fat, you are correct. But I think we need to gain a bit of perspective when we define high fat. If you are comparing soybeans to other plants, it comes out on top. However, if you are substituting tofu for meat or milk, it is appreciably lower in saturated fat and has no cholesterol. In addition, all soy products are not high in fat. Texturized vegetable protein (TVP) contains absolutely no fat, and more and more companies are manufacturing lowfat versions of tofu, soy flour, and soy milk. If you are interested in cutting out fat, relax—the little fat you get from tofu or tempeh will help you more than it will harm you.

## A Nutritional Guide for Soy Products

($^1$/$_2$ cup unless stated otherwise)

| SOY FOOD | PROTEIN | CALCIUM | FIBER | FAT |
|---|---|---|---|---|
| Soy beans, boiled | 14.3 gm. | 88 mg. | 1.80 gm. | 7.70 gm. |
| Soy flour, defatted | 47.0 | 188 | 4.0 | 1.2 |
| Soy protein isolate (1 oz.) | 22.6 | 50 | 0.07 | 0.95 |
| Texturized vegetable protein | 11 | 85 | 6.00 | 0.4 |
| Soy milk | 5.0 | 80 | 0.92 | 2.0 |
| Miso | 16.3 | 80 | 3.40 | 8.40 |
| Tempeh | 17 | 80 | 7.00 | 7.0 |
| Tofu, firm | 12.8 | 118 | 1.0 | 7.10 |
| Tofu, soft | 9.4 | 130 | 0.83 | 5.60 |

## Introducing Soy Products

If I conducted a survey on the street and asked people where they could find soy, I expect most would reply soy sauce and tofu. Well, this is partially correct. The tofu part is right, but there is actually little soy in the soy sauce we douse over our moo goo gai pan. Tofu is without a doubt the most popular of the soy foods, but let me introduce you to a wider range of possibilities. Be on the lookout for miso, tempeh, fresh soybeans, soy milk, and soy flour in your local market. Many of you may have tried miso soup or stir-fried tofu and vegetables at your favorite Japanese restaurant. Some brave souls have tested tofu burgers and tofutti, a tofu-based ice cream. There is a plethora of manufactured soy products filling the deli section and frozen food aisles of our markets, such as soy-milk yogurt, soy cheese, tempeh burgers, soy-flour pancakes, bakery products, pizza toppings, frozen dinners, tofu dogs, and veggie burgers. Finding soy is no longer a scavenger hunt.

## Tofu

Tofu is derived from soy-milk curd in much the same way that cheese is made from milk. The curds are compressed in blocks, some firm, some soft and spongy, and sold packaged in water or sealed vacuum-packed. By itself, tofu is odorless and tasteless, but in recipes, it acts like a sponge that soaks up the flavors of the foods around it. If this seems foreign to you, think about how chicken or pasta tastes without seasoning—neither is very distinctive without the sauce.

Tofu is extremely versatile. You can serve it mashed, marinated, grilled, or added to soups, chili, dips, casseroles, and soups. You can substitute it for meat or cheese or just add it to a tried-and-true recipe. You can blend it into drinks with fresh fruit, honey, and vanilla. The soft, silken tofu makes a light, creamy shake.

## Tempeh

Tempeh (pronounced "tem-pay"), an exotic-sounding soy product, is made from whole cooked soy beans infused with a starter mold for fermentation. Like tofu, it is compressed into dense blocks of soy, but it is distinctively different because it is mixed with a grain such as rice or millet. The flavor is somewhat smoky or nutty; some describe it as mushroomlike. Tempeh is wonderful marinated and then grilled until brown. Chunks of tempeh can easily be integrated into spaghetti sauce (like meatballs), sloppy joes, or chili mix. You can pan-fry it with onions and mushrooms and add it to stuffing or your favorite casserole.

## Miso

Miso is a thick paste made from soybeans, salt, a fermenting agent, and usually a grain such as rice or barley. It is a favorite condiment of Japanese and Chinese cooks because just one tablespoon can create intense flavors for broths, sauces, dressings, and marinades. Miso is very low in calories but high in salt, so if you have hypertension or are salt-sensitive, you may want to avoid this soy enhancer.

## Texturized Soy Protein

Texturized vegetable protein (TVP) is a dried, granular product primarily used as a food extender and often added to meat dishes like meat loaf, tacos, or chili. It is manufactured from defatted soy flour that is compressed, giving it a rough, grainy texture. There is no change in flavor if you substitute TVP for about one-fifth of the meat in recipes calling for ground beef.

## Fresh Soybeans

Fresh green soy beans are relatively new to the produce section of the market and may not have reached your store yet. Cooked like lima beans or peas, they can be eaten hot or cold. A serving of $1/2$ cup is equal to an 8-ounce glass of milk and has the iron content of two eggs. I find they serve nicely as a snack or added to a fresh green salad.

•   •   •

Soy products are entering mainstream markets. You no longer have to search them out in health food or specialty stores. Also check your local deli for salads including tofu and tempeh, and bakery products made from soy flour. If you are really serious about eating soy products, cookbooks with tasty recipes calling for soy flour, soy milk, tofu, and tempeh are now filtering into the bookstores. Check the appendix for recommendations.

We all need ample protein to survive, but the kind and the amount we should eat depend on the individual. Generally speaking, the proteins that appear to strengthen the heart can be found in plants, soy, fish, and small amounts of poultry and red meats. Eating a variety of these, rather than singling out one, may be the most prudent approach to ensuring we get enough protein in our diet.

# Part Three

# SUPER SUPPLEMENTS

# 10

# ANTIOXIDANTS: THE SECRET WEAPON

I always wanted to be somebody,
but I should have been more specific.

—LILY TOMLIN

The spotlight is on antioxidants these days, with front-page headlines reading "Vitamin E Lowers Heart Disease," "Beta-Carotene Cuts Women's Heart Risk," and "Vitamin C Saves Arteries." An arsenal of evidence points to the fact that antioxidants, when taken both individually and collectively, can slash the risk of heart disease and reverse the damage to an already ailing heart.

Most heart-health programs are aimed at reducing fat in the diet, yet when we read about the high-fat Mediterranean diet and the fact that the locals rarely die from heart problems, we can't but wonder if our energies are misplaced. We live in fear that our daily croissant puts us one step closer to the grave, while the French and Italians cavalierly douse their bread in oil and wash it down with a glass of red wine. There must be more to this situation than meets the eye. One explanation could be that the people in these areas eat foods that contain substances that also guard against heart disease.

The Mediterranean locals do eat differently from Americans and from people in most other Western countries. They regularly eat significant quantities of fresh fruits and vegetables, foods that contain plentiful amounts of antioxidants such as vitamin E, vitamin C, and beta-carotene. But let us not quickly adopt antioxidants as the single cure for heart disease. The entire story of what keeps us healthy evolves continually, and we should keep our minds open to additional studies and new possibilities. The theory that foods rich with antioxidants are as important to the heart as a low-fat diet has been proven, so it is something to consider when planning your healthy heart diet, but antioxidants should not be the sole factor you rely on.

Antioxidants in their many forms contribute to reversing the biological processes that result in clogged and hardened arteries. Key antioxidants, and those that have been most studied, are vitamin E, vitamin C, and beta-carotene. Supporting antioxidants that may be found to be equally beneficial in the future include selenium, copper, zinc, manganese, coenzyme Q-10, quercetin, lipoic acid, and certain sulfur-containing amino acids such as cysteine. Even this list is incomplete, because there are virtually hundreds of known antioxidants whose properties have yet to be evaluated in terms of their specific health benefits. They may play equally vital roles in the prevention of heart disease, but until they have been time-tested, we can only make recommendations based on the information at hand.

## HOW ANTIOXIDANTS PROTECT THE HEART

Heart disease is partly caused by, or at least greatly aggravated by, oxygen turned bad. It is hard to believe, but the substance that gives us life can also turn against us. One of the most important recent discoveries in science is the dark side of oxygen, which often wreaks havoc in our bodies by attacking our cells, clogging our arteries, causing cancerous mutations, and accelerating the aging process.

Deep within the molecules of the human body, two formidable forces wage an intense battle. On one side stand rampaging free radicals, renegade oxygen molecules whose primary goal is to destroy cell membranes. Opposing them are the stalwart defenders of the cell structure, the antioxidants, and it is their purpose to deactivate the free radicals in order to maintain cell integrity. Our bodies weaken when the highly volatile free radicals attack the arterial wall and leaving it vulnerable to fat and cholesterol accumulations,

| FREE-RADICAL INITIATORS | FREE-RADICAL FIGHTERS |
|---|---|
| Ultraviolet light | Vitamin E |
| Radiation | Vitamin C |
| Air pollution | Beta-carotene |
| Toxic industrial chemicals | Selenium |
| Cigarette smoke | Zinc |
| Pesticides | Coenzyme Q-10 |
| Alcohol | Lipoic acid |
| Rancid fats | Cysteine |

which can harden into plaque. It may take decades before signs of this process become evident, but eventually the cumulative damage creates recognizable symptoms of disease, including chest pains, inflamed joints, or cancerous mutations.

Free radicals enter the body from many outside sources, such as ultraviolet light, radiation (including X-rays), air pollution, toxic industrial chemicals, cigarette smoke, pesticides, alcohol, drugs, and rancid fats. Obvious ways to keep them under control are by avoiding all of the above. But I cannot imagine staying indoors every day so as not to breathe unhealthy air, or growing all my own foods to be sure not to take in pesticides. This is unrealistic for most of us. A more pragmatic option is to fortify our cell defenses by ingesting a healthy supply of antioxidant food compounds. Not only can they stop the rampaging oxygen molecules in their tracks—they can also repair some of the damage already done.

## COMBINING ANTIOXIDANTS

The evidence supporting the effectiveness of individual antioxidants in diminishing heart disease is impressive. Having them work as a team confers even greater protection. Separately they are helpful, but together they are our secret weapon against heart disease. In a Harvard study, women who took vitamin E, vitamin C, and beta-carotene on a regular basis experienced a remarkable 50 percent decrease in heart disease risk, and their stroke risk fell by 54 percent.

## VITAMIN E: FREE-RADICAL FIGHTER

Vitamin E is considered the most potent antioxidant. Over six thousand studies show that it guards against heart disease primarily by preventing LDL cholesterol from being oxidized by free radicals. When vitamin E is lacking in the cells, LDL fats are susceptible to oxidation. When researchers mix LDLs with vitamin E in a test tube, oxidation does not occur. The susceptibility of LDLs to oxidation is inversely related to the presence of antioxidants in the body, most notably, vitamin E. In other words, when vitamin E is low, LDL oxidation occurs spontaneously, but when vitamin E intake is high, oxidation is reduced and so are the level of LDL cholesterol and the initiation of cholesterol-forming plaque.

Many researchers believe that an inadequate vitamin E blood level is a better predictor of heart disease than elevated cholesterol. In October 1991, a World Health Organization study showed that low blood readings of vitamin E were predictive of heart attacks 62 percent of the time, while elevated blood cholesterol was predictive only 29 percent, and elevated blood pressure only 25 percent of the time.

## The Compelling Case for Vitamin E

Data from two large-scale independent studies coming out of Harvard University show that vitamin E reduced the risk of heart disease in women as well as in men. In the women's study, researchers followed over eighty-seven thousand nurses for a period of eight years. The risk of coronary disease in the women who took more than 100 IU of supplemental vitamin E daily was 34 percent lower than in those who did not supplement. The men's results were similar. Even taking vitamin E for two years lowered heart disease risk by 40 percent in women and 26 percent in men. The researchers found no protective effect in women who derived their vitamin E from food alone (see the chart that follows) or those who took a multivitamin containing the RDA levels of 30 IU of vitamin E.

The strongest and most convincing evidence so far that vitamin E can be used to treat an existing heart problem comes from a 1996 study done in Cambridge University in England. The Cambridge Heart Antioxidant Study (CHAOS) involved two thousand women and men with confirmed heart disease. Half of the participants were given either 400 or 800 IU daily of natural vitamin E and the other half a placebo. After eighteen months, the vitamin E users were found to have reduced their risk of heart attack by a whopping 77 percent. The somewhat astonished researchers hailed vitamin E as more powerful in harnessing heart disease than aspirin or cholesterol-lowering drugs. They emphasized that the health-giving effects of vitamin E were apparent about six months after beginning the program.

The bulk of the research on vitamin E suggests that people achieve optimal results in preventing artery-clogging plaque when taking supplemental doses in the range of 100 to 400 IU a day. Since the best sources of vitamin E are high-fat foods like oils and nuts, it is next to impossible to get that quantity from your diet alone. If you would like to try, consider that to get just 100 IU of vitamin E a day, you would have to eat the following amounts of the foods that contain it:

## Can You Eat Your Vitamin E? (100 IU/day)

1 cup sunflower seeds

1/2 cup soybean oil

5 cups peanuts

2 cups almonds

19 cups spinach

8 cups coleslaw

7 cups raw cucumber

7 sweet potatoes

Vitamin E performs other functions that relate to heart health. It has the potential of controlling inflammation, an initial stage in the chain of events leading to weakened arteries and plaque buildup. It is instrumental in thinning the blood and keeping it from forming dangerous clots. This can be lifesaving for women who easily form vein clots or are at high risk for stroke. A remarkable decrease in blood stickiness (platelet adhesion) was observed after supplementing with vitamin E for only two weeks. In subjects taking 200 IU of vitamin E, platelet adhesion was reduced by 75 percent. Those taking a double dose of 400 IU saw an 82 percent reduction. Vitamin E may be a safer alternative for women who cannot tolerate the daily dose of aspirin for blood thinning.

Vitamin E also prevents cells from self-destruction and may actually help to prolong the life of the cell. Late-breaking news suggests that a daily dose of 200 mg of vitamin E bolsters immune function, especially in older people. It was recently found to slightly decrease the progression of midstage Alzheimer's disease. Research is exploding in all areas regarding the aging process, and at the center you will usually find vitamin E.

## To Take or Not to Take

Each time a new study verifies the existing data about a vitamin or mineral, many nutritionists eagerly look for acknowledgment and support from the scientific community. Despite the evidence, however, the medical mantra continues: "We need more studies." What is so ironic is that many of these well-known researchers and physicians who withhold their blessings from vitamin E take it themselves. When a roomful of scientists were asked if they took vitamin E, half of them raised their hands. More shocking than the first response was the second. When the scientists were asked if they would recommend it to their patients, most raised hands fell.

It appears that cardiologists supplement with antioxidants but do not recommend them to their patients. The June 1997 issue of the *American Journal of Cardiology* reported an interesting survey conducted by a ninth-grade Florida student, Jason Mehta. It is not a normal practice for prestigious medical journals to include articles by such young authors, but Mehta's father is professor of medicine at the University of Florida's College of Medicine, so maybe that helped to get the article published. In any case, the survey results reported that 44 percent of 181 American cardiologists admitted to taking supplements—vitamin E, vitamin C, and/or beta-carotene—yet only 37 percent recommended supplements to their patients.

There are doctors and scientists who stand behind their decision to supplement. Jeffrey Blumburg, M.D., chief of the Antioxidant Research Lab at Tufts University Medical School, takes 400 IU of vitamin E daily and says he is comfortable with not having definitive results. "In this country we have hundreds of thousands of people dying from heart disease and cancer. I think the evidence suggesting vitamin E can curtail the suffering and cause of these diseases is very strong, and there appears to be no downside to me; therefore, I elect to supplement."

Gladys Block, M.D., an epidemiologist at the University of California at Berkeley and an antioxidant researcher, also supports her position in favor of taking vitamin E. In a recent interview she was quoted as saying, "Looking at the whole body of literature, even without exact clinical trials, I believe we can say antioxidant vitamins reduce the risk of cancer and heart disease."

The doses in the studies may seem high (between 100 IU and 400 IU) if you are comparing them to the RDA of 30 IU. The weight of the research clearly shows that vitamin E from food alone, or even the amount you can get from a regular multiple vitamin, is not sufficient for combating heart problems. The most recent research from the University of Texas found the higher dose of 400 IU to be most beneficial for lowering amounts of oxidized LDL cholesterol. Less was not effective.

I don't want to confuse you or send mixed messages, but it is my intention to present all the research, not just what I feel will best support my case. Vitamin E in food was in fact found to provide substantial benefit to the heart. A recent study coming out of the University of Minnesota, under the supervision of Dr. Lawrence Kushi, examined the diets of more than thirty-four thousand postmenopausal women and assessed, among other factors, their intakes of vitamins A, E, and C from food sources and supplements. By the end of the follow-up, 242 of the women had died of coronary heart disease. After analyzing the data it was suggested that in postmenopausal women the intake of vitamin E from food is inversely associated with the risk of death from coronary heart disease. The specific statistics show that those who ate roughly 5 to 8 IU a day appeared to reduce their risk of dying from heart disease by about 30 percent; women who ate more than 8 IU a day seemed to cut their risk by more than 60 percent.

Researchers are cautious about commenting on this data, because it is the only study that has observed a lower risk of heart disease in women who consume such low levels of vitamin E. The problem that is inherent in observational studies like this one is that the research does not show whether it was the vitamin E that lowered the risk or something else in the diet. Scientists admit they need far more evidence before they can assess whether small amounts of vitamin E in foods can reduce the risk of coronary disease.

## Official Approval for Antioxidants

One public health organization has officially come out and recommended vitamin supplements for the purpose of warding off life-threatening diseases such as heart disease and cancer. The Alliance for Aging Research, a Washington, D.C.–based health advocacy group, advises that Americans take specific antioxidants to protect against the diseases of aging. The Alliance came up with ranges for vitamin E, vitamin C, and beta-carotene, based on more than two hundred studies on antioxidants conducted over the last twenty years. The panel that evaluated the data consisted of respected scientific experts from reputable research and academic institutions around the country.

## How Much Vitamin E Is Effective Yet Safe?

The Alliance for Aging Research recommended 100 to 400 IU daily of vitamin E—the equivalent of three to thirteen times the USRDA. In case you are concerned about the toxicity of higher levels of nutrients, vitamin E has been found safe, with no adverse side effects, in levels up to 1,200 IU for several months. There are precautions for certain individuals. Please, first check with your doctor if you have high blood pressure, rheumatic or ischemic heart disease, or diabetes, are on blood-thinning medication, or have a condition contributing to vitamin K deficiency, such as liver disease or malabsorption syndrome.

## Choosing the Right Vitamin E Supplement

Vitamin E is a generic term for a group of related compounds. It occurs naturally in four major forms—alpha-, beta-, gamma-, and delta-tocopherol. While gamma is the primary tocopherol in foods, it is alpha that we find in the body and in supplements. The most biologically active form of vitamin E in supplements is the natural d-alpha tocopherol. It has been shown to be more efficiently absorbed and more available to the body than the synthetic version, dl-alpha tocopherol. Unfortunately, it is also the most expensive. Mixed tocopherols are also available, and personally I like to vary d-alpha with the mixed tocopherols and get the best of both worlds. It is also a good practice when buying vitamins and minerals to avoid extra additives, preservatives, yeast, and fillers.

Deciphering supplement labels is somewhat akin to decoding a doctor's prescription slip; they can appear unintelligible and meaningless. Since vitamins and minerals often come from chemical mixtures rather than direct from foods or plants, the names are difficult to decipher and pronounce. Vitamin E, for example, is derived from many substances, some of which are water-soluble and some fat-soluble; thus, next to d-alpha tocopherol we find in parentheses further descriptions of the source. The most absorbable varieties of vitamin E that you want to look for on the bottle are succinate, acetate, or free d-alpha tocopherol.

Vitamin E is a fat-soluble nutrient; therefore, it is absorbed from the intestinal tract in the presence of fat. To ensure you are getting the most from your vitamin, take E with meals, dividing the dose. For example, if your intention is to supplement with 100 IU a day, take 50 IU at breakfast and another 50 IU at dinner. You may be able to find adequate levels of vitamin E in your multiple vitamin/minerals tablet. If not, a separate antioxidant could be a good idea.

Vitamin E can be destroyed and rendered inactive when combined with certain substances. Two forms of iron, ferric chloride and inorganic iron, should not be taken together with vitamin E. There is no problem in mixing vitamin E with the ferrous fumerate or chelated iron, however, so check your multivitamin/mineral tablet to see which source of iron is present. Another caveat: don't take vitamin E with your contraceptive pill. Like the iron, contraceptive pills can interfere with the availability and action of vitamin E, in which case you won't benefit from it, so take the two pills several hours apart. In case you were wondering, vitamin E will not affect contraception.

A segment of the population may require additional vitamin E. People who take supplemental fish oils or have a diet rich in polyunsaturated oils need more vitamin E to protect them against rancidification of the oils. Vigorous exercise and smoking also create a heightened need for vitamin E.

## Food Sources of Vitamin E

| FOOD | VITAMIN E (IU) |
| --- | --- |
| General Mills Total (1 cup) | 30* |
| Kellogg's Product 19 (1 cup) | 30* |
| Almonds (3 tbsp.) | 11 |
| Safflower Oil (1 /tbsp.) | 9 |
| Kellogg's Complete Bran Flakes (³/₄ cup) | 8* |
| Kellogg's Low-Fat Granola (¹/₂–²/₃ cup) | 8* |
| Wheat germ, toasted (¹/₄ cup) | 8 |
| Sunflower seeds (1 tbsp.) | 7 |
| Sweet potato, cooked (¹/₂ cup) | 7 |
| Canola oil (1 tbsp.) | 5 |
| Soybeans, boiled (1 cup) | 5 |
| Papaya (1) | 5 |
| Corn oil (1 tbsp.) | 4 |
| Peanuts (3 tbsp.) | 3 |
| Spinach, cooked (¹/₂ cup) | 2 |
| Mayonnaise, full-fat (1 tbsp.) | 2 |
| Margarine (1 tbsp.) | 2 |
| Bread, whole-wheat (2 slices) | 1 |
| Broccoli, cooked (¹/₂ cup) | 1 |
| Asparagus, cooked (5 spears) | 1 |
| Avocado (¹/₂) | 1 |
| Prunes, dried (8) | 1 |

*Vitamin E added by manufacturer

## Food May Not Be Enough

We know from scientific studies that specific nutrients in specific amounts can decrease our probability for heart disease. Food will always remain the first choice for our vitamin and mineral intake, and you can use the preceding list to add natural sources of vitamin E to your diet but it will be not enough.. The chances are slim that you are going to get more than 10 to 15 IU of vitamin E daily from sources like whole grains, eggs, vegetable oils, spinach, asparagus, and avocados.

## SELENIUM: SMALL BUT MIGHTY

Inadequate selenium levels have been correlated with an increased risk of heart disease and other chronic diseases associated with aging. A trace mineral, which means that it is required by the body in minute quantities, *selenium* is part of a crucial enzyme, *glutathione peroxidase,* which defends against oxidant damage to cellular membranes. When selenium and vitamin E levels are not up to par, glutathione peroxidase cannot adequately protect the body from the chemical destruction that sometimes results in heart and circulatory diseases. When present, this dynamic duo also guard against tissue damage related to restricted oxygen supply or blood flow. In a double-blind, placebo-controlled study, twenty-two of twenty-four patients receiving one milligram of selenium and 200 IU of vitamin E daily enjoyed significant relief from angina (pain) while only five of twenty-four patients taking sugar pills were reported to have benefited. Selenium has also been shown to inhibit platelet aggregations, demonstrating anticlotting tendencies.

In population studies in the United States and other nations, we find that many forms of cardiovascular disease increase as selenium in the soil decreases. In Finland, where heart disease reaches the highest levels worldwide, a long-term case-controlled study showed that the blood levels of selenium in eleven thousand Finns measured below normal, as did the selenium levels of the soil of that country. The death rate from acute coronary disease was nearly three times higher there than in areas where selenium content was higher, and the rate of nonfatal heart attacks was twice as high. Here in the United States we have a "stroke belt," an area in the South encompassing part of Georgia and the Carolinas. It has both the highest stroke rate and a very high incidence of heart disease compared to the rest of the country, and correspondingly, a very low selenium soil content. China and Germany also report a similar correlation between selenium in the soil and a greater number of heart patients.

Selenium plays a pivotal role in bolstering the immune system. It is capable of detoxifying heavy metals such as mercury and cadmium, as well as various drugs, alcohol, cigarette smoke, and peroxidized fats. It is also known to protect against different types of cancer, coronary artery disease, peripheral vascular disease, and arthritis.

The range of selenium intake recommended for an adult is 0.05 mg to 0.2 mg, which is usually expressed as 50–200 mcg. Most people who consume meat regularly are

## Food Sources of Selenium
(3 oz. unless indicated)

| FOOD | SELENIUM IN MCG |
|------|----------------|
| **SEAFOOD** | |
| Lobster | 66 |
| Tuna | 60 |
| Shrimp | 54 |
| Oysters | 48 |
| Fish | 40 |
| **MEAT AND EGGS** | |
| Liver | 56 |
| Egg (1 medium) | 37 |
| Ham | 29 |
| Beef | 22 |
| Chicken | 21 |
| Lamb | 14 |

likely to get enough selenium. See the chart above. If you are a vegetarian and don't eat meat, fish, or eggs, you may need to supplement. The elderly could be at risk for selenium deficiency if they aren't taking in enough meat protein and also because, generally speaking, they do not absorb nutrients as well as they did at a younger age. If you are taking a full-spectrum multivitamin/mineral tablet, you should be covered.

## VITAMIN C: MORE THAN A COLD REMEDY

Countless numbers of health-conscious people ward off pesky colds by popping vitamin C and ascorbic acid tablets, and they may be inadvertently protecting their hearts, too. Like other antioxidants, vitamin C neutralizes free radicals before they attack the artery wall. Additionally, this popular vitamin heals already weakened arteries, making them less vulnerable to cholesterol buildup. Vitamin C helps regulate cholesterol production in the liver as well as the conversion of cholesterol to bile. Adequate amounts help move cholesterol easily through the body and remove unwanted excess. Some studies suggest that vitamin C might lower total blood cholesterol, reduce LDL cholesterol, and raise HDL cholesterol. Vitamin C, by reducing the amount of a dangerous fat called *lipoprotein(a)*, makes blood cells less sticky so clots are less likely to form.

Vitamin C has been used therapeutically in the treatment and follow-up of heart attack victims to deal with existing blood clots. Supplements of 2,000 mg of vitamin C have been shown to facilitate the chipping away of clumps that have already formed on critical arteries. And, in a double-blind study, patients coming out of surgery who were given 1,000 mg of ascorbic acid developed significantly fewer blood clots later on than did a control group who did not receive any vitamin C.

## Meeting Your Vitamin C Needs

Individuals with coronary artery disease characteristically have diminished levels of ascorbic acid in their blood. The Nurses' Health Study, which examined close to ninety thousand women between the ages of thirty-four and fifty-four, found this to be the case. Women who had ingested less vitamin C had a 42 percent greater risk of developing heart disease than the women with sufficient amounts.

The Alliance for Aging Research considers a daily dose of 250 to 1,000 mg an appropriate range for warding off diseases of the heart. It is likely that you can find a solid dose of the lower range in your food if you work at it. I would strongly urge you to do your best to incorporate fresh fruits and vegetables in your diet, not only for the vitamin C benefits but to provide you with other antioxidants and nutrients that are equally health enhancing.

To maximize your vitamin C intake, eat fresh rather than frozen foods. If you can't find top-quality fresh fruits and vegetables in the winter, eat frozen vegetables, which retain more vitamin C than canned

### Sources of Vitamin C

| FOOD | VITAMIN C (MG) |
| --- | --- |
| Pepper, red (3 oz.) | 163 |
| Pepper, green (3 oz.) | 110 |
| Broccoli, cooked (1 cup) | 98 |
| Orange juice, frozen (1 cup) | 98 |
| Papaya, (1/2) | 95 |
| Cranberry juice cocktail (1 cup) | 90 |
| Strawberries (1 cup) | 85 |
| Orange (1) | 80 |
| Cantaloupe, cubed (1 cup) | 67 |
| Grapefruit (1/2) | 42 |

ones. For maximum nutrition, eat your fresh produce soon after picking or purchasing. Vitamins are easily lost when fresh foods are handled, bruised, cut up, overcooked, or reheated. Slicing, dicing, and chopping exposes a greater surface area to the air, and more of the nutrients are lost. Cut and shredded vegetables lingering for hours in a salad bar lose significant amounts of vitamin C as well as other important nutrients.

As diligent as you may be about meeting your needs through food, it is likely that you will still need to take vitamin C supplements. Check the following chart to see how close you can come to reaching 1000 mg/day.

## Can You Eat Your Vitamin C? (1000 mg/day)

15 oranges

25 green peppers

10 cups strawberries

22 tomatoes

34 potatoes

7 cups cooked broccoli

## Supplementation: Some Need More, Some Need Less

Vitamin C is water-soluble, and excesses are excreted in the urine, so even in large amounts (up to 10 grams) it is relatively innocuous. The exact dosage one should take seems to be best determined individually. There is a tried-and-true method to determine when you have assimilated more than your body can handle: it is called bowel tolerance. If you experience diarrhea, you've exceeded your limit. Some people may find they can match Linus Pauling's notorious 10 grams per day of vitamin C, while others can tolerate only 250 mg.

The need for vitamin C varies considerably from one person to another. If you are a smoker, your vitamin C requirements shoot up. Smokers have been found to have lower levels of vitamin C both in their blood and in their white blood cells. These levels are lowered up to 40 percent in individuals who smoke more than twenty cigarettes a day and by 25 percent in those who smoke less than this.

Smoking increases the risk for heart disease, but if you are not yet prepared to quit, take vitamin C for extra protection.

Exposure to environmental pollutants and other factors such as alcohol and caffeine use, various drugs, infection, surgery, trauma, advanced age, and stress bolster your requirements for vitamin C. If you are taking any of the following medications, you may want to up your daily dosage: aspirin, barbiturates, birth control pills, cortisone, levodopa, sulfonamides, and tetracycline. There may be others not on this list, so please consult your doctor or pharmacist.

If you are taking more than 200 mg per day of vitamin C, it may reduce the effectiveness of tricyclic antidepressants such as Elavil, Triavil, Asendin, Norpramin, Tofranil, and Vivactil. Again, this may not be a complete list, so if you are taking any antidepressants, you should inform your doctor that you are taking supplements. Also, if you are about to have a blood or urine test, it is a good idea to stop taking vitamin C, or anything but a multivitamin, for a few days before; it may give a false reading.

## Which Vitamin C?

When it comes to supplemental vitamin C, the choices are staggering. It really doesn't matter whether you choose natural or synthetic forms or whether they are derived from rose hips or acerola. The body readily absorbs them all. You can buy vitamin C in tablets, granules, or chewables, timed-released or regular. Take your pick. If you find vitamin C hard to stomach, palm-derived ascorbate or calcium ascorbate may be best for you. As with most vitamins, it is best taken in divided doses and with meals or snacks.

## BETA-CAROTENE: FOR BETTER OR WORSE?

Researchers discovered rather accidentally that beta-carotene helps protect against cardiovascular disease. A group of Harvard scientists setting out to establish whether beta-carotene had a protective effect against cancer serendipitously found that men taking a supplement of beta-carotene suffered one-half the number of strokes, heart attacks, and sudden cardiac deaths as those ingesting an inert sugar pill. Another study found that beta-carotene along with vitamin E reduced the risk of a first heart attack. Quoting from the Nurse's Health Study, women who took in 11,000 IU a day of beta-carotene had a 22 percent lower risk of heart disease and a 37 percent lower risk of stroke than women ingesting only a few thousand IU a day.

## Cautions Regarding Beta-Carotene

After a long series of optimistic reports about beta-carotene, two major controlled, randomized trials raised a red flag, dampening the enthusiasm for this antioxidant. The CARET study (Beta-Carotene and Retinol Efficacy Trial) came to a halt ahead of schedule because the beta-carotene supplements appeared to be doing more harm than good. The over eighteen thousand individuals (6,289 of whom were women) being observed were already at high risk for lung cancer—they were heavy smokers, former heavy smokers, and asbestos-industry workers. After four years, those taking vitamin A (25,000 IU) and beta-carotene (30 mg) showed a higher lung cancer rate and overall higher mortality rate than the control group. This was particularly alarming in light of a 1994 study from Finland, which also found that beta-carotene supplements increased the risk of lung cancer in male smokers.

Further evaluation from Finland and the United States seems to confirm that women and men who are not heavy smokers need not be concerned. Finnish researchers point out that the supplements increased the risk of lung cancer only in those who smoked more than a pack of cigarettes a day and/or drank "above average" amounts of alcohol. Beta-carotene did not increase the risk for lighter smokers or former smokers.

The mechanism that might explain the puzzling association between beta-carotene and lung cancer in heavy smokers is as yet unclear, but there is one strong suspicion. In the January 1997 issue of the *Journal of the American Chemical Society*, English researchers proposed that the problem is not so much the presence of beta-carotene as the absence of vitamin C. Normally, beta-carotene enhances the antioxidant effect of vitamins C and E. However, smoking depletes the body's supply of both these vitamins, and, without an adequate amount of vitamin C, a potentially harmful form of beta-carotene may accumulate.

Antioxidants can have both protective (antioxidant) as well as adverse (prooxidant) effects. They work most effectively as a team, some countering the adverse effects of others. Cigarette smoking is a particularly harmful behavior and is a major source of free radicals. When vitamins C and E are not available in adequate amounts, beta-carotene acts as a prooxidant, possibly compounding the harmful effects of heavy smoking.

The bottom line here is, if you smoke, don't take beta-carotene supplements on their own. Make sure you also are getting adequate amounts of vitamins C and E. It is especially important that you eat several portions of fruits and vegetables each day, even more than the prescribed four or five.

## Other Carotenoids

Beta-carotene is not the only antioxidant carotenoid. Scientists have identified more than six hundred varieties of carotenoids in plants and other foods, yet only about four hundred of these have been chemically isolated and classified. So far, virtually all show antioxidant properties, but only thirty to fifty are converted into vitamin A in the body. Different carotenoids work on different parts of the body, and generally, high blood levels are associated with lowered risk for various diseases. Beta-carotene seems to stand out as the star carotenoid, probably because it is the easiest to measure in the blood and thus the one with which scientists have experimented the most. The question that seems obvious to me and many other health educators is, Are the health benefits we ascribe to beta-carotene due solely to this one carotenoid or could they be caused by one or more of the others or the synergistic effect of the mix?

Included in the family tree of carotenoids identified so far are alpha-, beta-, and gamma-carotene, beta-cryptoxanthin, lycopene, lutein, and zeaxanthin. Even though we may not have the research to verify it, there is every reason to believe that some of these futuristic-sounding carotenoids may be partly responsible for the health benefits ascribed to beta-carotene. And, so far, we don't have supplements that incorporate the full spectrum of carotenoids found in foods. Therefore, the best advice to date is to eat heartily of your fruits and vegetables, emphasizing the ones with the brightest colors.

The following chart provides a list of various carotenoids and the foods that contain them. They offer a range of antioxidants and nutrients that support a strong and healthy heart.

| CAROTENOID | FOOD SOURCES |
| --- | --- |
| Alpha-carotene | Pumpkin, carrots, cantaloupe, guava, yellow corn |
| Beta-carotene | Pumpkin, carrots, cantaloupe, sweet potatoes, apricots, spinach, other leafy greens |
| Gamma-carotene | Tomatoes, apricots |
| Beta-cryptoxanthin | Tangerines, papayas, oranges, mangoes, peaches, nectarines |
| Lycopene | Watermelon, tomatoes, guavas, pink grapefruit |
| Lutein and zeaxanthin | Kale, spinach, collards, chicory, beet and mustard greens, sweet red peppers, hot chili peppers, corn |

## Beta-Carotene Supplements

The reality is that very few women eat two to three fruits and four to five vegetables a day, and therefore supplementation is a logical choice. A tablet that includes 6 to 15 mg of beta-carotene mixed with vitamins C and E is reasonable insurance for good health. If you eat a carrot a day (a carrot has about 12 mg of beta-carotene), you may not have to worry, but, confess, how many of you are doing that? Even if you are taking antioxidants in pill form, continue to conscientiously eat as many fruits and vegetables as possible. There are other unidentified antioxidants and phytochemicals yet to be discovered hiding under the surfaces of these powerful foods.

## COENZYME Q10: NOT SO NEW

Many scientists from around the world have branded the vitaminlike antioxidant compound coenzyme Q10 a miracle nutrient because of its inextricable link to oxygen and ultimately to life itself. Your body cannot survive without coenzyme Q10. Researchers estimate that once the body becomes more than 25 percent deficient, it suffers in any number of ways, ending up with a panoply of diseases ranging from high blood pressure and a lowered immune system to heart failure and cancer. Deficiency is found in 50 to 75 percent of individuals with heart disease.

## What Is This Coenzyme Q-Something?

Coenzyme Q10 was discovered in the 1940s but wasn't isolated or named until 1957, when it was originally called *ubiquinone*, because it is ubiquitous in nature and because it belongs to a class of compounds called *quinones*. CoQ10, as we now know it, is found in a variety of foods: notably, beef (especially the heart), chicken, fish (primarily salmon, sardines, and mackerel), eggs, nuts (peanuts are especially good), vegetable oils (the highest amount is found in rapeseed oil), broccoli, spinach, and wheat germ. The body also manufacturers CoQ10 from the raw materials mentioned and with the help of specific vitamins like vitamins B-2, B-3, B-6, C, folic acid, and pantothenic acid. Because it is so abundant in nature, one would not suspect people would have deficiencies, but they do occur for a number of reasons. Genetic error or an acquired defect in CoQ10 synthesis is one of these. Or we simply may not be ingesting the foods that have either adequate CoQ10 or the cofactors needed to produce it. And as is true for most nutrients, with age we are less likely to efficiently absorb CoQ10.

## What Does CoQ10 Do?

At the most basic level, coenzyme Q10 helps to create energy within the heart of a cell. It is an essential component of the mitochondria, which is known as the powerhouse of the cell, and its primary job is to protect the cell from oxidative stress. CoQ10 is instrumental in the synthesis of the basic energy molecule within the cell, *adenosine triphosphate* (ATP). Without coenzyme Q10, ATP fails, energy fails, and production fails. Many health educators have called CoQ10 the spark that ignites the mitochondrial engine. In its absence, the body may "short-circuit," letting free radicals loose into the mitochondria. Eventually, the energy dissipates and the cell ultimately fails altogether.

Coenzyme Q10 rescues tissues in need by regulating the flow of oxygen into the cells. It can improve any organ or tissue that is damaged by oxidative stress, and it has been specifically useful in reenergizing heart cells and rejuvenating weakened heart muscles so that they pump blood more efficiently throughout the body. Studies from both the United States and Japan show that supplemental CoQ10 can lower the blood pressure of high-risk patients without additional medication. Many conditions associated with heart disease—heart failure, angina, hypertension, mitral valve prolapse, enlarged heart, and ischemic heart disease—show marked improvement with CoQ10.

## An International Body of Research

Fifty to sixty major investigative studies in the past decade have clearly documented a variety of cardiac-related conditions that are helped with supplemental CoQ10. Scientists at several international conferences have attested to the value of this relatively unknown antioxidant in fighting cardiovascular disease. In Japan it has been used for three decades to treat congestive heart failure, and it is widely prescribed throughout Asia and Western Europe. Yet, in the United States, most doctors remain uninformed about its potential healing qualities.

Research from around the world has confirmed the fact that CoQ10 reduces major and minor symptoms of heart disease. Extensive Japanese research has shown that about 70 percent of heart patients are helped with supplemental CoQ10. An Italian study involving 2,664 patients with heart failure showed that after three months of taking an average of 100 mg of CoQ10, there were improvements in the classic signs and symptoms of congestive heart failure: less edema, relaxed breathing, normal coloring, fewer heart palpitations, and better sleeping patterns.

The United States isn't totally absent from the medical literature when it comes to CoQ10. The research that has appeared in American journals has been done primarily under the supervision of Dr. Karl Folkers, director of the Institute for Biomedical Research at the University of Texas. Dr. Folkers is considered one of the foremost pioneers in the field for his work on CoQ10 in the United States, Japan, and Europe. In one of his many studies on patients with congestive heart failure, he found that three-fourths of the patients taking CoQ10 survived for three years, while only one-fourth lasted that long with conventional therapy. The researchers boldly suggest that heart disease can be a direct result of CoQ10 deficiency.

## Dosage and Safety

Board-certified cardiologists have been utilizing CoQ10 for years to treat people who have major heart conditions or are at risk for heart disease. Stephen Sinatra, M.D., has been treating patients for twenty years at the New England Heart Center in Manchester, Connecticut, and he has found that it works more than 70 percent of the time. He adds that some patients taking CoQ10 cut their dosage of medications in half after a few months.

Before I give you dosage information, I want to make it clear that I am not a doctor, nor do I prescribe nutrients therapeutically. I am providing information alone. If you have a heart condition, please do not stop taking your medication to try CoQ10 or any other nutritional remedy. Talk to your doctor first and work together with him or her. You may want to use CoQ10 as an adjunct to your standard treatment, but do not replace your treatment without first discussing it with your doctor.

Dr. Sinatra suggests a dosage range between 90 mg and 180 mg for patients with angina, cardiac arrhythmia, or hypertension, and for those who have undergone angioplasty. He ups the dosage to 180 mg to 360 mg for people with more severe problems of coronary heart failure or cardiomyopathy. To protect your heart, a safe amount falls between 30 mg and 60 mg a day. You do not need to check with your doctor for this "insurance" support, as long as you don't use it to replace your regular treatment. This is a very safe compound. No toxicity has been reported in the literature, even at levels considerably higher than the ones recommended.

Because CoQ10 is a fat-soluble nutrient, it is best taken with meals. So divide your dosage into 10-mg to 20-mg portions. CoQ10 comes in both a dry form and a softgel oil-based preparation. The latter is preferred, because it enhances bioavailability throughout the body.

## CoQ10 Holds Promise for the Future

The ubiquitous quinone is a versatile nutrient and might be useful for other conditions as well as for heart disease. It has been shown to protect against tissue inflammation, such as that found in periodontal disease; it bolsters the immune system; it thwarts the damaging effects of aging; it may be helpful in weight loss; and it is currently being studied as a treatment for breast cancer, Huntington's disease, Parkinson's disease, and multiple sclerosis.

## ALPHA LIPOIC ACID: A RISING STAR

*Alpha lipoic acid* assumes the title of Universal Antioxidant because of its unique ability to rejuvenate worn-out antioxidants like vitamins E and C and glutathione. Replenished, these critical nutrients continue their job of protecting LDL cholesterol from oxidation. Usually the body makes an adequate supply of alpha lipoic acid, but under certain circumstances deficiencies could occur, in which case, supplementation might be useful. The primary source is red meat, and since many of us have taken to eating more conservative amounts of animal products, we fall short. Levels also decline with age.

Research shows that this vitaminlike nutrient may be especially helpful in combating diabetes, a significant risk factor for heart disease. It improves sugar metabolism and sensitivity to insulin. Excess blood sugars damage proteins, blood vessels, connective tissue, and myelin surrounding the nerve cells. By reducing the effects of glycation, alpha lipoic acid may lower the risk of heart disease and other complications of diabetes. In Germany it is approved for the treatment of diabetic neuropathy (nerve damage). By improving blood flow to peripheral nerves, it actually stimulates the regeneration of new nerve fibers.

## PYCNOGENOL: NEW ON THE SCENE

*Pycnogenol* is probably a new word in your vocabulary. It is a bioflavonoid that works as an antioxidant and specifically protects vitamin C from being oxidized as it is absorbed. It strengthens the circulatory system by reducing free-radical damage and inflammation at the cell site. Pycnogenol protects blood platelets from clumping and forming clots and keeps them from sticking to the arterial walls.

You can find pycnogenol in fruits (especially grapes and cranberries), vegetables, and beans. Should these selections not find their way to your dinner plate, a recommended protective dosage is 30 mg/day. Supplements are made from the bark of European coastal pine trees or from grape seeds.

# 11

# BOLSTERING THE B VITAMINS

We can do no great things—only small things with love.
—MOTHER TERESA

T he time has come for *all* women to seriously evaluate their nutrient intake, especially when it comes to three B vitamins—B-6, B-12, and folic acid. This seemingly insignificant trio may be our best protection against the top three killers—heart disease, stroke, and cancer. Equally important, any woman who is considering having a child should know that folic acid can prevent many of the devastating birth defects known as neural tube defects, such as spina bifida and anencephaly.

## THE OVERWHELMING RESEARCH ON HOMOCYSTEINE

*Homocysteine* is a new term associated with heart disease that may soon be as familiar to us as cholesterol and high blood pressure. Strong and remarkably consistent data have linked this amino acid, which is produced from meat and dairy foods, with hypertension, stroke, and clogged arteries. Of particular interest are the data that show that dangerously elevated homocysteine levels can usually be controlled with three innocuous B vitamins that are found in most multiple vitamin supplements.

Homocysteine is a normal constituent of cells, an amino acid that is formed in the body from the breakdown of another nontoxic amino acid called *methionine*. After a person eats a protein-rich meal of meat, dairy, or beans, methionine is metabolized and homocysteine levels rise in the blood. Responding to unhealthy levels of homocysteine, the body either converts it back to methionine with the help of vitamin B-12 and folic acid or converts it to the nontoxic amino acid cysteine with the help of vitamin B-6 (see illustration).

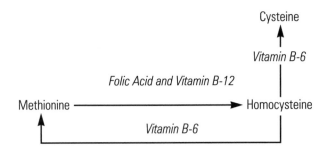

Cysteine

↑

*Vitamin B-6*

*Folic Acid and Vitamin B-12*

Methionine ⟶ Homocysteine

↑

*Vitamin B-6*

If the conversion does not take place because of a genetic defect or vitamin deficiency, elevated homocysteine levels may build up inside the cell and initiate the process that ends with clogged arteries.

The mechanism by which homocysteine specifically damages cells and results in heart disease is still open to conjecture. A leading theory proposed by scientists at the Harvard School of Public Health is that excessive homocysteine levels actually initiate the process itself by damaging the inner lining of the arteries. Another possibility is that once the cells are compromised, homocysteine fuels the fire by fostering the proliferation of unhealthy cells. Homocysteine appears to thicken the blood, increasing the risk not only of heart disease but also of stroke. And finally, it may facilitate the conversion of LDL cholesterol into free radicals, which are known culprits in atherosclerosis.

The risks associated with homocysteine may help explain why estrogen seems to protect women from heart attacks. Until menopause, women run a decidedly lower risk of heart disease than men. Around menopause, when estrogen is waning, homocysteine concentrations rise, and so does our risk for heart disease. There is also speculation that high homocysteine levels might contribute to bone loss in women past menopause. It is an interesting theory and one that obviously needs more research, but the fact that women have higher levels of homocysteine after menopause and concomitantly experience heart disease and osteoporosis may just be more than coincidence.

The history of homocysteine is interesting and demonstrates how slowly the medical process of discovery progresses from the time of theory or recognition through the labyrinth of scientific testing to knowledge within the medical community and finally to public understanding and implementation.

The research began in the late 1960s when Dr. Kilmer McCully (then of Harvard and now of the Veteran's Medical Center in Providence) conjectured that this obscure amino acid might somehow be connected to heart disease. As a novice pathologist at Massachusetts General Hospital, Dr. McCully came across a case of a two-month-old child who had died of homocysteinuria, a rare genetic disease characterized by extremely high levels of homocysteine in the urine and blood. When he examined the boy's arteries, he found they were clogged and hardened, much like those of seniors with advanced vascular disease. But traditional medicine sometimes resists new discoveries, and for some time Dr. McCully's groundbreaking research was either ignored or ridiculed.

It took fourteen years and a massive research project studying three hundred physicians before Dr. McCully was vindicated. The now-classic study, which compared doctors who had suffered a heart attack with another group who showed no indication of a heart condition, found that the men with homocysteine levels above the ninety-fifth percentile were three and a half times more likely to have a heart attack than those in the bottom 90 percent (less than 14.1 nmol/mL).

It is not difficult to build the case against homocysteine in relation to heart disease. In 1991 a team of doctors in Ireland and Great Britain found homocysteine to be an independent risk factor for vascular disease. They found that 28 to 42 percent of patients with vascular diseases affecting the heart, brain, or legs had elevated levels. Their conclusion was that individuals with high blood homocysteine levels were nearly twenty-eight times more likely to develop premature vascular disease than those with normal levels.

Nearly two dozen reports point out that patients with clogged arteries have higher concentrations of homocysteine in their blood than people with healthy arteries. Early in 1995, a Tufts University team led by Dr. Jacob Selhub connected elevated homocysteine to stroke. Nearly 40 percent of the women and men in the study had clogged neck arteries (carotid stenosis), which is known to lead to stroke. After the researchers eliminated other risk factors, they found that the patients with high homocysteine levels were twice as likely to have clogged arteries in their neck as those with normal levels.

Convincing research keeps on flooding in. In June 1997, a report from the Adelaide Hospital in Dublin, Ireland, published in the *Journal of the American Medical Association*, announced that a study of fifteen hundred women and men in nineteen European medical centers found that those who ranked in the top 20 percent for homocysteine levels doubled their risk for heart disease. On the other hand, people in the study who were supplementing with folacin, B-6, and B-12 curtailed their risk substantially. A Dutch study reported in *Arteriosclerosis, Thrombosis, and Vascular Biology* found that every 10 percent rise in homocysteine levels brought a corresponding increase in heart disease risk. A *New England Journal of Medicine* article in July 1997 uncovered more than seventy-five clinical and population studies that demonstrated a relation between total homocysteine level and coronary artery disease, peripheral artery disease, stroke, or venous thrombosis.

## THREE B'S TO THE RESCUE

Homocysteine overload is easily remedied with adequate amounts of the B vitamins—folic acid, B-6, and B-12. Wouldn't you expect that all this research would trigger a nationwide alert and family doctors and cardiologists would be handing out B vitamins like they do sample drugs? Nope—we're told to wait for more proof. Meanwhile, thousands of women and men are dying from a disease that could possibly be stopped with a mere multivitamin pill that is not harmful and costs pennies a day.

### Folic Acid

Folic acid, folacin, or folate (they are all used interchangeably), appears to be the principal B vitamin that regulates homocysteine levels and prevents birth defects. It is generally accepted that it takes 400 mcg of folic acid to lower homocysteine levels and to prevent neural tube defects. Ironically, the RDA once was set at 400 mcg, but in 1989 the National Academy of Sciences cut it in half because it was not deemed practical for most people to get this much from their diet. What were they thinking? Do we lower our standards to make people feel less guilty about not eating better? Or do we let them know that if they can't get what they need from their diet, they should supplement? Guess where I stand on this issue. I can't help but wonder where

### Folate Sources

| FOOD | MICROGRAMS OF FOLATE |
|------|----------------------|
| Product 19 cereal (1 cup) | 400 |
| Total cereal (1/2 cup) | 400 |
| Brewer's yeast (1 tbsp.) | 310 |
| Liver, cooked (3 oz.) | 185 |
| Lentils, cooked (1/2 cup) | 180 |
| Oatmeal, fortified (3/4 cup) | 150 |
| Pinto beans, cooked (1/2 cup) | 145 |
| Sunflower seeds (1/2 cup) | 136 |
| Avocado, medium | 113 |
| Orange juice (1 cup) | 110 |
| Spinach, cooked (1/2 cup) | 102 |
| Asparagus (4 spears) | 88 |
| Romaine lettuce (1 cup) | 75 |
| Peas, broccoli or Brussels sprouts (1/2 cup) | 50 |
| Orange, medium | 40 |
| Banana, medium | 22 |

else in life, politics, and religion we have lowered the bar to make life easier and what that will do to the health of our bodies and souls.

The same question keeps cropping up: Should we try to get as much of our vitamins as we can from food, or just go ahead and supplement? Usually I would go with the first choice, but in the case of folic acid, I would choose to supplement. One study I found showed that we are better off with a supplement or fortified food than with nonfortified folate-rich foods. Geraldine Cuskelly from the University of Ulster in Northern Ireland assembled sixty-two women and provided them with different types of folic acid: some were given regular folate-rich foods, some fortified-rich folate foods, and others supplements. Following standard procedure, she matched them with women who ate what they would normally eat and took no supplements. After three months, blood levels of folate increased significantly only in the women who got the folic acid supplement or the fortified foods. It appears that folate is not absorbed well from foods, so if you go that route, you need to compensate for poor absorption and eat more than the chart suggests. Take a look. Are you getting 400 mcg from regular food or folate fortified foods?

Many health advocates are screaming for revision of the RDA as it applies to folic acid, especially for women of childbearing age and older adults, who do not absorb nutrients as efficiently as they did when they were younger. Others who may be at risk for folic acid deficiency include adolescents, alcoholics, those infected with HIV, and AIDS patients. In a study from Tufts University, the women who consumed one and a half times the RDA or 270 mcg for folate still had relatively high homocysteine levels. Those taking in only about 400 mcg daily of folate had the lowest concentrations of homocysteine in their blood.

In January 1998, Americans' folate levels got a boost when a U.S. Food and Drug Administration mandate for folate fortification took effect. The B vitamin is now added to most enriched breads, flours, pastas, rice, and grain products. The rule was enacted to ensure that women of childbearing age will be protected from having a child with birth defects. I think this is an excellent decision in light of a March of Dimes survey of more than two thousand women that found only 15 percent of the women knew that folic acid was instrumental in preventing birth defects. Half had never even heard of folic acid before—a sad commentary on how slowly vital information filters down to the public for application. Folate fortification may ultimately help fight a deadly disease that affects a large segment of the population—heart disease. One prominent researcher estimated that such increased consumption may save fifty thousand lives per year in the United States.

If you are eating fortified cereals and breads regularly, you may not require additional supplementation with folic acid. While it is unlikely that you can overdose on the supplement in cereal and bread, there is a potential of getting too much if you are taking more than 400 mcg a day, which is a common dosage for a multitablet. There is risk associated with exceeding 1,000 mcg a day of folic acid for a length of time: it can mask a type of anemia sometimes seen in people with a B-12 deficiency.

## Vitamin B-12

Vitamin B-12, or cobalamin, works together with the team of B's to metabolize homocysteine levels. Older adults, the ones who are especially at risk for heart disease, typically have lower B-12 levels. One reason this may occur is because they simply don't eat enough B-12-rich foods—meat, fish, poultry, eggs, and dairy products. Another possibility is that they produce too little stomach acid

### Food Sources for Vitamin B-12

| FOOD | VITAMIN B-12 (MICROGRAMS) |
|---|---|
| Oysters (3½ oz.) | 18.0 |
| Liver (6 oz.) | 13.6 |
| Trout (6 oz.) | 7.2 |
| Beef (6 oz.) | 4.4 |
| Crab (6 oz.) | 3.6 |
| Tuna (½ cup) | 1.8 |
| Halibut (6 oz.) | 1.6 |
| Nonfat milk (1 cup) | 1.0 |
| Yogurt (1 cup) | 1.0 |
| Egg (1) | 0.6 |
| Cheddar cheese (1 oz.) | 0.2 |

to extract the vitamin from food proteins. Finally, they may be low in a substance called the intrinsic factor, which is vital to B-12 absorption. Let's face it—as we age, we don't fully benefit from the food we eat. Body processes slow down and nutritional deficiencies are much more prevalent.

Other groups of individuals at risk for B-12 deficiency include pregnant women, strict vegetarians (those who eat no meat, fish, eggs, or dairy products), long-term antacid users, individuals with Crohn's disease or chronic pancreatic insufficiency, those with a genetic inability to metabolize B-12, individuals infected with the HIV virus, and AIDS patients. Most multivitamins contain between 20 and 50 mcg of vitamin B-12, which is generally adequate. Disease conditions may require larger doses, and you and your doctor may decide that vitamin B-12 should be administered through intramuscular injections rather than as an oral supplement.

Textbooks list pernicious anemia as the classic result of long-term vitamin B-12 deficiency. However, not everyone with a deficiency of B-12 ends up with anemia, because it takes decades to deplete the body's stores. It is still a good idea to be cognizant of the potential signs, because we are all different and some may use up their limit earlier than others. Symptoms of a B-12 deficiency are an unpleasant feeling, tingling, or burning pain in the hands or feet, numbness below the knees, loss of muscle strength, confusion, memory loss, and dementia.

A bunch of articles have appeared in medical journals calling for food to be fortified with vitamin B-12 along with folic acid. A handful of clinicians believe we are missing the boat by not looking at the whole picture. Balance is important in nature and chemistry, and adding vitamin B-12 to the mix would create the best of both worlds. If you can add folic acid to cereal, why not throw in vitamin B-12 as well? Look for this in the future.

## Vitamin B-6

The final vitamin in this trio is B-6, or pyridoxine, a vitamin that poses a real challenge to most Americans. In a large national survey (NHANES II), it was found that 90 percent of females and 71 percent of males did not meet the study's suggested allowance of 3.0 mg for vitamin B-6. The ability to absorb vitamin B-6 from foods declines almost steadily with age, becoming critically low among the elderly. Other groups at risk for declining levels include teenagers, pregnant women, vegetarians, and heavy drinkers.

The evidence is clear that vitamin B-6 can lower homocysteine levels, but there is another phenomenon regarding B-6 and heart attacks that leaves doctors perplexed. It is known that after a heart attack, patients often have very low blood levels of vitamin B-6, and when provided supplemental B-6, they improve more quickly than patients who are not taking the vitamin. Some doctors suggest that a low measurement of vitamin B-6 following a heart attack can be useful in predicting how quickly a heart patient will recover. The higher the blood levels, the faster the recovery period.

Research on animals and humans links a vitamin B-6 deficiency to a host of problems. Some studies show that diabetes may be aggravated by a B-6 deficiency and that supplemental doses of B-6 may normalize glucose metabolism and reduce the need for insulin.

Other studies suggest that supplemental vitamin B-6 can enhance carbohydrate tolerance during pregnancy, when diabetes poses a special risk. Tracking vitamin B-6 levels by means of a glucose tolerance test prior to pregnancy may signal which women are at risk and avert the dangers of gestational diabetes.

Women who take the oral contraceptive pill may have a greater need for vitamin B-6 than women not on hormones. There is evidence that women on the pill sometimes experience carbohydrate (sugar) intolerance similar to what one finds

### Sources of Vitamin B-6

| FOOD | VITAMIN B-6 (MILLIGRAMS) |
| --- | --- |
| Baked potato (1) | 0.7 |
| Banana (1) | 0.7 |
| Chicken, light meat (3 oz.) | 0.5 |
| Carrot juice (6 oz.) | 0.4 |
| Strawberries (½ cup) | 0.4 |
| Beef (3 oz.) | 0.4 |
| Tuna (3 oz.) | 0.3 |
| Spinach, cooked (½ cup) | 0.2 |
| Corn on the cob (1) | 0.2 |

in diabetes. This situation has been somewhat corrected by supplemental vitamin B-6 in levels as low as 5 mg per day.

Vitamin B-6 is required for the proper functioning of more than sixty enzyme systems; it is essential for normal protein breakdown and regulation; it plays a pivotal role in the multiplication of all cells and the production of red blood cells, as well as the cells of the immune system. Vitamin B-6 can have a profound effect on a variety of health conditions that affect women. Some of them include premenstrual syndrome (PMS), asthma, carpal tunnel syndrome, diabetes, cancer (possibly breast and bladder), sickle-cell anemia, aging, and dementia.

Vitamin B-6 is safe in moderation—that is, up to 100 mg per day. Doses over 200 mg per day have proven toxic in some individuals. Even though it is water-soluble and excesses are flushed out of the body, high doses have produced neurological disturbances resulting in numbness of the feet, hands, and mouth, and instability in walking. Some women take megadoses for relief of PMS and water retention and end up with frightening symptoms. The damage is usually not permanent, but it is better to maintain doses between 10 and 40 mg per day unless a health professional recommends something different. One more caution: if you are taking levodopa to treat Parkinson's disease, restrict your supplement to less than 5 mg per day. Vitamin B-6 converts the drug into a form that cannot pass the blood/brain barrier, rendering it ineffective.

# NIACIN: A VITAMIN AND A DRUG?

Niacin, or vitamin B-3, a common B vitamin, is by far the oldest and least expensive cholesterol-lowering drug on the market. It has been touted as being as effective in lowering total and LDL cholesterol as any prescription drug available, and its ability to raise HDL levels is unparalleled. In a study of women and men given a sustained-release form of niacin (meaning that it is released into the bloodstream relatively slowly), LDL cholesterol went down by an average of 50 percent. Those taking a fast-action or immediate-release niacin saw their LDL cholesterol drop by only 22 percent. The dosage to achieve this dramatic effect was 3,000 mg of niacin per day. The researchers commented that even at levels as low as 1,500 mg a day, both forms of niacin cut LDL cholesterol appreciably and raised HDL as well. Moreover, these doses produced reduction in blood triglycerides of 40 to 60 percent.

Niacin has passed the second test as an aid to heart disease: it can reduce the rate of recurrent heart attacks in patients who have had atherosclerosis. This evidence comes from a huge study started in 1966 called the Coronary Drug Program. This major collaborative project involved fifty-three research centers throughout the United States and recruited 8,341 patients (all men) who had suffered at least one heart attack. After fifteen years, the men who took niacin experienced an 11 percent reduction in total mortality compared with patients in the four other groups taking various drugs. Remarkably, in a 1986 follow-up, it was determined that the men supplementing with niacin sustained protection nine years after the study ended and even after they had stopped their niacin treatments.

## The Downside of Niacin

Niacin should be taken only under the supervision of a doctor. In moderate to large doses, between 1,500 and 3,000 mg, it can result in hepatitis, peptic ulcers, intestinal bleeding, and kidney and liver failure. In some patients it may elevate blood sugar levels, so it would be a poor choice for diabetics.

The toxicity of niacin, like that of most medications, is dose-related. People who take a dose of about 500 mg of regular niacin experience flushing and a tingling sensation accompanied by red skin rash. This is not harmful, but it is uncomfortable enough to force some people to give it up. When my husband tried it, he turned beet-red in the face and neck and couldn't tolerate the itching under his shirt and tie. Some people also report nausea, headache, and fatigue.

There are several kinds of niacin: nicotinic acid, nicotinamide, and niacinamide. Nicotinic acid is the form that improves your blood cholesterol profile. Nicotinic acid comes in two major forms: regular, also called rapid-release, and sustained release. The preparations that allow the vitamin to enter your bloodstream more slowly are much more pleasant to take; unfortunately, they are also more likely to produce internal side effects, most particularly hepatitis.

# 12

# THE MIGHTY MINERALS

*It's a funny thing about life; if you refuse to accept
anything but the best, you very often get it.*
—SOMERSET MAUGHAM

S pecific minerals are emerging as strong defenders in the fight
to protect our hearts. During the past several years, a credible
body of evidence has grown supporting the idea that maintaining a daily dietary intake of minerals protects against high blood
pressure and therefore coronary vascular disease. Studies of all varieties, observational and interventional, in humans and in extensive
laboratory tests, have found that low levels of calcium, magnesium,
potassium, and phosphorus are partly responsible for salt sensitivity
in some adults.

The most consistent dietary advice for lowering blood pressure
we have heard over the past decade is to reduce salt in our diets or
eliminate it altogether. But a review of several large databases of
observational studies contradicts this long-standing rule. When
adults meet or exceed the recommended daily requirements of calcium, magnesium, and potassium, the intake of a diet high in salt is
*not* associated with elevated blood pressure. According to a top
researcher in this field, David A. McCarron, M.D., "Educating individuals to maintain, on a daily basis, adequate intakes of calcium,
potassium, and magnesium rather than limit their sodium chloride is
a viable health recommendation that individuals can implement to
reduce their risk of sodium-chloride induced hypertension."

# CALCIUM: NOT JUST FOR THE BONES

Our mothers cajoled us as children to drink milk so we would grow up with healthy, strong bones—and they were partly right. The calcium found in milk and other sources does protect our bones from deteriorating as we grow older. For more details about the specifics of calcium and osteoporosis, read my book *Menopause Without Medicine*. What these sage women (along with scientists) did not realize at that time was that this important mineral also preserves our muscles, nerves, colons, and hearts. Did you know that calcium may relieve leg cramps, calm jittery nerves, prevent colon cancer, lower high blood pressure, and possibly reduce blood cholesterol as well?

Studies gathered from around the world strongly suggest that diets adequate in calcium are associated with lower blood pressure readings. While the studies don't agree unanimously, most report that people who eat an ample supply of calcium-rich foods have lower blood pressure and a reduced risk of developing hypertension.

The extensive Nurses' Health Study, which has provided so many clues concerning diet and atherosclerosis, found that inadequate dietary calcium was associated with a 22 percent increase in the risk of hypertension. Women who had been diagnosed with osteoporosis, and were thus suspect for being deficient in calcium, were more than twice as likely to have high blood pressure as women of the same age without osteoporosis. Some researchers found that up to 45 percent of people with hypertension were deficient in calcium and therefore responded positively to calcium-rich foods or supplemental calcium.

A most convincing study published in the *New England Journal of Medicine*, April 17, 1997, acknowledged that individuals with high blood pressure who adopted a diet rich in dairy products, as well as fruits and vegetables, lowered their blood pressure an average of 5.5 points. Those participants who were careful about the produce but left out the dairy had only a 2.8-point reduction. Those who started with the highest blood pressure saw the greatest improvement, with an average drop of 11.4 points (a reduction competitive with that achieved with medication). The authors concluded that if everybody in the United States adopted this healthy diet, our country's incidence of heart disease would fall by 15 percent and of strokes by 27 percent.

Some scientists feel that calcium may be as important as or possibly more important than sodium in regulating blood pressure. Just as some individuals are sensitive to excess salt, others are calcium-sensitive. In fact, these two groups may be one and the same. A review summarizing information from several large observational databases offered indirect evidence that sodium and calcium metabolism are inexorably linked. What the researchers found in analyzing the information was that the people who had high blood pressure and consumed high-salt diets made up the same segment of society that consumed the least amount of dietary calcium, and to a lesser degree magnesium, potassium, and phosphorus. Could salt sensitivity be an indicator of calcium deficiency? Some researchers think so.

Several clinical studies clearly demonstrate that supplemental calcium has a blood pressure–lowering effect. It is generally agreed that a dose between 1 and 2 grams is effective in depressing blood pressure in one-third to one-half of people. In one study, conducted by cardiologist Dr. John Laragh of Cornell University in New York State, 60 percent of hypertensive patients showed a decline in blood pressure with 2 grams of calcium carbonate pills per day. The average drop was from 160/94 to 128/81. In another controlled double-blind study, people were given 1,500 mg of calcium for twelve weeks. The drop in blood pressure, called modest but significant, further supports the blood pressure–lowering effects of supplemental calcium.

People with mild hypertension (diastolic readings around 100) may be able to lower blood pressure by eating foods high in calcium. Granted, it is not easy to consume even the new recommended amounts of 1,000 mg to 1,200 mg per day. Consider the following:

## Can You Eat Your Calcium? (1,000 mg/day)

3 1/2 cups milk

8 cups cottage cheese

5 ounces cheese

5 cups almonds

7 cups broccoli

8 ounces sardines

2 cups tofu

Most people have difficulty eating their quota of calcium, so supplementation is necessary. I caution you to stay within the recommended guidelines unless you are under the care of a health professional. Heavy doses of calcium may initiate a boomerang effect in some individuals and actually raise blood pressure. Your goal is to rectify any gaps that you have in your diet, so stay within the suggested range for your age group. We do know that some hypertensives (usually those with the greatest elevations) respond better than others do, and some do not see any movement in their levels at all. It is worth giving it a three-month trial before starting on drugs that carry unpleasant side effects.

## Establishing Calcium Goals

American women fall a bit short in attaining the minimum goals for calcium in the diet. We average about 565 mg per day, which, according to the new standards, is less than half of what our bodies demand for strong bones and a healthy heart. The National Research Council (NRC) has recently revamped the recommendations for calcium and other minerals based on optimal levels required for good health. In place of the recommended daily allowances (RDAs), we now have the new and improved dietary reference intake (DRIs) for specific nutrients. For calcium, the current standard has been raised to 1,000 mg per day of calcium for women before age fifty and 1,200 mg per day after age fifty. The National Institute of Health ups the target even more, to 1,500 mg for postmenopausal women.

For the first time, the NRC has placed a ceiling on certain nutrients. The upper limit for calcium is 2,500 mg per day. No side effects are known to occur at doses below 2,500 mg of calcium. However, intakes far over this level can result in constipation and nausea and may increase the risk of high blood pressure in certain people. Megadosing over long periods can lead to a rare disorder called hypercalcemia, which means there is more calcium in the

## Calcium Content
## of Selected Foods

| FOOD | CALCIUM (MILLIGRAMS) |
|------|----------------------|

### DAIRY PRODUCTS

Milk (1 cup) . . . . . . . . . . . . . . . . . . . . . . 300

Yogurt (1 cup) . . . . . . . . . . . . . . . . . . . . . 415

Cottage Cheese (1 cup) . . . . . . . . . . . . . 140

Swiss Cheese (1 oz.) . . . . . . . . . . . . . . . 270

Mozzarella (1 oz.) . . . . . . . . . . . . . . . . . . 205

American Cheese (1 oz.) . . . . . . . . . . . . 174

Feta Cheese (1 oz.) . . . . . . . . . . . . . . . . 140

### VEGETABLES

Spinach, cooked (1 cup) . . . . . . . . . . . . . 245

Broccoli, cooked (1 cup) . . . . . . . . . . . . . 200

### FISH

Sardines, canned (3½ oz.) . . . . . . . . . . . 240

Salmon, canned (3½ oz.) . . . . . . . . . . . . 240

Crab (1 cup) . . . . . . . . . . . . . . . . . . . . . . 140

Oysters (1 cup) . . . . . . . . . . . . . . . . . . . . 110

### SOY

Tofu, firm (1 cup) . . . . . . . . . . . . . . . . . . 515

Tofu, regular (1 cup) . . . . . . . . . . . . . . . . 260

blood than can be deposited in the bones. Since the excess cannot stay in the blood, it is deposited in the kidneys and soft tissues. In extreme cases, an overdose of calcium over time can result in kidney failure and vision problems.

Older studies cite kidney stones as a serious result of too much calcium. This is no longer considered an issue. A study in 1993 of over forty thousand men found that the higher their calcium intake, the fewer kidney stones they developed. Another myth shattered.

## Food Sources of Calcium

The most concentrated sources of dietary calcium are dairy products. However, not everyone can obtain calcium from dairy products, because some people have lactose intolerance or sensitivities to other milk proteins. Some individuals are allergic to milk, some are genetically predisposed to have adverse reactions to it, and others simply dislike it. Fortunately, there are ways to get natural dietary calcium without relying on dairy products. Fish such as canned sardines, mackerel, and salmon have good amounts of calcium, as do tofu and vegetables such as broccoli and spinach. Examine the list above to see how much calcium you get from your favorite food sources.

## How Much Calcium Do You Absorb?

If you feel relatively comfortable that you are obtaining your daily allotment for calcium from food, you may want to reconsider after you factor in your absorption rate. Our bodies do not utilize 100 percent of the calcium taken in via our diet; all you can really expect to utilize is between 20 and 30 percent. The actual percentage depends on your individual body requirement, diet, lifestyle factors, and supporting nutrients. Look over the following lists, and add or subtract as you check off depleters and enhancers of calcium uptake.

## Depleters of Calcium

Smoking

Alcohol (two or more drinks a day)

High-sugar and high-fat diet

High salt intake

High-protein diet

Little sunlight

Low activity (less than four hours per day on feet)

Drugs (steroids and thyroid meds, Cholestyramine, Furosemide, Tetracycline)

## Nutrients Involved in Calcium Absorption

Magnesium ($\frac{1}{2}$ calcium total)

Vitamin C (200–1,000 mg)

Vitamin D (400–600 IU)

Zinc (15–30 mg)

Boron (3 mg)

Phosphorus (700–1,200 mg)

Potassium (4,000 mg)

### Supplemental Sources

The array of calcium supplements on the market can drive a consumer right out of the store, empty-handed and dizzy. There is calcium carbonate, chloride, citrate, lactate, gluconate, phosphate, and micronized calcium. It can be partnered with magnesium, zinc, vitamin C, and a variety of individual nutrients. Labels advertise "no sugar," "no starch," "no additives," "free of milk," "yeast-free," "natural," "physician-recommended"—any number of claims that only confuse an already frustrated shopper.

Let's see if I can help make your choice somewhat easier. Calcium carbonate is by far the most popular source, as well as the most concentrated and cheapest form. Not only is it included in up to 90 percent of the supplements, it is also the main ingredient in antacids such as Tums and Rolaids. Most carbonates are derived from ground limestone (specified on labels simply as "calcium carbonate"), or ground oyster shell. Unless calcium carbonate from oyster shell is purified, it may contain heavy metal contaminants such as lead, and is not recommended. Also because of the possibility of lead contamination, bone meal is another popular supplement that should be avoided. Calcium phosphate, like calcium carbonate, is a highly concentrated formulation, but it is difficult for the body to break down and therefore should be avoided. Calcium gluconate and calcium lactate are more soluble but are less concentrated, which means you will require more tablets to get your daily dosage.

Calcium citrate is one of the best-absorbed forms of supplemental calcium and, unlike most of the others, it is utilized by the body whether it is taken with meals or not. To further ensure bioavailability, some companies are combining calcium citrate with malate, which you might notice listed on the label. Absorption of calcium, along with other nutrients, decreases with age, and calcium citrate is the preferred supplement for the older woman. It generally takes two to three tablets to total the 1,200 mg daily requirement. Calcium chelates and micronized versions also work well.

Absorption varies considerably from supplement to supplement, and you can't tell by how you feel if your body is breaking it down. But there is a way you can actually test your supplement at home to see if it can dissolve in your stomach. Put the tablet in a small cup of vinegar and wait for it to dissolve. If the calcium doesn't completely disintegrate in half an hour, throw it out. Your stomach acid is not going to break it down either.

Calcium is best taken in divided doses with food, because the body doesn't absorb large amounts as efficiently as small ones. This is true of food as well as supplements. If your calcium is carbonate, splitting the dosage over two to three meals cuts down on the possibility of constipation, a problem for some people who choose this formulation.

People who have conditions that cause high concentrations of calcium in the blood, such as an overactive parathyroid gland or cancer, should avoid calcium supplements.

# MARVELOUS MAGNESIUM

Magnesium is frequently overlooked as essential to heart function, even though magnesium deficiency shows up consistently in patients suffering from atherosclerosis, angina, congestive heart failure, stroke, cardiac arrhythmias, heart attack, and hypertension. An electrolyte, magnesium regulates the balance of calcium and sodium in the cells, particularly in the heart and blood vessels. Adequate amounts help to keep blood vessels elastic and relaxed and ensure that the heart beats smoothly and regularly.

Magnesium is not a minor mineral; it is a major cofactor in over three hundred enzymatic reactions in the body, including the metabolisation of glucose, conversion of carbohydrates, protein, and fats to energy, manufacture of proteins, synthesis of the genetic material within each cell, electrical stability of cells, maintenance of membrane integrity, muscle contraction, nerve conduction, and regulation of vascular tone.

## Relationship to Calcium

Magnesium works in tandem with calcium. Together, they regulate the contraction and relaxation of blood vessels. Too much of one or too little of the other can upset the balance and lead to a number of heart-related problems. If there is much more calcium than magnesium in the blood, the arteries might constrict more than they relax. Prolonged constriction of the coronary arteries reduces the blood and oxygen supply to the heart, resulting in hypertension and possibly heart attack.

Magnesium functions as the gatekeeper for calcium, potassium, and sodium. If magnesium is low in the cells and calcium levels are high, calcium floods the cells, making them more susceptible to muscle spasm. A heart attack may be triggered when the coronary arteries fail to provide adequate oxygen to the heart because of involuntary contractions in the smooth muscles of the artery wall. Inadequate magnesium may predispose individuals to potentially fatal disruptions of normal cardiac rhythm, *cardiac dysrhythmia.*

Clinicians have successfully treated cardiac dysrhythmias with magnesium. Recent studies have indicated that people who have experienced an acute heart attack have a much better chance for survival if given magnesium intravenously immediately after the attack. Sometimes blood levels of magnesium appear normal even when the cells are undeniably deficient, which has been demonstrated by researchers who report successful treatment with magnesium of heart dysrhythmias in patients taking diuretics. If your serum levels for magnesium test below normal, then it is highly probable that the magnesium levels in your heart are below normal, too.

## Relationship to Cardiovascular Disease

Compelling evidence ties sublevels of magnesium to cardiovascular problems such as ischemic heart disease, hypertension, stroke, irregular heartbeat, and angina, or chest pain. Early population studies noted a higher incidence of sudden death from heart attack in areas where people consume soft water. Conversely, in areas where people drink hard water, there exist lower rates of heart disease, stroke, and high blood pressure. Hard water contains both calcium and magnesium; however, it is the magnesium that appears to be the more important of the two in protecting against ischemic heart disease, the medical term referring to reduced blood flow to the heart.

Several studies by Dr. Lawrence Resnick, a cardiologist from Cornell University in New York, show that people with high blood pressure characteristically test low for magnesium, and that raising cell levels of magnesium often results in a drop in blood pressure. Most individuals taking diuretics to lower their blood pressure see improvements when they increase their levels of magnesium, since the medication depletes magnesium and other minerals. But please don't stop your medication on your own. You must talk this over with your doctor and together decide on your course of action.

Magnesium may reduce the pain and cramping in the legs called *intermittent claudication*, a condition caused by reduced blood flow to the lower limbs. Magnesium levels are generally low in the muscles of patients with this disorder, and supplementation has been shown to effectively alleviate their discomfort, making walking easier and more enjoyable.

## Who Might Be Deficient in Magnesium?

Magnesium affects all tissues, especially those of the heart, nerves, and kidneys. Symptoms of magnesium insufficiency run the gamut from very minor and subtle signs to dangerous disease states. Consider the following list for signs of deficiency. Having one or two does not necessarily indicate a problem, but if several of these are true for you, you might have a deficiency.

## Possible Signs of Magnesium Deficiency

Muscle twitching

Muscle spasm

Muscle weakness

Myoclonic jerks (often during sleep)

Restless legs syndrome

Lack of coordination

Growth failure

Loss of appetite

Nausea

Stomach upset

Swollen gums

Loss of hair

Depression

Confusion

Personality changes

Magnesium deficiency can result from inadequate amounts of magnesium in the diet, excessive vomiting or diarrhea, long-term use of diuretics, diabetes, alcohol abuse, excessive caffeine use, protein malnutrition, chronic stress, excessive exercise, too much calcium, and kidney disease. Over many years without this singular mineral, major, devastating health problems can arise, lowering our quality of life and sometimes leading to premature death.

## Health Conditions Linked to a Lack of Magnesium

Hypertension

High blood cholesterol

Cardiac dysrhythmia

Ischemic heart disease

Congestive heart failure

Diabetes (Type 2)

Depression

Migraines

Premenstrual syndrome (PMS)

Kidney stones

### Supplemental Magnesium

Most American women take in approximately half of the magnesium they need on a daily basis. The recommended supplemental dosage to prevent deficiency is in the range of 200 to 500 mg per day, depending on how much you get in your diet. Most women average 200 mg per day, but estimate for yourself. How do you register on the magnesium scale? Magnesium is considered safe up to 6,000 mg, but I don't recommend anywhere near this dosage unless a physician is treating you. High doses can be harmful, especially to individuals with kidney problems and with certain heart irregularities. An unusually high dose can also upset the balance of other nutrients.

Magnesium supplements are poorly absorbed and can cause diarrhea in sensitive people. For this reason, the favored source is magnesium aspartate. It appears to be better absorbed than the more popular magnesium oxide and also is easier on the gastrointestinal tract. Magnesium is best taken in combination with calcium in a 2:1 ration, 2 parts calcium to 1 part magnesium. If your calcium intake is 1,000 mg, then 500 mg of magnesium is an appropriate balance. Before you buy separate calcium and magnesium supplements, check to see how much is included in your daily multi-vitamin, so you don't run the risk of taking more than you need.

## POWERFUL POTASSIUM

Potassium acts as an electrolyte in the body, which means it actually carries a tiny electrical charge that regulates muscle functioning, including that of the heart. The third most abundant element in the body, potassium helps to maintain the heart's electrical impulses and is vital in the regulation of heart rhythm. A deficiency or an imbalance in potassium can shut down the heart in a beat.

### Food Sources of Magnesium

| FOOD | MAGNESIUM (MILLIGRAMS) |
|---|---|
| Lentils, cooked (½ cup) | 134 |
| Split peas, cooked (½ cup) | 134 |
| Tofu (½ cup) | 130 |
| Peanuts (¼ cup) | 63 |
| Banana (1) | 58 |
| Peanut butter (2 tbsp.) | 56 |
| Avocado (½) | 56 |
| Chicken (6 oz.) | 50 |
| Spinach, cooked (½ cup) | 48 |
| Beef and pork (6 oz.) | 40 |
| Milk, low-fat (1 cup) | 40 |
| Wheat germ (2 tbsp.) | 40 |
| Haddock, baked (6 oz.) | 40 |
| Oysters (6) | 27 |
| Whole-wheat bread (1 slice) | 19 |
| White bread (1 slice) | 5 |

### Potassium/Sodium and Hypertension

Potassium and sodium play antagonistic roles in the body, specifically in the regulation of blood pressure. Sodium is highly concentrated in the plasma and fluids that surround the body's cells, called the extracellular spaces, while potassium is more comfortable living inside the cells. We upset the balance of the two minerals when we flood our bodies with sodium and curb our dietary potassium. Excessive sodium chloride coupled with insufficient potassium induces an overload in fluid volume and an impairment of the blood pressure–regulating mechanism. The result: high blood pressure.

High dietary sodium raises blood pressure, while high dietary potassium brings it down. We tend to focus only on the excessive use of salt in our daily diets, when too low an intake of potassium may be as important as sodium in creating hypertension. People who eat plenty of foods rich in potassium appear to be protected from hypertension and stroke-related deaths. Moreover, increasing potassium intake, through either diet or supplementation, can be helpful in treating existing high blood pressure.

As we have progressed from a hunting-gathering lifestyle to our modern industrial society, we have witnessed a reverse in the sodium/potassium ratio in our diets and, subsequently, runaway blood pressure levels. When we look at cultures that have no processed, salt-laden products and eat heartily of fresh fruits and vegetables, we rarely find elevated blood pressures.

In our attempt to normalize blood pressure levels, we have focused primarily on restricting salt in the diet. Even though this is a good idea for many reasons, it is not the only course of action and possibly not even the best way to gain control over raised blood pressure levels. When populations within industrialized societies are compared, the link between salt intake and high blood pressure is not as strong; rather, the correlation between potassium intake and hypertension appears more significant.

Many population studies demonstrate a definitive potassium–blood pressure connection. Vegetarians generally have lower blood pressures than meat eaters. This relationship was examined in two groups of adults living in Israel in the 1980s. After noting that only 2 percent of the vegetarians had hypertension compared with 26 percent of the nonvegetarian group, the researchers examined the contributing factors to determine the primary differences. Of all the data considered, including family history for hypertension, obesity, smoking, coffee consumption, and sodium and potassium intake, only potassium consumption was found to be significant. The investigators concluded that the most protective antihypertensive factor in the vegetarian diet was the presence of higher amounts of potassium.

Independent studies from the United States, England, Scotland, Japan, China, Belgium, and Israel have collectively agreed that high intake of dietary potassium is associated with lower blood pressure readings. A monumental international effort called the INTERSALT Study has been tracking the blood pressures of over ten thousand women and men in thirty-two countries around the world to determine possible factors related to a rise in blood pressure. Researchers found that even after considering body mass index, dietary sodium, and alcohol consumption, high potassium levels were highly predictive of low blood pressure readings.

If you think that you can pig out on salt and counteract it with potassium pills, think again. Whether supplementing with potassium works is not clear-cut at this time. Just as sodium restriction doesn't work for all individuals with high blood pressure, the outcome of potassium chloride supplementation is likewise mixed. It lowers blood pressure in some and raises blood pressure in others. Apparently, considerable variation exists in individual sensitivity with respect to both sodium chloride and potassium chloride. Some researchers surmise it is the chloride part of the supplement that may be the confounding factor responsible for these confusing results, but as of this date we don't really know for sure.

Balance in Nature and in life is something with which we need to be concerned. How much potassium you ingest in relation to your sodium intake is important to your blood pressure and overall health. The Food and Nutrition Board of the National Academy of Science recommends eating less sodium than potassium. They feel a balanced ratio is 0.6 gm of sodium for every 1.0 gm of potassium. Americans generally reverse the numbers and end up eating twice as much sodium and half the amount of potassium. Reversing the ratio would greatly lower the blood pressures of many high-risk individuals.

The interaction between levels of potassium and sodium as well as other minerals such as calcium and magnesium is very important to cardiovascular health. Too little or too much potassium in the cells can shut down muscle contraction and electrical nerve impulses, resulting in irregular heartbeats, muscle inactivity, and cardiac arrest. Heart failure linked to potassium depletion and electrolyte disturbances can result in sudden death, and can be brought about by fasting, very low calorie diets, or severe diarrhea. Women suffering from anorexia or bulimia are most definitely at high risk.

## Protection Against Stroke

High potassium intake is an independent risk factor for stroke-related death: less potassium raises the risk; more lowers the risk. This was the conclusion of a twelve-year study of residents in an affluent community in southern California. The dietary habits of over eight hundred women and men between the ages of fifty and seventy-nine were carefully scrutinized by dieticians. During the twelve years, twenty-four deaths occurred from stroke. When the subjects' diets were compared, it was found that the stroke victims had significantly lower potassium intakes than the survivors. It was noteworthy that the results were independent of blood pressure, obesity, cholesterol level, cigarette smoking, alcohol, blood sugar, and also levels of the other minerals. The most significant finding was that even one serving of fresh fruits or vegetables (high-potassium foods) conferred a 40 percent reduction in risk.

## How Much Potassium Is Too Much?

There is no RDA for potassium. The Food and Nutrition Board of the National Academy of Sciences suggests that people consume at least 2,000 mg of potassium each day and adds that it is safe to consume three times that amount. The upper limit has been set at 18,000 mg per day. Over this amount, potassium spills into the blood and can cause alterations in fluid balance and disturbances in heart and kidney function. Unintentionally, some people overcompensate and totally eliminate salt, replacing it with potassium substitutes. Do not overuse salt substitutes; this can be just as dangerous as dousing your food with salt. Two more caveats: if you are taking potassium-sparing diuretics, don't use potassium salt substitutes, and if you have kidney disease, potassium is out.

Caveat: People taking blood pressure–reducing medications should consult their doctors before using products high in potassium. Some diuretics force the body to retain potassium, and too much can cause heartbeat irregularities. The same advice applies to anyone with kidney problems, who may not be able to filter excess potassium from the blood.

The following list will help you determine just how much

additional potassium you are getting by using potassium as a substitute for salt.

## Potassium Deficiency: A Greater Problem

Inadequate dietary potassium combined with any number of conditions that block the absorption of potassium or deplete potassium stores results in the more common problem of potassium deficiency. People at high risk for inadequate potassium

## Potassium Replacement in Some Salt Substitutes

| SALT SUBSTITUTE | POTASSIUM IN mEQ* PER TEASPOON |
|---|---|
| Morton's Salt Substitute | 70 |
| No Salt | 68 |
| Adolph's Salt Substitute | 65 |
| Nu-Salt | 55 |
| Morton's Seasoned Salt Substitute | 50 |
| Adolph's Seasoned Salt Substitute | 33 |
| Morton's Lite Salt | 40 |

* mEQ=milliequivalent. A unit used as a measurement for electrolytes; it is the weight in milligrams of an element that combines with or replaces 1 mg of hydrogen.

levels in their bodies include those with chronic diarrhea, chronic vomiting, diabetic acidosis, kidney disease, overuse of certain diuretics (Thiazides, Furosemide, Ethacrynic), overuse of certain laxatives (Senna, Phenolphthalein, Bisacodyl), chronic alcoholism, and chronic magnesium deficiency. Dehydration is a danger; many of these conditions or behaviors lead to loss of body fluids, and a potassium deficiency can blunt a person's desire for water.

## Symptoms of a Potassium Deficiency

Muscle weakness

Slowed growth

Bone fragility

Sterility

Mental apathy and confusion

Kidney damage

High blood pressure

## Food Sources

For the majority of people, the best way to get natural potassium is through food, primarily fruits and vegetables. Your goal is a minimum

| FOOD | POTASSIUM (MILLIGRAMS) |
|------|------------------------|

### FRUITS

| | |
|---|---|
| Dates (1/2 cup) | 575 |
| Banana (1 med.) | 440 |
| Apricots, dried (1/4 cup) | 318 |
| Cantaloupe (1/4 melon) | 341 |
| Peach (1 med.) | 308 |
| Orange (1 med.) | 263 |
| Raisins (1 oz.) | 210 |
| Apple (1 med.) | 182 |
| Strawberries (1/2 cup) | 122 |

### VEGETABLES

| | |
|---|---|
| Potato (1 med.) | 782 |
| Avocado (1/2) | 680 |
| Tomato, raw (1 med.) | 444 |
| Spinach, cooked (1/2 cup) | 292 |
| Carrot, raw (1 med.) | 225 |
| Asparagus (1/2 cup) | 165 |

### DAIRY PRODUCTS

| | |
|---|---|
| Milk (1 cup) | 370 |
| Yogurt (4 oz.) | 220 |

### MEAT, POULTRY, FISH

| | |
|---|---|
| Salmon (6 oz.) | 756 |
| Chicken, light meat (6 oz.) | 700 |
| Cod (6 oz.) | 690 |
| Roast beef (6 oz.) | 448 |
| Tuna (3 oz.) | 225 |

of 2,000 mg each day. Add up the numbers to see how close you come.

## Supplemental Potassium: Yes or No?

Potassium supplements are available, but most require a doctor's prescription and thus are recommended only for someone who is taking diuretics or has a health problem that needs medical supervision. Even though there are some potassium supplements available in doses of 99 mg per tablet, I don't recommend them unless you are one of those high-risk individuals. Even then, it is a much better idea to get your potassium from food. There is no chance of overdosing on bananas and avocados.

## SODIUM AND HYPERTENSION

Salt is necessary for maintaining the fluid balance of cells and blood. There is no doubt that we need it for life. But how much is too much? Some suggest that *no* salt is ideal; others are more lenient and feel that as long as we don't go overboard and upset our potassium balance, there is no problem with eating salt. Our personal salt requirement depends to a great degree on our physiological response to salt. It is clear that in some individuals, excess salt does indeed raise blood pressure, while others can enjoy greater latitude with the shaker. Only by eliminating it from your diet and retesting in a few months can you determine to which group you belong.

Studies of world populations show a direct correlation between diets high in salt and high blood pressure. The Japanese diet, as healthy as it is in some respects, is loaded with salt in the form of soy sauce, miso, and salted fish. A range of 25 to 50 grams of salt (up to 10 teaspoons) per day likely contributes to the high percentage of hypertension in the Japanese population (40 to 60 percent) and their astronomical stroke rate (170 percent above U.S. numbers). Conversely, in what we would call "primitive" cultures that do not have access to salty foods, high blood pressure is virtually nonexistent. For those of you who are thinking it is genetics, not so. When these non–salt eaters move to developed areas and gain an appreciation for salty fast-food items and chips and dip, they too wind up with the same high rates of blood pressure as we who grew up with a penchant for salty foods.

English doctors reporting in the *British Medical Journal* in the early 1990s combined the findings of studies from twenty-four communities around the world. Dietary sodium and blood pressure were evaluated in more than forty-seven thousand people from both industrialized and underdeveloped countries. The results clearly established that dietary salt was directly related to blood pressure; for each 2,400 mg of daily sodium in the diet, blood pressure increased by about 10 points. This striking effect was strongest in people who were hypertensive and in the elderly, both groups already highly vulnerable to heart attacks and strokes.

The evidence is strong that cutting down on salt lowers blood pressure in some individuals. A landmark study conducted at London's Charing Cross Hospital by Dr. Graham MacGregor found that moderately restricting salt intake could lower blood pressure by an average of 6 percent, which is about the same amount one would expect if taking a diuretic or beta blocker.

For some individuals, *salt* is a four-letter word. Experts estimate that up to 20 percent of the population is salt-sensitive, meaning they have a reduced ability to excrete excessive salt, which means that salt triggers elevated blood pressure in them. Such people would benefit greatly from monitoring their salt intake. Unfortunately, there is no test for this hyperreaction to salt other than trial and error. It is not a difficult test; all you need do is restrict your salt for two to three months and retest your blood pressure. If it goes down, you are salt-sensitive; if it doesn't, you probably are not.

## How Much Salt Is Too Much?

How much you can get away with depends on whether or not you already have high blood pressure. Some major studies have indicated that when salt is cut in half from 4,000 mg per day to 2,000 mg, a significant reduction in blood pressure follows. Considering that the average diet in the United States includes 2 to 3 teaspoons of salt each day, those with hypertension will be looking at dramatic changes in their eating patterns.

There is no RDA for salt; instead of establishing a minimum amount required for good health, national authorities now offer maximum targets for sodium intake. The National Academy of Sciences and several other large interest groups propose that the ceiling not exceed 2,000 mg (1 teaspoon of salt contains 2,000 mg sodium). Some people find this relatively easy to follow once they become aware of their salting habits; others see it as a monumental challenge.

Salt is an acquired taste, but once you get accustomed to it, food tastes bland without it. I recommend changing habits slowly. You are more likely to succeed in tapering off than if you go cold turkey and totally ban salt from your diet. Start by lightening up on the shaker so you get used to the taste. Then slowly replace salt in your recipes with more inventive spices or salt substitutes. Read labels and note how much salt there is in the products you regularly eat. Be aware of other sources of sodium in processed foods besides salt: sodium nitrite, sodium phosphate, sodium bicarbonate or baking soda, monosodium glutamate or MSG, sodium bisulfite, sodium propionate, and sodium saccharine. Here is a rule of thumb: if a product contains less than 135 mg of sodium per serving, it is considered safe.

About 75 percent of the salt we eat comes from processed foods such as soups, broths, sandwich meats, canned vegetables, frozen foods, hot dogs, smoked poultry, and pizza. Condiments are also killers: go light on catsup, prepared mustards, pickles and olives, tomato sauce, soy sauce, teriyaki sauce, and commercial salad dressings. Chips, pretzels, and popcorn, and the diet sodas we wash them down with, go without saying.

## Salt Alternatives

If you absolutely cannot live without sprinkling something saltlike on your food, there are alternatives on the market that have less sodium than table salt. Researchers at Tufts University have evaluated the amount of sodium and potassium in some of the latest salt substitutes; and equally important, their findings include how they taste.

### Salt Killers

| FOOD | SODIUM (MILLIGRAMS) |
|---|---|
| Pickle (1 large) | 1,428 |
| Soup, freeze-dried (1 pkg.) | 1,350 |
| Soy sauce (1 tbsp.) | 1029 |
| Soup, creamed, canned (1 cup) | 996 |
| Smoked salmon (1 oz.) | 890 |
| Ham, cured (3 oz.) | 860 |
| Cheeseburger (1) | 823 |
| Pepperoni (5 slices) | 560 |
| Roquefort cheese (1 oz.) | 513 |
| Apple pie (1 piece) | 482 |
| Cottage cheese (4 oz.) | 459 |
| Bacon (2 slices) | 440 |
| Total cereal (1 oz.) | 352 |

| PRODUCT | SODIUM (MG) | POTASSIUM (MG) | TASTE TEST |
|---|---|---|---|
| (Values: ¼ tsp.) | | | |
| Regular salt | 590 | 0 | |
| Diamond Crystal | 390 | 0 | Close to salt |
| Morton Lite Salt | 290 | 340 | Bitter to some |
| Cardia | 270 | 180 | Close to salt |
| No Salt | 0 | 659 | Bitter |

## CHROMIUM

Consistently consuming a diet deficient in the trace mineral chromium is associated with blood sugar abnormalities and coronary heart disease. Several studies have noted that patients with advanced heart disease have lower chromium levels in their tissues; heart disease rarely emerges when chromium levels are optimal. Chromium is thought to protect the lining of the arteries from damage, thereby preventing invasion and buildup of cholesterol. Insufficient chromium in the diet raises blood cholesterol, and conversely, augmenting dietary chromium lowers total cholesterol in the blood while raising HDL levels.

## Chromium and Cholesterol

Chromium improves the HDL/LDL ratio by lessening the amount of artery-clogging LDL particles and by raising the number of cholesterol-scavenging HDLs. Studies from the early 1980s showed that chromium reduced LDLs by 17 percent, increased HDLs by 17 to 23 percent, and lowered total cholesterol by 10 to 36 percent. A study a decade later, conducted by Dr. Raymond Press and his colleagues at Mercy Hospital and Medical Center in San Diego, California, used updated, more sophisticated technology and confirmed the cholesterol-lowering effects of chromium picolinate, one of the more bioavailable sources of the mineral. Two groups of patients with poor cholesterol profiles were observed and compared. One group was given supplemental chromium and the other a placebo; then the procedure was reversed. The patients who took chromium first experienced a healthy change in their cholesterol profile and continued to see benefits until they were switched to the placebo. No benefit was apparent with placebo treatment. The group that started with the placebo first saw no change in their cholesterol numbers until they received the chromium, when they too witnessed a significant positive difference. In both groups, once the chromium was discontinued, the health benefits faded with time as chromium levels fell.

Chromium may exert greater benefits when combined with other nutrients than as an independent agent. Dr. Jeffrey Gordon, another researcher from southern California, used a combination of chromium picolinate, niacin (the B vitamin), and dietary changes to achieve a 24 percent reduction in total cholesterol, a 27 percent reduction in LDL-cholesterol, a 43 percent reduction in triglycerides, and an improvement in the HDL/LDL ratio. The sample group was small but the results impressive.

The amount of chromium used to achieve cholesterol-lowering effects ranges between 200 and 600 mcg. Dr. Press used the lower amount in his study, and Dr. John Roeback of the University of

North Carolina found that 600 mcg daily of a high-chromium yeast raised HDL levels by 16 percent. Others clinicians have quoted elevations of HDLs up to 25 percent after supplementing with chromium for two to sixteen weeks.

## Chromium as It Relates to Diabetes and Hypoglycemia

The most studied function of chromium is to regulate the metabolisation of sugar in the blood. Chromium supplements may help to temper both high blood sugar, a condition associated with diabetes, and low blood sugar, the state characteristic of hypoglycemia. This important trace mineral is a component of the *Glucose Tolerance Factor* (GTF), a substance that works intimately with insulin to facilitate the absorption of blood sugar (glucose) into the cells and regulate blood sugar levels. A deficiency of chromium can result in impaired insulin activity, insulin insensitivity, and elevated blood sugar.

While there is no direct evidence that chromium prevents diabetes, there is evidence that it does increase glucose tolerance, and therefore it should be included in a diabetic's dietary program. Poor dietary intake of chromium results in limited availability of GTF and impaired insulin activity, resulting in blood sugar elevation and a diabetes-like condition similar to adult-onset diabetes. Four decades ago, when tests were conducted with rats fed a chromium-deficient diet, it was found they developed the symptoms of diabetes. When they were nourished with chromium, the rats' symptoms quickly vanished.

In 1990, the United States Department of Agriculture (USDA) reported that adequate chromium levels are important in the treatment of Type 2 diabetes or the non-insulin-dependent version. The same researchers who investigated chromium and cholesterol at Mercy Hospital in California also studied the effect of chromium picolinate on Type 2 diabetics. The scientists measured both fasting blood sugar levels and glycosylated hemoglobin levels in adult-onset diabetics. Fasting blood sugar levels are routinely used as a measurement of blood sugar status; however, since both blood sugar and insulin levels can fluctuate appreciably in diabetics, glycosylated hemoglobin provides a better indicator of what is happening to the sugar in the blood over a longer period of time. The researchers found that 200 mcg of chromium in a picolinate form reduced fasting blood sugar levels by 18 percent and glycosylated hemoglobin levels by 10 percent in just six weeks.

If you are diabetic and want to experiment with chromium supplementation, please notify your doctor first and have your blood sugar monitored, because it may alter your serum glucose levels and change your medicinal needs.

A USDA study group has shown that chromium not only aids in lowering high blood sugar but also jump-starts the blood sugar of subjects sensitive to low blood sugar, a condition known as *hypoglycemia*. Rather than the elevated surge of sugar in the blood characteristic of diabetes, hypoglycemia causes a drop in blood sugar levels. Dr. Richard A. Anderson and his research team gave hypoglycemics 200 mcg of supplemental chromium for three months in a double-blind crossover study in which neither patients or doctors knew who was getting the mineral and who the placebo. Chromium supplementation alleviated the hypoglycemic symptoms and significantly raised minimum blood sugar levels, which, according to the researchers, suggests that impaired chromium nutrition and/or metabolisation may be a factor in causing hypoglycemia.

## Chromium and Weight Loss

Several studies have found that chromium picolinate decreases body fat and builds muscle without dieting or increased exercise. One study at a weight-loss clinic in Texas reported that, after seventy-two days, the group taking chromium in a nutritional drink lost an average of 4.2 pounds of fat and gained an average of 1.4 pounds of muscle. Two groups were provided chromium in different dosages. Those taking 400 mcg per day averaged a 27 percent better response than those taking 200 mcg. The groups receiving no chromium in their drinks experienced no change in fat or muscle.

Some doctors claim that chromium deficiency facilitates fat production because without adequate chromium the metabolism gets sluggish. Anything eaten above what the body can use will be quickly stored in the fat tissues—which, by the way, is true whether or not you are chromium deficient. A lack of chromium can cause persistent hunger, uncontrolled cravings, and serious mood swings. When there is insufficient chromium, insulin is inefficient and the blood sugar doesn't get into the brain cells that control appetite and mood. A vicious circle of erratic blood sugar levels sends the most disciplined women hunting for crumbs in the cabinet.

Chromium works to pare fat from the body in two principal ways: it indirectly boosts the metabolism and thus enables the body to burn more calories, and it signals the brain to turn off the hunger mechanism. Chromium helps insulin increase energy production in muscle cells, and together they work to build muscle tissue. The more muscle mass you have, the more calories you burn at rest. Exercise is the best way to build your muscles, but even without exercise, chromium can slightly increase skeletal muscle.

If you lack adequate chromium in your diet, it may make a difference. Chromium supplementation may improve the results you derive from exercise by increasing your muscle mass, but it will not magically melt away pounds. To lose weight, you will still need to reduce caloric intake, and you will have to exercise.

## Chromium Deficiency

There is reasonable evidence that marginal chromium deficiency is common in Americans of all ages. The statistics report that at least 90 percent of all Americans have below-average chromium levels. Dr. Richard Anderson from the USDA found that 100 percent of thirty-two adults tested in one study consumed less than the 50 to 200 mcg recommended by the National Academy of Sciences. Women specifically scored around 25 mcg a day, which is abysmally low when you consider how important it is as a potential contributor to preventing heart disease and blood sugar abnormalities. Deficiency is likely in pregnant women, the aged, people who exercise strenuously, and those who favor highly refined foods over whole grains and lean meats.

As we rely more on highly processed refined foods that are packed with sugar and fat, we are heading for nutritional disaster. Not only do these foods not include chromium, but a high-sugar diet causes the body to use up even more than the miniscule amount received. Unfortunately, even when we choose healthy vegetables, our diet may still suffer, since the soil in which they were grown is not always rich in this vital nutrient.

## Symptoms of Chromium Deficiency

The body provides clues to nutrient deficiencies. Early signs are usually so general that it is difficult to determine whether we have a full-blown deficiency or are just overworked, underfed, or both. Signs that might lead you to consider your chromium status include the following:

> Fatigue
> Difficulty losing weight
> Ease in gaining weight
> Food cravings
> Numb toes and fingers
> Elevated blood sugar
> Mood swings
> Reduced muscle coordination
> Type 2 diabetes
> Heart disease

## Food Sources of Chromium

Chromium is found in small amounts in Brewer's yeast, wheat germ, whole-grain breads and cereals, lean meats, cheese, molasses, thyme, and black pepper. If these are not a regular part of your diet, I suggest a multivitamin and mineral formula that includes at least 200 mcg of chromium.

## Supplemental Chromium

The dietary form of chromium is extremely safe, even in amounts greater than needed for nutritional purposes. Chromium found in nutritional yeasts and chromium picolinate is well received by the body and far superior to inorganic chromium or chromium chloride, which can also be found in supplement form. Take chromium together with the B-complex vitamins found in a high-quality nutritional supplement.

Optimal intake has yet to be decided, but governmental agencies and clinicians generally agree that a range between 50 and 200 mcg is both effective and safe. The need for chromium appears to be related to body size; bigger people require more than smaller people. Consuming sugar, candy, soft drinks, and convenience foods substantially ups the demand, as does strenuous exercise.

Toxicity from supplementation has not been recorded. When overdose does occur, it is generally related to consuming excessive levels of chromium in foods contaminated with chromium. A sign of overdose is a metallic taste in the mouth, diarrhea, and cramping.

# 13

## QUASI-SUPPLEMENTS AND HEALING FOODS AND HERBS

*Nothing in life is to be feared. It is only to be understood.*

—MARIE CURIE

C omplementary medicine is a burgeoning field in health care. Many people are embracing a variety of nontraditional disciplines because they are cheaper and safer than some drugs that have potentially harmful side effects, as well as being as effective. It has been proven repeatedly that specific nutrients, herbs, and spices can play an important role in lowering blood pressure, improving the blood cholesterol profile, and regulating the circulatory system. The list of natural substances that positively affect the heart is growing, and new products with exotic-sounding names are entering the mainstream literature. Some of the foods and herbs have been widely used and studied in other countries and have only recently begun to gain respectability in the United States. This chapter explores some of the old and new remedies that may (or may not) be beneficial for the heart.

### DHEA: QUESTIONABLE

*Dehydroepiandrosterone,* or *DHEA,* is growing in celebrity status. You see it everywhere—crowding the entrances to heath food stores, covering rows of shelves in popular discount stores, crammed in with the vitamins at your local market. Given the claims for what

DHEA can do, it is not difficult to see why this stuff is so hot. Advertisers package it as an antiaging remedy, the latest fountain of youth. It is said to enhance well-being, boost energy, promote weight loss, heighten sexual libido, support cardiovascular health, rev up the immune system, and combat diseases such as AIDS, lupus, Alzheimer's, and some types of cancer. That is quite a reputation to live up to, considering the bulk of the research to date has been conducted in the lab on small, furry animals.

DHEA is not a vitamin or mineral but rather a natural hormone that is produced in the brain, skin, and adrenal glands. It is sometimes referred to as the "mother steroid," because it is the most abundant steroid in the body and because it is used to produce other hormones, including estrogen, progesterone, and testosterone. For reasons that are not clear at this time, our production of DHEA declines as we get older. By age forty-five, we produce only half of the DHEA we produced at age twenty. Many researchers have noted that along with declining levels come a host of diseases, one being cardiovascular disease. Is this coincidence or cause?

The topic at hand is heart disease, so let us look at the data thus far. In a study from the late 1980s, conducted by Dr. Elizabeth Barrett-Connor from the University of California at San Diego, men with high blood levels of DHEA suffered half the incidence of heart disease as those with low levels. Sounds good. Unfortunately, women with high levels of DHEA showed the reverse, an increase in heart disease. Follow-up studies with a larger sample over a longer period of time again connected low levels of the hormone with heart attack incidence for men, but once again, no positive or negative effect was established for women. Preliminary studies suggest that DHEA may help lower blood cholesterol in men, but in women the results are less clear and much less convincing.

It appears at this time that DHEA does not protect women's hearts. That is the bad news. The good news is that a few studies have suggested DHEA may help bolster the immune system. In a study of postmenopausal women, a 50 mg daily dose of DHEA was associated with a significant increase in the activity of natural killer cells associated with preventing the development of tumors. Preliminary research in postmenopausal women has found that DHEA may also protect against obesity and adult-onset diabetes, two risk factors for heart disease. In one of the investigations, the same dosage of 50 mg a day appeared to reduce insulin resistance and lower serum triglyceride levels.

What do we do with this conflicting information? Unless you are working with a doctor who is monitoring your blood levels of DHEA, I would say hold off. There is serious scientific interest in this adrenal hormone, and studies are under way right now, but so far the research is limited and inconclusive and the long-term risks unknown, especially for women.

No one knows yet how DHEA works, when it works, or if the benefits come from the hormone itself or from the sex hormones and other steroids the body converts it into. Side effects from DHEA are not entirely known. Researchers have found that it can have a masculinizing effect on women when taken in doses from 50 to 100 mg. An increase in facial hair and acne has been reported, as has a higher incidence of ovarian cancer in women with high DHEA levels. Since neither the risks nor the benefits have been proven, I recommend that you avoid using DHEA at this point in time. There are so many other proven ways to strengthen the heart. We don't have to try things that are questionable.

## If You Are Already Taking DHEA

Some cardiologists who treat heart disease therapeutically with nutrition are currently using DHEA as one of their tools. Working with a doctor who is monitoring your blood levels, hormone status, and other markers on a regular basis is very different from haphazardly ingesting a potent hormone as if it were a multivitamin pill. Julian Whitaker, M.D., former surgeon and founder of the Whitaker Wellness Institute in Newport Beach, California, stresses that before you even start taking DHEA, it is important to have a blood test for DHEA-sulfate or a saliva hormone test. After taking it for three months, get checked again to make certain your levels aren't too high.

The dose recommended for women is 25 mg per day; any more than this should be taken only under the supervision of a physician. Dr. Stephen Sinatra, cardiologist at the New England Heart Center in Manchester, Connecticut, calls for smaller doses and recommends that premenopausal women over 30 take 5 to 10 mg of DHEA every other day and that postmenopausal women, whether or not they have heart disease, take the same amount unless they have a family history of breast cancer or ovarian cancer, in which case they should not take it at all.

Dr. Whitaker also warns about the purity of the products sold. Don't settle for anything less than 100 percent pure DHEA. Do not take any of the products that claim to be precursors to DHEA, as there is no evidence that they will elevate DHEA in the body. He also recommends that the hormone contain ascorbyl palmitate, a fat-soluble form of vitamin C, to enhance the body's absorption of it.

## L-CARNITINE : FULL OF SURPRISES

*L-carnitine* is an amino acid that transports fatty acids into the mitochondria, the energy center of the cells, where they are burned for energy. Our bodies produce L-carnitine (the biologically active form found in our tissues) naturally as long as there is an adequate supply of two other amino acids, lysine and methionine, both found abundantly in fresh vegetables. Vitamin C, vitamin B-6, and niacin, plus the mineral iron, are also necessary for this reaction to take place. Without any of these ingredients, a deficit could result in a lowered level of fatty acid concentrations in the cells and reduced energy production.

L-carnitine is responsible for keeping the heart and other muscles vital. Fatty acids are the major sources for production of energy in the heart and skeletal muscles, structures that are particularly vulnerable to L-carnitine deficiency. Clinical trials have demonstrated positive effects of L-carnitine supplementation in patients suffering from various forms of cardiovascular disease. It has been reported for some time that supplemental L-carnitine can significantly reduce total blood lipids, lower blood triglycerides, and raise HDL levels. In clinical trials, the positive effects of lowered triglycerides continued as long as L-carnitine was supplied; when it was withdrawn, triglyceride levels rose again.

L-carnitine improves tolerance to exercise for patients with coronary heart disease. When given L-carnitine before an exercise stress test, heart patients experienced more efficient heart function.

L-carnitine allows the heart muscle to utilize its limited oxygen supply more efficiently. It pumps blood with greater ease and fewer beats, and there is less tendency for oxygen deprivation.

Deficiency of L-carnitine can lead to muscle weakness, severe confusion, angina or heart pain, cardiac enlargement, congestive heart failure, and cardiac myopathies, all of which respond to L-carnitine supplementation. Individuals who are particularly at risk include kidney patients on hemodialysis and those with liver failure. Strict vegetarians and pregnant or nursing women may also be at risk.

Claims continue to surface promising that L-carnitine can build muscles, increase physical endurance, bolster energy, and aid in weight loss. At this time, there is no proof that it can accomplish any of these goals if you have normal L-carnitine levels. The story may be different if you are deficient, but the same can be said of almost any nutrient.

The dietary intake of L-carnitine for optimal health has not been established, but a cadre of physicians and nutritionists recommend 500 to 1,000 mg daily as a protective amount, especially if you don't eat any of the following foods: beef, lamb, tofu, tempeh, or avocado. If you decide to supplement, use only the L-carnitine form, not the DL. The L-form has not produced any unpleasant or toxic side effects, even when taken in doses over 1,600 mg for more than a year.

## GARLIC: GOOD FOR WHAT AILS YOU

Garlic (*Allium sativum*) is one of the oldest and most popular herbal medicines, mentioned in ancient Chinese, Greek, Roman, Indian, and Egyptian writings. According to Egyptian papyruses, it was used in over eight hundred potions to cure twenty-two different ailments, from worms to weakness. Throughout history, garlic has found a niche in the medical realm. Louis Pasteur brought garlic to the world's attention in 1858 when he discovered it contained potent antibacterial properties. Albert Schweitzer treated amoebic dysentery with fresh garlic, and it was used in two world wars as an antibiotic to prevent infection in open wounds, saving the lives of thousands of soldiers.

Once thought to keep evil spirits and vampires at bay, the pungent clove has generated current interest based on a growing body of evidence that garlic contains formidable medicinal properties that may protect us from a host of chronic illnesses, including heart disease and cancer. Since 1960, some one thousand research papers have been published on the herb, and many more are in progress.

Some of garlic's most dramatic effects are on the cardiovascular system. It lowers blood cholesterol and triglycerides, reduces the susceptibility of LDL cholesterol to oxidation, and increases the levels of protective HDLs. It lowers blood pressure and reduces the clotting tendency of the blood that often leads to heart attacks and strokes. Researchers who study population groups suspect that garlic consumption may contribute to the especially low incidence of atherosclerosis in countries like Spain and Italy.

## Garlic Lowers Cholesterol Levels

Reports from international journals during the past twenty-five years have suggested that garlic may be effective in decreasing total cholesterol levels by as much as 15 to 20 percent, often accompanied by improvements in HDL/LDL ratios. When Stephen Warshafsky and his colleagues at the New York Medical College in New York carefully reviewed the world literature, they found that eating one-half to one clove of garlic a day decreased total cholesterol levels by about 9 percent. The number seems small, but according to researchers it is by no means insignificant, considering that medications are deemed effective if they reduce blood cholesterol levels by 15 percent.

The studies used a variety of garlic sources—fresh cloves, dried powder pills, garlic in oil, and aged garlic extracts. In a German study, a dried garlic powder, Kwai, was tried in a double-blind test of forty-two women and men with high cholesterol. The supplemental dosage of 900 mg/day produced an average drop of 12 percent in blood cholesterol levels in a four-month period. When scientists from England and Australia combined the results of sixteen studies, they calculated the same average, a 12 percent reduction.

## Garlic Lowers High Blood Pressure

Garlic is widely used in Germany to bring down elevated blood pressure. In a double-blind study using a powdered supplement that was equivalent to two cloves a day, blood pressure went from a high of 171/102 down to 152/89 after ninety days. The placebo group showed no improvement. It is thought that the mechanism at work in tempering blood pressure is a relaxing effect that garlic has on the smooth muscles of the blood vessels.

## A Clove, a Pill, or a Powder?

Garlic contains a variety of vitamins, minerals, and amino acids, and it is a rich source of sulfur-containing compounds that have biological activity. Which one or combination of these imparts the heart-healthy effects is unclear. Some speculate it is *ajoene*, one of the sulfur-containing compounds, which has a potent anticlotting action. Others suggest garlic's most active ingredient is another of the sulfur-rich substances, *allicin*, because of its antibiotic qualities. So far, six compounds in garlic have been identified as having potential cholesterol-lowering tendencies. But most of us don't feel the need to know which specific substance to credit, as long as garlic works.

What works most effectively—fresh or fake? We know for sure that fresh cloves provide health benefits. Many garlic enthusiasts believe that uncooked garlic, chopped or mashed (allicin is released only after garlic is cut) offers the greatest benefits, but reliable sources also say that cooking the garlic doesn't affect it all that much. You can easily add it to salads, pasta, sandwiches, and vegetable dishes just before serving. Or take it straight, the way centenarians Sarah and Elizabeth Delany describe in their wonderful book, *Having Our Say, The Delany Sister's First 100 Years:* "Every morning, after we do our yoga, we take a clove of garlic, chop it up, and swallow it whole."

Garlic is not tolerated well by everyone. Some find that after eating a wonderful Italian dinner, they are socially unacceptable. Bad breath, indigestion, body odor, and gas are common aftereffects.

Garlic in pill form may be better tolerated by some individuals; however, there may be a downside. While it is clear that the herb form is safe, we have no data on the long-term safety of concentrated extracts. High doses may lead to bleeding problems in people taking anticoagulant drugs, including aspirin. Certain substances in garlic appear to exert a blood-thinning effect, so if you are taking a medication that thins your blood, you may be getting a double dose. To be on the safe side, let your doctor know.

Garlic supplements have been enjoying a boom in the market. In 1993, grocery store sales of garlic supplements rose 67 percent, reaching $9.3 million. And each year since then, new products have crowded the shelves. Like other dietary supplements, garlic pills are not characterized as drugs according to government regulators, so they are not scrutinized as long as their manufacturers do not make any health claims on the label. As a result, there is tremendous variation in composition among the various garlic supplements.

So, how do we choose? Powdered pills are made from fresh garlic that has been dried, ground, and compressed. Processed carefully, they contain the same ingredients as the fresh clove, although something is always lost in the manufacturing. The amount of allicin and other ingredients released by the different powder products has been shown to vary as much as eighteenfold. Since manufacturers are not required by the government to post amounts on the label (although some do), comparing is a challenge. The Center for Science in the Public Interest (CSPI) has evaluated popular garlic supplements for their allicin content and also for *S-allyl cysteine* (SAC), another compound in garlic that has been shown to protect against some cancers. Highest on the list for allicin content, surprisingly, was McCormick (Schilling) garlic powder. One-third of a teaspoon provides 5,000 mcg of allicin and costs about a nickel a serving. Ingesting a third of a teaspoon of garlic powder is probably not a reasonable option for most of us, but using it in our cooking is.

Another option is enteric-coated supplements. According to some researchers, this coating keeps the allicin from being released before it reaches your small intestine. Top products listed by CSPI, which include both allicin and SAC, include KAL Beyond Garlic, Garlique, and Garlicin. The best-selling garlic supplement on the market, Kyolic, contains a fair amount of SAC but no allicin.

## ONIONS: THEY DON'T JUST MAKE YOU CRY

Early Egyptian writings hail onions as a tonic for the blood. Modern data confirm that, like garlic, onions counteract the platelet aggregation or clumping seen after eating a high-fat meal, and they also increase fibrinolytic activity. Inhibiting fibrin formation and breaking up and dissolving unwanted and dangerous clots is crucial to preventing heart disease. It might be a good idea to add raw onions to a fatty meal. Don't discard onions, like my kids do; keep them on the hamburger, because they may help to counteract the clot-promoting action of the meat and the mayo.

Crude extracts of onion have been shown to exert antihypertensive as well as cholesterol-lowering effects. In one study, the juice of a single white or yellow onion taken daily raised HDL levels by 30 percent in people with abnormally low HDL readings. Harvard cardiologist Dr. Victor Gurewich tested this folk medicine cure and found that about 70 percent of his patients who added onions to their diet were successful in lowering their blood pressure.

A raw onion or the equivalent in juice can be an important component of a heart-healthy plan. Cooking seems to inhibit the HDL-raising effects, but cooked onions fight heart disease in other ways. Even one-half of an onion may effectively push up your HDLs, so try it if that is all the onion you can enjoy. Some is better than none at all.

## CAYENNE PEPPER: SPICES UP YOUR LIFE

*Capsicum,* the ingredient in red peppers that makes them sizzle in your mouth, may be another "hot" remedy for the heart. Believed for centuries to be a general stimulant and energizer, capsicum has also shown promise in preventing blood clots from forming and in helping to break up potentially dangerous clots. Researchers from Thailand and the United States have found that capsicum stimulates fribrinolytic activity, a natural process that helps resist the formation of large clots by dissolving them when they are small.

You don't have to douse your food with red peppers to benefit from their anticlotting effects. You could visit Thai and Indian restaurants more often or experiment by incorporating fresh or dried red peppers in your familiar family recipes. I don't think there is much worry about overdosing on red peppers. Given the hotness, moderation is easily enforced. Actually, you don't have to chew and swallow the pepper to enjoy the benefits. Even when you hold it in your mouth and suck on it for a short time, it works.

Fears that spicy foods might aggravate duodenal ulcers have been grossly exaggerated. Ironically, capsicum protects and rebuilds the stomach lining and is used by some clinicians to treat digestive problems. Parenthetically, this hot spice is rich in vitamins A and C, calcium, iron, and potassium, and it contains smaller amounts of the B-complex vitamins, magnesium, phosphorus, and sulfur.

## SWITCH TO GREEN TEA

Tea is second only to water as the most common drink in the world. Both black and green tea originate from the same source, the leaf of *Camellia sinenis*, but green tea is processed in a way that protects its important *polyphenols*, phytochemicals known to possess potent antioxidant properties. Just one of these polyphenols, known as EGCg and found in no other plant, constitutes half of all green tea polyphenols and is one of the strongest antioxidants yet discovered (even stronger than vitamin E).

Studies suggest that green tea may guard against heart disease in the following ways:

+ Protecting against free-radical damage.

+ Reducing total cholesterol.

+ Inhibiting oxidation of LDL cholesterol.

+ Elevating HDL cholesterol.

+ Reducing high blood pressure.

+ Inhibiting abnormal clotting in blood vessels.

In Asia, tea consumption is much higher than here in the United States—five to ten cups a day is common. This level may be optimal to reap the full protective rewards of the tea, but it is unlikely most of us will aspire to drinking this much tea. I think, though, that we could easily replace some of our diet drinks and sugary fluids with green tea, and, as an adjunct to other dietary and lifestyle changes, it may help promote a healthy heart. The flavonoids and antioxidants in green tea may also have a salutary effect against several cancers.

# HERBS FOR THE HEART

Herbal medicine was with us long before written documents ascribed healing qualities to specific plants and herbs. It is probably the oldest form of healing on earth, yet it is still considered a part of folklore—mystical, ineffective, and a waste of money. Whether you believe in botanical remedies or not, there are a number of herbs reported to protect and support the cardiovascular system.

There are a variety of ways to prepare herbs. I prefer the simplicity of teas and capsules, but you can buy tinctures and extracts or boil your own mix of fresh roots, flowers, and seeds. You can drink them, apply them topically, or inhale them for different medicinal effects. You should be aware that even though herbs are natural compounds, they can be potent and even harmful when improperly used. Always consult a health care specialist and follow directions before self-diagnosing and self-medicating. The table lists some of the herbs that can be used to maintain and heal the heart.

## Herbs for the Heart

| Herb | Effect |
|------|--------|
| Alfalfa | Inhibits platelet clumping |
| Bilberry | Strengthens capillaries<br>Improves circulation |
| Blessed thistle | Strengthens the heart<br>Improves circulation |
| Dandelion | Strengthens weak arteries<br>Promotes circulation<br>Diuretic (contains potassium) |
| Evening Primrose | Lowers cholesterol<br>Lowers blood pressure<br>Inhibits clot formation |
| Fenugreek | Lowers cholesterol |
| Ginkgo Biloba | Stops free radicals<br>Prevents blood clotting<br>Increases blood flow |
| Ginseng | Fights stress<br>Normalizes blood pressure<br>Lowers blood cholesterol<br>Improves circulation |
| Hawthorne | Used to treat heart palpitations, angina pectoris, heart valve defects, enlarged heart, and arteriosclerosis |

# Part Four

# DESIGNING YOUR PROGRAM FOR HEART HEALTH

# 14

# EATING AND DRINKING FOR HEALTH

Life itself is the proper binge.

—JULIA CHILD

D iet plays a pivotal role in preventing and reversing heart disease. The jury is in and the evidence is clear. What remains cloudy is which exact combination of macronutrients (fats, carbohydrates, protein) and micronutrients (vitamins, minerals, phytonutrients) offers the maximum protective effects. After immersing myself in the literature, I am still hesitant to choose and pass on to you one single plan; therefore, what I am presenting is a range of dietary recommendations based on three proven programs that have been evaluated and deemed protective against diseases of the heart.

One diet does not fit all. We are each unique in many respects, so to recommend that we all eat exactly the same foods in the same proportions seems ridiculous. Many roads lead to good health, and it is up to you to decide what makes sense to you.

## AN OVERVIEW OF
## THREE HEART-HEALTHY PLANS

### The Ornish Program for Reversing Heart Disease

The low-fat vegetarian diet proposed by Dr. Dean Ornish is the most radical approach to heart health and a challenge for many to follow, even when highly motivated. However, heart patients who have followed it along with moderate exercise and stress-reducing techniques have seen dramatic improvements, which is reason enough to look at what makes it work. The ultra low fat (10 percent) plant-based diet consists mostly of vegetables, grains, beans, and fruits. No meat, poultry, or fish is allowed. The primary sources of protein include a daily cup of nonfat milk and an occasional egg white. No caffeine, moderate salt, and moderate alcohol (less than 2 ounces per day) complete the guidelines. The diet is primarily adopted by individuals who have suffered a heart attack and are willing to take extreme measures. It is not for everyone; however, if you have had a close call with death, you may be interested in investigating the specifics of the diet, which are outlined in *Dr. Dean Ornish's Program for Reversing Heart Disease.*

Dr. Ornish feels that by adding another 5 percent of fat to the diet, his program can be used as a preventive measure. Many individuals still find 15 percent total dietary fat too spartan and are not likely to follow it as a way of life. Other researchers have shown that an ultra low fat diet may not be necessary to keep the heart fit and might actually be detrimental to women.

## DASH: Dietary Approaches to Stop Hypertension

In response to a troubling trend of increased incidences of heart failure, stroke, and kidney disease, in November 1997 the National Heart, Lung, and Blood Institute (NHLBI) issued an updated strategy for the prevention and treatment of hypertension. Basing its recommendations on a landmark study called the Dietary Approaches to Stop Hypertension Study (DASH), the NHLBI suggests that following a diet to lower blood pressure, which is a major risk factor for so many diseases, is just as effective as taking medications. For the first time, this governmental organization unreservedly advises individuals with an elevated pressure of 140–159 systolic and 90–99 diastolic, if they have no cardiovascular disease or other risk factors, to try dietary and exercise changes for a year before turning to medication. The NHLBI experts go a step further and recommend that all Americans adopt this program as a preventive measure to lower their risk of heart disease, diabetes, osteoporosis, and cancer.

A little background on the DASH study: It was conducted by eminently qualified American researchers from various medical schools and involved 459 adults enrolled at four centers around the country. The participants were randomly assigned to one of three groups. The control group followed a typically high-fat (40 percent total fat) American diet, group number two matched the control group in fat and cholesterol but included fruits and vegetables in their diet, and the third group reduced both their saturated fat and their cholesterol intake and ate a good amount of fruits and vegetables. Salt intake was held constant for all involved in the study at 3,000 mg a day, which is higher than most health experts advise. Calorie intake was the same in all three diets, so no one lost weight, and alcohol was limited to no more than two drinks a week. The diet that won hands-down was the *combination* diet, followed by the diet observed by the third group of volunteers. In eight short weeks, what is now called the DASH Diet lowered average blood pressure in those with high blood pressure by 11.4 points systolic over 5.5 points diastolic; and for those with normal or slightly high blood pressure, the diet reduced it by an average of 3.4 points over 2.1 points.

The DASH diet is more liberal with fat than the Ornish diet, allowing up to 30 percent fat in the diet. It also includes small portions of meat, chicken, fish, and eggs. Like the Ornish plan, the DASH diet emphasizes fruits, vegetables, whole grains, and beans.

According to the researchers, DASH is easy to follow: just cut the fat, double your intake of fruits and vegetables, and stick to low-fat dairy products. If you are interested in the specifics of this diet, see appendix B for the address of the National Heart, Lung, and Blood Institute; they will send you the information. The Web site for the DASH diet is also listed in appendix B.

## The Mediterranean Diet

Cardiologist Stephen Sinatra, among others, believes that the Mediterranean diet reduces your risk of heart disease and sudden death more than any other program available. Nutritionists and epidemiologists at the Harvard School of Public Health, the European office of the World Health Organization, and Oldways Preservation & Exchange Trust obviously agree, since they developed the Mediterranean pyramid as an alternative to the U.S. Department of Agriculture's Food Guide Pyramid, the one we frequently see on boxes of cereal and loaves of bread.

The Mediterranean plan is universally attractive because it allows the most liberal amounts of fat or oil in the diet (up to 40 percent); limits but doesn't exclude red meat; recommends fish and poultry a few times a week; emphasizes fruits, vegetables, beans, pasta, and low-fat dairy products; and allows up to two glasses of alcohol a day. Critics of this diet point out that a high-fat diet without sufficient exercise will add fat to the body, which is not good for the heart, and that two drinks a day may increase a woman's risk for breast cancer.

## FAT: HOW MUCH IS HEALTHY?

The range of what is healthy in terms of dietary fat seems to be quite broad. As we have seen, it expands to an upper limit of 40 percent of total calories in Mediterranean countries. While taking in almost half of one's total daily calories from fat may work in France because of a number of additional factors in the diet and lifestyles of people there, I think it would be irresponsible to suggest that as a possibility for Americans. It has taken us decades of health awareness to bring our total fat down from 42 percent to around 33 percent. To now inch our way back up would not be a positive step toward improved health, unless we also moved to a Mediterranean country and adopted their entire way of life.

I think it is safe to say that for most Americans, the absolute upper limit should not exceed the American Heart Association's recommendation of 30 percent total fat. The question many of us struggle with is how low must we go to prevent diseases of the heart. A report in the November 1997 issue of the *Journal of the American Medical Association* stated that reducing fat intake to below 30 percent did not provide further benefits and might pose an additional risk. In this study of over four hundred men with high cholesterol, a moderate reduction of fat lowered LDL cholesterol, but in the severely restricted diets (18 percent to 22 percent fat in the diet), the good cholesterol also came down.

In addition, a very low fat diet may not serve women as well as men. There is evidence that women who eat too little fat may both elevate their triglyceride levels and lower their HDLs. And the results of seven studies now conclude that an ultra low fat diet (less than 20 percent of total calories) is not effective in lowering breast cancer risk. And for those experiencing hot flashes, taking in less than 20 percent fat increases menopausal discomfort by reducing estrogen levels.

The bottom-line intake of total fat for women concerned with preventing heart disease should be somewhere between 25 to 30 percent of total calories. Most women think that you must stick to a regimented amount each and every day. I believe that we are allowed more leeway in our diets. Some days you may want to push your limit or even exceed it, and then the next day you can make it up by cutting the fat. I find it helpful to think more in terms of a weekly percentage than a daily routine. It also relieves some of the guilt associated with "blowing it" on certain days.

## Percentage of Fat and Fat Grams

When nutritionists talk about fat, they almost always speak in terms of percentage of total calories. The reason for this is to help you evaluate the relation of fat to calories both in specific foods and in the overall diet. For the consumer, though, this is difficult to visualize and impractical, so let us simplify the numbers and change the percentages into fat grams. This will give you some idea of how drastically your diet needs revamping. It is not meant to inflict guilt, just to provide information.

The following chart will help you nail down the range of grams that is appropriate for you depending on your food intake and energy needs. Some women make a science out of knowing exactly how many fat grams they take in on any given day. I don't think that is necessary. Once you have a sense of what is in the food you eat regularly, you can decide what changes you can realistically make.

The chart shows us that if we take in roughly 2,000 calories daily, the total fat grams in our diet needs to fall somewhere between 44 and 66 per

### Daily Fat Allowance in Grams

| TOTAL CALORIES | TOTAL FAT IN GRAMS 30% | 20% |
|---|---|---|
| 1,000 | 33 | 22 |
| 1,500 | 50 | 33 |
| 2,000 | 66 | 44 |
| 2,500 | 83 | 55 |

day. I would like to repeat that if on a special occasion you choose to splurge, finding yourself off the chart entirely, the rest of the week you can edge your way back. Lifetime changes are not made overnight.

## Keeping a Food Journal

In order to start slicing fat from your daily menu, it is important to know how much you are taking in. You don't want to go overboard and make your life completely miserable, but you do want to have a handle on the work that needs to be done. I am a great believer in keeping a food journal. It provides startling clues to the amount of food you consume, your tastes and cravings, how much nutrition you are getting, and when and why you eat. If you are serious about changing your diet, a food journal is very helpful, at least until you determine your dietary habits and define your goals.

Many of you are familiar with keeping a journal, so this isn't a totally new concept. To make it somewhat enjoyable, go out and buy a pretty, cloth-covered notebook, one that feels warm and friendly. Or if you don't want to carry around an obvious journal, mark a section in your day planner or keep track on your calendar. For an entire week, write down every piece of food and every liquid that enters your mouth. Try not to judge your eating patterns yet; work especially hard not to feel guilt or remorse about what you have eaten. This is an exercise, not an evaluation—yet. Approach it as if you were a journalist covering a story: just present the facts. After seven days, and with the help of a fat gram counter and food labels in your pantry and refrigerator, tally up your daily grams and average them. Match your numbers with the chart, and from there you will be able to determine the primary areas that need attention.

To help you begin your journey of self-discovery, I have provided an example of how you might set up your daily food intake journal. You can copy this one directly or alter it according to your specific desires or needs. You will notice that in addition to a section on the fat content of your diet, I have included a column for counting grams of fiber. You can use pages 113–114 to estimate total fiber as well as soluble fiber in your diet. Once you have completed a week of entries, sit down and total the numbers, and average them

## DAILY FOOD JOURNAL

| Time | Food | Fiber (gm) | Fat (gm) |
|------|------|------------|----------|
| | | | |
| | | | |
| | | | |
| | | | |
| | | | |
| | | | |
| | | | |
| | | | |
| | | | |
| | | | |
| | | | |
| | | | |
| | | | |
| | | | |
| | | | |
| | | Total___ | Total___ |

for the week. You should also look over your food choices and see how many fruits and vegetables you average a day and how many other foods that have been shown to contribute to heart health made it into your journal.

## Weekly Reflection

✦ What type of fat do I eat?

✦ How much fat?

✦ How much fiber?

✦ How many fruits?

✦ How many vegetables?

✦ How much fish?

✦ How many legumes or beans?

✦ How much soy?

### Estimating Percentages

It is also good to know how to read labels and compare fat grams and total percentages. Sometimes the grams may seem relatively innocuous, but the product may still contain a high percentage of fat. Frozen dinners are especially tricky. For example, say you have an entrée that has 350 total calories (sounds good for dinner) and fifteen fat grams listed. This doesn't seem unreasonable, but when you multiply it out, the total percentage of fat is 39 percent. Probably not the low-calorie, low-fat meal you thought you were buying.

If you want to figure out the percentage of fat in foods that you eat regularly, it is fairly simple. But you will need a calculator. First, multiply the fat grams that are found on the label of most foods by nine (each gram of fat has 9 calories). Next, divide the answer by the total calories and voilà, you have the percentage of calories from fat. Or,

(grams of fat times 9) divided by (total calories)
= percent of fat calories

In the example of the frozen dinner above:

15 grams of fat times 9 = 135 fat calories

135 fat calories divided by 350 total calories
= 0.385 or 38.5 percent of fat calories

Here is another example from a package of cookies. The total fat grams are 7 and the total calories 140. Just plug in the numbers.

7 grams of fat times 9 = 63 fat calories

63 fat calories divided by 140 total calories = .45 or 45 percent of fat calories

Not many of us take calculators to the market and check out each and every product, although occasionally you do see women doing this. If you would like to practice buying items that contain less than 30 percent of total calories as fat, here is any easy way to spot-estimate: allow 3 grams of fat per 100 calories. In the above example of 9 grams and 140 calories, it is obviously over 30 percent.

## Special Fats to Avoid

One point upon which all heart programs agree is that saturated fats (found in meats, dairy products, butter, and tropical oils), *trans* fats (found in margarine and commercial salad dressings, and hydrogenated fats (found in processed foods and bakery products) should be limited. I often wonder if the health benefits of the various programs really are about what you *don't* eat as opposed to what you *do* eat. In looking over your own dietary records or considering your daily food choices, working at limiting saturated fats is an excellent beginning to strengthening your heart.

## Fake Fats

Americans are so phobic about fat that manufacturers are driven to constantly come up with new fat-free products. These popular products that claim zero fat should also read "zero nutrition." Olestra (brand name Olean) is the first food additive with "negative nutritional value." And nutritionists are not pleased. The newest of the fake fats will be used in snack foods such as potato and tortilla chips, so for now it may not seem all that critical to the consumer. After all, how many chips can one eat? The truth be known, when we realize something is fat-free, we feel it gives us license to pig out. So we might gorge on enormous quantities of items that we would never consider if they contained a touch of fat. Fortunately, eating too many fake fats will cause enough discomfort that we are unlikely to repeat bingeing again. Olestra chips can cause nausea, bloating, and diarrhea. If Olestra doesn't bother you, you should still limit it to snacks. It has been proven to eliminate key nutrients from the body—carotenoids, phytochemicals, and the vitamins A, D, E, and K. The negatives could outweigh the positives in this case.

# CHOOSING THE BEST CARBOHYDRATES

Carbohydrates serve as the foundation of all heart-healthy diets. The Ornish program derives 70 to 80 percent of its calories from the carbohydrates in grains, fruits, and vegetables. Both the DASH and the Mediterranean diets draw more than half of their daily food recommendation from a variety of breads, cereals, rice, and pastas. On this one point everyone agrees: if our regular food intake revolves around whole, fresh foods grown in the ground, we are well on our way to preventing a host of debilitating diseases.

## Simple Versus Complex Carbs

Carbohydrates come to us in two forms: simple and complex. In a heart-healthy diet we need to downplay simple and emphasize complex. The problem is that most women have it reversed. Always in a hurry, we grab a cookie rather than a banana. When we need comfort, it is chocolate and pastry we turn to, not a piece of fruit or an oat-bran muffin. Without paying attention, we often make too many of the wrong choices when it comes to carbohydrates. If we are concerned about our hearts, we must learn to save the simple carbs for occasional treats and incorporate complex carbs into our daily eating pattern.

## Simple Carbohydrates

Simple carbohydrates include all the sugars. Not just the common white table sugar known chemically as sucrose, but a long list that includes glucose (blood sugar), fructose (fruit sugar), lactose (milk sugar), maltose (malt sugar), and sugar alcohols like sorbitol and xylitol. Simple carbohydrates occur naturally in fruits, vegetables, grains, and dairy products, but most of the sugars we eat daily come from processed foods found in a box or a can. Of the total amount of sugar produced, 65 percent is used by the food and beverage industry in the manufacture of bakery products, cereal, candy, frozen foods, soups, sauces, condiments, sodas, beer, and wine.

You can inspect the nutrition labels on the back of a box or can to get a sense of how much sugar is in a product. Since ingredients are listed on labels in the order of greatest weight, the closer the sugar source is to the beginning of the list, the more sugar you can expect to be getting. Also, be aware that there are many hidden sources of sugar, with names that are not easily recognizable. When you add them together, you realize the quantity of sugar in the product is probably more than you had anticipated. Here are some of the names under which sugars are added to foods:

| | | |
|---|---|---|
| Brown sugar | Glucose | Molasses |
| Confectioner's sugar | Lactose | Powdered sugar |
| Corn syrup | Levulose | Raw sugar |
| Dextrose | Maltose | Sorbitol |
| High-fructose corn syrup | Maltodextrin | Sorghum syrup |
| Honey | Mannitol | Sucrose |
| Fructose | Maple syrup | Xylitol |

Simple sugars and highly refined carbs excite our taste buds but provide little health value, and they may go a step further and cause us harm if eaten daily and in large enough quantities. Our challenge isn't getting the allotted number of total carbohydrate servings; it is choosing complex carbohydrates that provide adequate fiber and nutrition. We have grown accustomed to white bread, white rice, pasta, and potatoes, and these simple starches behave just like sugar when digested. Too many, too often, can upset our blood sugar regulating mechanism, add fat to our bodies, and trigger adult diabetes in susceptible individuals.

White table sugar, disguised in candies, cakes, pies, muffins, cereals, and sodas, should play a minor role in our daily diet, because it contributes only calories to our body. Whether or not it directly promotes heart disease is debatable. We know that concentrated sugar may interact with other nutrients to produce a deficiency of copper, a condition associated with heart disease. And too much sugar may create a chromium deficiency, which is linked to diabetes. There are so many other reasons why too many sweets are not advisable that I don't think we necessarily have to prove a direct link to heart disease. I am not saying *no* sweets should ever touch your lips—I am saying sugar should remain in the background.

## Fructose

I want to single out one simple sugar because it is so ubiquitous in food processing, and is now thought to alter cholesterol profiles. *Fructose* is the natural sugar found in fruit, and it has been considered a logical choice to replace sugar in sweetening any number of products on the market, from diet drinks to pastries. Because it is cheap to make, it has crept into our diets in the form of high-fructose corn syrup. In small doses, fruit sugar is quite wholesome, but the concentrated quantities we are getting from so many sources are giving nutritionists cause for concern.

Fructose, like glucose, can aggravate copper deficiency and profoundly affect the cardiovascular system. In animal studies, large doses of fructose were associated with heart disease. A 1993 USDA study found that fructose increased LDL cholesterol. Fruit sugar, like plain white table sugar, can easily be converted into triglycerides, an unhealthy fat that is particularly linked to heart disease in women. If you are overweight and can't seem to lose the extra pounds or if your triglyceride levels are high, consider the amount of fruit juices, fruit-flavored drinks, diet sodas, and fruit-sweetened snacks you eat and drink.

## Complex Carbohydrates

Complex carbohydrates are made up of chains of simple sugars; chemically, they are more complex than simple carbohydrates, which explains their name. They include the heavier, starchy grains and vegetables. The ones that contain the largest amounts of dietary

### Healthy Complex Carbohydrates

| Whole grains | Brown rice |
|---|---|
| Oatmeal | Barley |
| Millet | Rye |
| Kasha (buckwheat) | Cornmeal |
| Peas and beans | Quinoa |
| Tortillas | Couscous |
| Orzo | Polenta |

fiber are considered the most complex.

Complex carbohydrates are the all-stars in most healthy diets and the ones we want to particularly focus on to provide the bulk (no pun intended) of our calories. This means that each meal should include some grain: rice, oats, wheat, barley, or corn. Unrefined whole grains are high in fiber and loaded with vitamins, minerals, antioxidants, and plant chemicals, each benefiting the heart and body. Six to eleven servings daily are recommended, which sounds a bit more extravagant than it actually is, considering a serving size is one slice of bread or half a cup of cereal, rice, or pasta. To both increase your enjoyment of grains and introduce a wider variety of nutrients to your diet, it is a good idea to challenge your taste buds and try some grains that you have noticed only from afar. Open your mind and your mouth to fresh nutritional experiences, and fill you diet with an array of health-giving complex carbohydrates.

## Fruits and Vegetables

There is an overwhelming agreement among researchers that fruits and vegetables absolutely must find their way to our plates on a more regular basis. It is easy to understand why fresh produce rates so high, but, in case you need a gentle reminder, fruit is packed full of nutrients—vitamin C, beta-carotene, potassium, iron, fiber—and a host of phytonutrients that have barely been identified. We should include a minimum of two or three pieces of fruit in our diet daily. Review the past week: How many days did you come close to the recommended quota?

If you are at a loss for new ways of incorporating fruit into your daily diet, consider these suggestions: Most people find breakfast the most convenient time of the day to get in one or two portions. Just about any fruit goes well with cereal—bananas, blueberries, raspberries, or strawberries. Grabbing juice on the run instead of coffee might serve as a healthy alternative. Carry fruit in the car for a quick snack, add pears and apples to your green salads, make a side dish of cut-up fresh fruit, or mix fresh fruit with unsweetened canned fruit in the winter when choices are sparse. Juice bars are everywhere now, so a quick stop can provide a tasty fresh fruit drink or smoothie. Even bottled fruit juice has come a long way since cranberry cocktails. Now you can get mango, papaya, or watermelon for a change.

Vegetables are a harder sell but are just as important. They provide complex carbohydrates, fiber, calcium, iron, beta-carotene, vitamin C, and phytochemicals. It is a good idea to choose a variety of colors of vegetables in order to get an assortment of nutrients. Vitamin A is found in deep green, yellow, and orange vegetables, and vitamin C is in green peppers, cauliflower, tomatoes, spinach, and cabbage. Raw, cooked, fresh, or frozen—anyway you can conceive of other than French-fried—is acceptable. The daily recommendation of four to five is a bit daunting unless you have a juicer and make veggie cocktails.

Let me offer a few suggestions other than the obvious lightly cooked or stir-fried vegetables. Salsa made from fresh tomatoes and onions counts as a serving—just be careful what you are dunking in it. Corn tortillas or pita bread are good, but try to avoid the high-fat and high-sodium tortilla chips. Did you know that the pumpkin in pumpkin pie counts as a vegetable? Just remember not to eat the crust. Spaghetti sauce is especially nutritious when you throw in onions, garlic, and green peppers. Have you tried *baba ghanoush* (pulverized eggplant) on pita bread? Squash soup, vegetarian stew, and pureed yams are some of the new ways to eat vegetables that I have tried in restaurants lately. Items such as low-fat coleslaw, carrot-raisin salad, potato salad, orzo and cucumbers, kashi and cranberries are finding their way into the deli section of many markets, so the challenge isn't as great as it was years ago. You just have to be aware of what is available and allow yourself to experiment with new taste sensations.

I believe that it is healthier to buy organic produce that is grown without synthetic pesticides, fertilizers, or growth regulators and processed without the use of chemicals, additives, or preservatives.

## Sizes of Fruits and Vegetables per Serving

| VEGETABLES | FRUITS |
|---|---|
| 1 cup raw, leafy vegetable | 1 medium fruit |
| 3/4 cup vegetable juice | 3/4 cup fruit juice |
| 1/2 cup cooked vegetable | 1/2 cup fresh, frozen, or canned fruit |

Although nutritionists do not agree on this point, and some claim organic produce is not necessarily nutritionally superior to conventionally grown produce, we do know that the fresher a fruit or vegetable is and the less it is handled, the better the chance it contains a richer supply of vitamins and minerals. And my subjective opinion is that it tastes much better.

## Carbohydrate Sensitivity

Many individuals are hypersensitive to sugar and starches and cannot metabolize them efficiently. A governmental survey found that about one-third of the U.S. population has trouble processing sugar. Some may have been born this way; others develop the problem with age and weight gain. Immediate signs of carbohydrate sensitivity can be subtle, such as fatigue or anxiety following a starchy meal. Long-term repercussions can be weight gain, elevated blood fats, and diabetes in predisposed individuals.

Traditional wisdom had it that pure, white sugar is responsible for sending blood sugar off the chart, while complex carbohydrates temper the reaction, doling out sugar more slowly into the blood. It turns out that sugar metabolism is not that simple. Nutritionist Phyllis Crapo from the University of Colorado and David Jenkins, Ph.D., at the University of Toronto, have found that carbohydrates differ in how rapidly they are broken down into glucose for absorption into the bloodstream.

This revolutionary discovery led to the development of what is called the *glycemic index* of foods. Foods with a high glycemic index cause the greatest elevation of blood sugar; those at the lower end have less adverse effect on blood sugar. Dr. Jenkins found that foods measuring low on the index minimize the need for the pancreas to secrete insulin to control blood sugar and help lower the level of blood fats like cholesterol and triglycerides in people with a genetic tendency to develop diabetes or heart problems. This research has served as an important tool for those who are diabetic or at risk for heart disease, suggesting that such individuals can modify their blood sugar levels by choosing the right kind of carbohydrate.

The following list of simple and complex carbohydrates may surprise you. Certain starches, like carrots and potatoes, send blood sugar soaring higher than plain table sugar or a Mars bar. It also appears that ice cream is better for you than wheat bread. We should be careful not to carry this to an illogical extreme. The only thing the chart really indicates is that all starches are not created equal and that some will trigger a more immediate blood sugar jolt in sensitive individuals than others. If you are overweight, hypoglycemic, diabetic, or have high triglyceride levels, then you need to monitor more closely the foods that are closest to the top of the index, as well as simple sugars.

## Glycemic Index of Specific Foods

| FOOD | MEAN VALUE |
|------|------------|
| **SUGARS** | |
| Glucose | 138 |
| Honey | 126 |
| Sucrose (table sugar) | 83 |
| Lactose | 57 |
| Fructose | 26 |
| **BREADS, CEREALS, GRAINS** | |
| Millet | 103 |
| Bread, wheat and white | 100 |
| Rye (crispbread) | 95 |
| Rice, brown | 81 |
| Buckwheat | 78 |
| Rye, whole grain | 68 |
| Pasta, white | 67 |
| Pasta, whole meal | 61 |
| **BREAKFAST CEREAL** | |
| Puffed rice | 132 |
| Cornflakes | 121 |
| Puffed wheat | 110 |

Shredded wheat . . . . . . . . . . . . . . . . . . . . . . . . . . . . . . . . . . . 97

Muesli . . . . . . . . . . . . . . . . . . . . . . . . . . . . . . . . . . . . . . . . . . 96

Oatmeal . . . . . . . . . . . . . . . . . . . . . . . . . . . . . . . . . . . . . . . . . 89

All Bran . . . . . . . . . . . . . . . . . . . . . . . . . . . . . . . . . . . . . . . . . 74

## LEGUMES AND LENTILS

Baked beans, canned . . . . . . . . . . . . . . . . . . . . . . . . . . . . . 60

Pinto beans, dried . . . . . . . . . . . . . . . . . . . . . . . . . . . . . . . 60

Kidney beans, dried . . . . . . . . . . . . . . . . . . . . . . . . . . . . . . 43

Chickpeas (garbanzos) . . . . . . . . . . . . . . . . . . . . . . . . . . . . 46

Peas, canned . . . . . . . . . . . . . . . . . . . . . . . . . . . . . . . . . . . 50

Lentils, dried . . . . . . . . . . . . . . . . . . . . . . . . . . . . . . . . . . . 36

Soybeans, canned . . . . . . . . . . . . . . . . . . . . . . . . . . . . . . . 22

Peanuts . . . . . . . . . . . . . . . . . . . . . . . . . . . . . . . . . . . . . . . 15

## ROOT VEGETABLES

Potatoes, instant . . . . . . . . . . . . . . . . . . . . . . . . . . . . . . . 120

Potatoes, baked . . . . . . . . . . . . . . . . . . . . . . . . . . . . . . . . 116

Potatoes, mashed . . . . . . . . . . . . . . . . . . . . . . . . . . . . . . . 98

Potatoes, sweet . . . . . . . . . . . . . . . . . . . . . . . . . . . . . . . . 70

Parsnips . . . . . . . . . . . . . . . . . . . . . . . . . . . . . . . . . . . . . . 97

Carrots . . . . . . . . . . . . . . . . . . . . . . . . . . . . . . . . . . . . . . . 92

## FRUIT

Raisins . . . . . . . . . . . . . . . . . . . . . . . . . . . . . . . . . . . . . . . 93

Banana . . . . . . . . . . . . . . . . . . . . . . . . . . . . . . . . . . . . . . . 84

Orange juice . . . . . . . . . . . . . . . . . . . . . . . . . . . . . . . . . . . 71

Orange . . . . . . . . . . . . . . . . . . . . . . . . . . . . . . . . . . . . . . . 59

Apple . . . . . . . . . . . . . . . . . . . . . . . . . . . . . . . . . . . . . . . . 52

Apple juice . . . . . . . . . . . . . . . . . . . . . . . . . . . . . . . . . . . . 45

## DAIRY PRODUCTS

Ice cream . . . . . . . . . . . . . . . . . . . . . . . . . . . . . . . . . . . . . 69

Yogurt . . . . . . . . . . . . . . . . . . . . . . . . . . . . . . . . . . . . . . . . 52

Nonfat milk . . . . . . . . . . . . . . . . . . . . . . . . . . . . . . . . . . . . 46

Whole milk . . . . . . . . . . . . . . . . . . . . . . . . . . . . . . . . . . . . 44

## SNACK FOODS

Corn chips . . . . . . . . . . . . . . . . . . . . . . . . . . . . . . . . . . . . . 99

Shortbread cookies . . . . . . . . . . . . . . . . . . . . . . . . . . . . . . 88

## EMPHASIZING VEGETABLE PROTEIN

The three heart-healthy programs are most in agreement on the amount of protein required for a healthy body. They recommend that 15 to 20 percent of the total diet be in the form of protein; most of us achieve this without too much difficulty.

If you are curious about how much protein you should take in daily, it is easy to determine using a simple formula. The RDA standard for protein is based on weight and can be individually determined by multiplying your weight in kilograms by 0.8 grams of protein. First, determine your weight in kilograms by dividing your weight in pounds by 2.2. Then, just multiply the result by 0.8. Here is the example of a 130-pound woman:

130 divided by 2.2 = 59 kilograms, multiplied by 0.8 = 47 grams of protein

This number isn't written in stone, and most bodies can handle a fairly wide fluctuation in either direction. If you are overweight, you may require less protein than the number you calculated, because the amount necessary is based on your ideal weight. Heavy bouts of regular exercise may alter the average, and you may want to go a little higher. If you are over sixty-five years of age, your body fails to utilize protein as efficiently as it did in earlier years. That does not mean that eating more protein would be beneficial. Supplementing your diet with an enzyme that helps assimilate the protein, such as betaine hydrochloric acid (HCl), papain, or prolase, may be a good idea.

American women consume around 65 to 70 grams of protein a day, which is well above the suggested range. Does this mean that we are mistreating our bodies with a few more ounces of chicken? According to the National Research Council, consuming up to twice the RDA for protein, which takes us close to 100 grams a day, is acceptable, but going over 120 grams per day is not. I would like to add that if the additional protein is laden with fat, it would definitely not be healthy, and for some women, inching close to the upper limit may not be the wisest choice.

Eating too much protein is a much greater problem in the United States than elsewhere in the world. There is evidence that an overabundance of protein, primarily animal protein, may be partially responsible for clogged arteries, high blood pressure, high cholesterol, and heart disease. Women need to be wary of red meat for other reasons. A study of more than fourteen thousand women found that those who ate red meat every day had nearly twice the risk of developing breast cancer as did those who regularly ate fish, poultry, and dairy products. An earlier study from data analyzing women's habits showed that the incidence of colon cancer was also more than twice as high among women who ate red meat daily as among those who ate it only a few times a week. Other suspected protein-related cancers include those of the uterus, rectum, pancreas, prostate, and kidney. Excess protein results in storage of body fat, calcium loss, and possibly kidney damage.

The term *protein* is derived from the Greek word *protos*, meaning first. An essential structural component of all living matter, it makes up more than half the dry weight of most of our cells. In other words, take the water out of our bodies, and half of the rest is protein. It is a basic substance found in every cell from the skin to the bones. We need it for healthy bones, healthy muscles, and tissue growth and repair. It is crucial to the enzyme systems that power the body's metabolism. It forms neurotransmitters in the brain, regulates fluid balance, and strengthens the immune system. Protein is so vital to life that it is part of almost everything we eat.

We associate protein with meat, but it is also found in dairy products, beans, grains, nuts, and, even broccoli. For most people, 3 ounces of lean meat, half a cup of beans, and a cup each of pasta, yogurt, and milk supply more than enough protein for a day's supply. This is why deficiency is rare in the United States, except in extreme cases of dieting and malnutrition. The following chart further breaks down protein sources into grams to help you determine where you fall in your daily requirements.

## Planning Your Daily Protein Intake

While the recommended daily amount of protein is not too different in the three heart programs, the methods for achieving the goal vary.

The Ornish vegetarian diet omits all meat, so the protein comes from grains, beans, egg whites, and nonfat milk. The Mediterranean plan limits red meat (beef, veal, lamb, and pork) to a few times a month but encourages weekly servings of fish, poultry, and eggs. The DASH diet allows up to 6 ounces a day of meat, poultry, and fish but also incorporates

### Sources of Protein in Grams (total around 40–70 gm/day)

Meat, chicken, fish (1 oz.) . . . . . . . . . . . . 6–8

Milk (1 cup) . . . . . . . . . . . . . . . . . . . . . . . 8

Yogurt (1 cup) . . . . . . . . . . . . . . . . . . 10–13

Egg (1) . . . . . . . . . . . . . . . . . . . . . . . . . . 6

Beans (½ cup, cooked) . . . . . . . . . . . . . . 7

Nuts (1 oz.) . . . . . . . . . . . . . . . . . . . . . . . 6

Grains (1 slice bread, ½ cup pasta) . . . . . . 3

Broccoli (½ cup) . . . . . . . . . . . . . . . . . . . . 2

low-fat and nonfat dairy products, and small amounts of nuts and seeds.

I think it is clear that no matter which plan we choose, we all need to be more careful about eating huge servings of red meat every day. This is going to challenge many who thrive on deli sandwiches that offer 7- to 10-ounce meat portions, and those who often eat out and select almost any kind of meat, which usually comes in 8- to 12-ounce servings. We need to save our prime rib and steak dinners for anniversaries and other infrequent celebrations. Another suggestion is to share a sandwich, or order one dinner and split the meat and order an extra side of vegetables or grains.

Individuals who eat more plant protein than animal protein have a lower risk of heart disease and are generally healthier. This may be the year you attempt experimenting with vegetarian meals based on a variety of grains, beans, nuts, seeds, and soy products. If this idea is new to you, try starting out with one nonmeat day or dinner a week.

## DRINKING TO YOUR HEALTH

### Alcohol

Moderate alcohol consumption increases HDL cholesterol levels and cuts the rate of heart disease in half. More than one or two drinks a day for women may harm the liver and breasts and shorten our lives. The definition of one drink is 5 ounces of wine, 12 ounces of beer, or 1¹/₂ ounces of hard liquor. All appear to confer a similar benefit—but red wine contributes additional antioxidants that you will not find in beer and hard liquor. Moderation is healthy for many women; however, if you are taking medication and if alcoholism is part of your family history, consider that even small amounts may not be for you.

## Grape Juice

You can enjoy the benefits of wine without the alcohol by going directly to the source, the grape. One study found that 8 to 10 ounces of purple grape juice has a potent effect on the blood platelets, making them less likely to form the clots that lead to heart attacks. The team leader, Dr. John Folts of the University of Wisconsin Medical School, said grape juice might even be more potent than aspirin, which is widely recommended for the prevention of heart problems.

## Caffeine

Coffee may keep you awake at night and cause your heart to race, but it will not directly put you at risk for heart disease. The ten-year Nurses' Study found no association between caffeine, blood cholesterol, and heart disease in women. There is a caveat, though: coffee beans contain *diterpenes,* chemicals that can slightly raise blood cholesterol and triglycerides, but they are removed when coffee is brewed by the drip-filter method. So if you stick with drip coffee made with a paper filter, you can continue to enjoy your morning brew.

Coffee lovers will be happy to hear that caffeine has other real benefits. It has been found to alleviate headaches, relieve asthma symptoms, improve memory, increase endurance, and boost your mood. A 1996 Harvard study even suggested that people who drank a few cups of coffee a day were 70 percent less likely to commit suicide than those who didn't drink any. Caffeine has been shown to have little effect on osteoporosis as long as calcium is adequate.

Don't think that I am giving a blanket endorsement for coffee; we still need to approach the subject with a certain amount of caution. There may be an indirect link between heart disease and heavy coffee drinking. Coffee has the potential for increasing homocysteine levels in the blood, which does promote the clogging of arteries. A Norwegian study found that women who drank more than nine cups a day had a 20 percent higher level of homocysteine in their blood. They were drinking the supposedly safe drip-filtered kind, so the culprit wasn't the oily diterpenes. Another reason to limit our intake is that caffeine acts as a diuretic and thus can result in loss of body fluid and important nutrients such as calcium and potassium. If you compensate by drinking extra water and replenishing your nutrients with a multivitamin mineral tablet, you can minimize this loss.

For some women coffee can be a downright unfriendly drink. Caffeine is a stimulant that reacts powerfully in some women, causing panic attacks, anxiety, and insomnia. It may cause heart palpitations or temporarily elevate blood pressure. Other women experience breast soreness after drinking coffee, even though the National Cancer Institute reassures us there is no relationship between caffeine intake and the incidence of fibrocystic breast disease.

If you drink coffee regularly, make sure it is filtered. Be cautious of espresso, Turkish-style coffee, and the unfiltered European coffees, such as the ones made in a French press (a carafe with a plunger). No matter how much you delight in your morning shot of caffeine, do not drink more than five cups a day.

## Tea (Black and Green)

Tea may provide many of the same antioxidants found in red wine, and therefore it may be as healthful as alcohol but without the side effects and dangers. Green tea contains one type of antioxidant, called catechins, thought to approximate the health-giving qualities of wine. Black tea (which is made from green tea leaves that have been dried and heated) provides other antioxidants, and its effectiveness in fighting free radicals parallels that of green tea. Studies suggest that green tea has cut strokes in half in Japanese women who drink at least five cups a day. Black tea—drunk in large quantities—may equal vitamin E in antioxidant activity, prevent blood clots, and cut the risk of fatal heart disease. If you are looking for a replacement for soda or coffee, how about tea?

## Water

People who drink hard water, rather than soft water, have lower rates of heart disease, stroke, and hypertension. The minerals calcium and magnesium, found in hard water, are favorable to heart health. Drinking eight glasses of pure filtered or bottled water between meals is generally a good idea for a healthy body. Water delivers nutrients to the cells, absorbs shock in your joints, muscles, and bones, enables your glands and hormones to operate more efficiently, allows your liver to break down more fat, and releases excess stored water.

Many of us are perpetually dehydrated without knowing it; such a state drains our basic energy. Signs of dehydration include dry hair, nails, and skin; a dry mouth; constipation; infrequent urination; a racing pulse; and the inability to sweat when exercising. Don't limit your water drinking to after exercising or when you are thirsty. Make it a habit to sip water throughout the day. Substitute some of those sodas and sugar-filled liquids with plain water and notice the difference in how you feel. Don't leave home without it; carry a water bottle with you everywhere.

## Other Healthy Drinks

+ *Fruit and vegetable juices:* Great sources of antioxidants, vitamins, minerals, and phytochemicals. Dilute if sugar content bothers you.

+ *Nonfat milk:* Good source of protein and calcium.

+ *Soy milk:* Excellent substitute for milk containing a rich blend of phytonutrients that lower blood cholesterol.

+ *Rice milk:* Good substitute for milk on cereal and in baking.

+ *Smoothies:* Good source of protein, calcium, antioxidants.

# 15

# FILLING IN THE BLANKS: SUPPLEMENTATION

Listen to your life. All moments are key moments.
—FREDERICK BUECHNER

I t is hard to get rid of the myth that healthy people do not require supplemental vitamins and minerals if they eat a balanced diet. Two parts of this pervasive belief are grossly in error. First, very few women eat the idealized diet that nutrition textbooks propose as healthy. And second, nutrition research over the past two decades has shown that supplemental nutrients above and beyond the recommended daily allowances (RDAs) *are* critical in preventing and treating chronic diseases such as heart disease and cancer.

As strongly as I believe that most individuals require more than food to meet their nutritional needs, I want to make it very clear that supplements are not a replacement for a nutritious diet. Researchers are continually identifying new substances in foods that promote health and protect against disease. Every day, scientists find more and more phytonutrients that may be just as important to our health as well-known vitamins and nutrients. To rely too heavily on only the nutrients of which we are aware is a mistake. Also, don't think that you can eat all the junk food you want and pop a pill as insurance. Certainly, it is better than doing nothing, but who knows what nutritious substances we are missing because they are not found in a multivitamin pill.

## WOMEN ARE NUTRIENT DEFICIENT

Most of us like to think that we eat a relatively healthful diet, and on some days we do. But if we were glaringly honest about our general habits, most of us would have to admit that we don't eat two to three fruits every day, rarely make the daily five-vegetable mark, and concentrate more on restricting calories and fat than on enhancing our nutrition. Because of these exclusions from our menus, we have been skimping on fiber, antioxidant nutrients, and precious phytochemicals. Governmental surveys of our eating habits and scientific studies comparing diets and disease prove that our diets are shamefully deficient in a variety of nutrients, including many important vitamins and minerals.

This is the result of not paying close attention to what we eat and not adding nutrients to our food supply. Nutritionists report that women are likely to be low in the following: vitamins A, D, C, and B complex (especially B-6, B-12, and folic acid), and the minerals calcium, magnesium, zinc, selenium, and copper. Women who are menstruating can add iron to the mix. The list expands with age, infection, disease, stress, smoking, and poor dietary habits such as drinking to excess or eating primarily processed, white nonfoods.

## OPTIMUM, NOT MINIMUM, NUTRITION

The recommended dietary allowances (RDAs) have been under attack for many years now. They were originally intended to provide suggested levels of minimum nutrition for healthy individuals below which classic deficiencies occur. This meant that if you were generally healthy and maintained the RDA levels for basic nutrients, you could be fairly certain you wouldn't contract the classic vitamin deficiencies such as scurvy or beri beri.

The RDA guidelines are obsolete and limited in many ways. They were not designed to enhance health, to address people who are in less than perfect health, to include an aging population, or for anyone with specific nutritional needs, such as people who suffer from chronic disease or periodic infection, or those who take medication.

The RDAs do not consider the potential for optimal health and the relationship between nutrient intake and protection from disease. Several private groups and governmental organizations have stepped in with dietary recommendations that exceed minimum levels and incorporate the latest research. For example, the National Institutes of Health found calcium levels inadequate across the board, but especially for postmenopausal women, and publicly recommended higher doses that will help prevent and treat bone loss.

Years of research have continued to confirm a strong association between vitamin E deficiency and heart disease. It has been called a better predictor of heart disease than blood cholesterol. Most of the research on vitamin E has found that people require supplemental doses in the range of 100 to 400 IU a day to prevent artery-clogging plaque, yet the RDA remains at a low 30 IU while those who set public policy await additional studies.

Other nutrients deserve recognition for their heart-protective qualities. The B vitamins, folic acid, B-6, and B-12, when in short supply, cause elevated levels of homocysteine, which may be responsible for one-third of all heart attacks. Many antioxidants and minerals like magnesium and calcium can strengthen our heart, prevent blood clots and cholesterol buildup, and potentially add years to our life and life to our years—yet we are still waiting for battling nutritionists to give us the okay.

## NUTRIENTS FOR A HEALTHY HEART

Nutrients above and beyond the RDA can keep our heart and circulatory system healthy, lower blood pressure, bring down LDL cholesterol and triglyceride levels, raise HDL cholesterol levels, and keep clots from forming and plaque from building. I recommend levels of specific vitamins and minerals that have been studied in reference to heart disease, basing my recommendations on the current medical literature at this time. All nutrients listed fall well within the safety range.

### Heart-Healthy Nutrients

| NUTRIENT | DAILY DOSAGE | HEART BENEFIT |
|---|---|---|
| *VITAMINS* | | |
| Beta-carotene | 5,000–20,000 IU | Prevents LDL oxidation |
| Vitamin E | 200–400 IU | Lowers LDL levels<br>Keeps platelets slippery<br>Improves circulation |

| | | |
|---|---|---|
| Vitamin C | 300–3,000 mg | Helps metabolize cholesterol |
| Folic Acid | 400–800 mcg | Lowers homocysteine |
| Vitamin B-6 | 20–60 mg | Lowers homocysteine |
| Vitamin B-12 | 20–60 mg | Lowers homocysteine |
| Niacin | 20–50 mg | Lowers cholesterol |

### MINERALS

| | | |
|---|---|---|
| Magnesium | 400–500 mg | Maintains blood vessels<br>May inhibit platelet clumping<br>Deficiency can cause spasms<br>of coronary arteries |
| Calcium | 1,000–1,500 mg | Supports magnesium |
| Selenium | 35–200 mcg | Antioxidant<br>May reduce platelet clumping |
| Chromium picolinate | 50–100 mcg | May lower total cholesterol<br>May lower triglyceride levels<br>May raise HDL levels |
| Potassium | 40–90 mg | Regulates heartbeat<br>Regulates blood pressure<br>Deficiency associated with<br>irregular heartbeat |

### OTHER NUTRIENTS

| | | |
|---|---|---|
| Coenzyme Q10 | 30–100 mg | Powerful antioxidant<br>Improves circulation |
| Omega-3 fatty acids | 3 gm | Cardioprotective |
| Pycnogenol | 25–50 mg | Antioxidant<br>May reduce platelet clumping |
| Garlic | 1–2 cloves | Lowers blood pressure<br>Lowers triglycerides and<br>cholesterol |

## TAKING SUPPLEMENTS

I have not provided a complete list of every nutrient found in a multivitamin/mineral supplement tablet; I mention only those that research has linked in some way to heart disease. This does not mean that the others are not important or that the ones mentioned in my list are superior to those excluded. Exposure to chemical and environmental pollutants causes the body to produce damaging free radicals, which further provoke changes that can result in heart disease. Adding a full-spectrum antioxidant team of nutrients will help to protect us from inevitable damage.

All nutrients are important, and heart disease patients and individuals at risk for heart disease (which is basically the rest of us) rarely get them at the levels we need from the food we eat. Therefore, I advise you to start with a complete multivitamin/mineral tablet. Try to find one that includes the nutrients in the preceding list at the suggested levels. You should be able to get something that closely approximates or falls within the various ranges. Nutrients work together, so it is not advisable to take individual supplements unless you are already covering yourself with an "insurance" multi. If your multi is lacking a nutrient, such as calcium (which is common), then add that particular supplement individually to your regime, but take care not to double up. If your multivitamin supplement contains 500 mg of calcium, you need a calcium supplement of only 500 mg. Quasi-nutrients like coenzyme Q10 may not be included in a multi formulation and may be taken as additional fortification, but not in place of your nutritional base.

## CHOOSING SUPPLEMENTS

Vitamin-mineral supplements line the aisles of pharmacies and supermarkets. They can be purchased at specialized health food stores, from catalogues or television, and through direct marketing companies. But are the different brands offered any different? Does the price reflect quality, or will any discount version provide the same nutritional benefits? This is a tough question to answer, and of course there are differing views.

I believe the quality of supplements does vary. Based on three decades of education and experience in nutrition, I am of the opinion that some supplements are better than others, just as is true of any other product. Having said this, it is not always easy to determine which ones excel and which ones are best left collecting dust on the shelf. The claims of "natural," "therapeutic," "organic," "buffered," or "time-released" don't provide realistic clues. Reading the sources of individual nutrients can be confusing even to the biochemically schooled. The vitamins most advertised are not necessarily the best.

Personally, what I do is choose from companies that I know keep abreast of the latest research, use top-quality sources, and provide the balance that is important for optimum absorption and utilization. I also listen to researchers, clinicians, and scientists who recommend products, because I know they have done their homework and use the same criteria that I do for determining quality, effectiveness, and safety. The mass-market brands that I recommend that are widely available in health food stores include Twin Lab, ANR, Thorne, Great Earth, and Shifts. Direct-marketing companies that I have investigated and like include Manatech, Rexall, and Shaklee. An excellent multivitamin formula that is available through the television infomercial market is called Comprehensive. And finally, two cardiologists whom I have quoted in this book offer their own brands: Dr. Stephen Sinatra's is called the Optimum Health Line, and Dr. Julian Whitaker's is Healthy Direction. Phone numbers for both are available in the appendix.

I think it is important to provide you criteria for determining for yourself whether or not a supplement is worth your money. The following will help you understand some basic terms that describe supplements, so it won't seem confusing.

## Natural Versus Synthetic Sources

Whether to by a natural product or a synthetic one is one of the most perplexing issues for a consumer. I know I am easily swayed by a label that advertises anything natural; however, when a vitamin supplement claims to be a *natural* product, the meaning is vague and often deceptive. For the most part, natural products undergo the same processing procedures as the "unnatural" synthetic versions, so except in the case of vitamin E, the distinction really doesn't matter.

Vitamins and minerals are manufactured from plants, yeast, and bacteria, or they are synthesized in a laboratory setting, or in many instances, both methods are used simultaneously. Sometimes only a small amount of an original source is used and processed into what manufacturers then advertise as natural. For example, in many of the natural vitamin C products, about 2 percent is from natural sources and the remaining comes from synthetic derivatives. A rose hip vitamin C is generally 90 percent or more synthetic, yet we are led to believe we are purchasing a natural product. Using pure, natural vitamin C (as is the case for many other nutrients) is not feasible because the end product would be much too large for us to swallow.

A few nutrients are formed by adding a synthetic vitamin or mineral to a yeast or some other natural base. The natural form of selenium, selenomethionine, is created when the synthetic mineral is cultivated in a natural yeast culture. Chromium in its natural form, GTF chromium, is produced this way, as are the B vitamins. They are marketed as natural, but are they really?

For the majority of nutrients, the advertisement ploy that vitamins are natural is meaningless. The one exception is vitamin E. Synthetic formulations of vitamin E have proven to be less effective than the natural d-alpha tocopherol form. The bottom line, when choosing between natural and synthetic, is that with the exception of vitamin E, it really doesn't matter.

## Chelated Minerals

A mineral is *chelated* when it is attached to another substance, usually an amino acid, for the purpose of enhancing its absorption. The reviews on chelation are mixed. Some researchers agree that it works for some nutrients better than for others. It is generally agreed that chromium picolinate, the chelated form of chromium, is better absorbed than some of the other chromium preparations. Two other minerals, iron fumarate and zinc gluconate, are less irritating to the stomach and intestine in chelated form, and thus are less likely to cause stomach distress and constipation than the sulfate forms of these minerals.

The bioavailability of minerals, whether chelated or not, greatly increases when they are taken with a meal. Both proteins and carbohydrates stimulate the release of digestive enzymes and juices that facilitate the breakdown and absorption of all nutrients. An exception to the rule is iron, which is better absorbed on an empty stomach.

## Buffered Vitamins

Acidic vitamins, such as vitamin C, can irritate the digestive tract, especially when taken in large doses. A substance that neutralizes or tempers the strong acidity can be added to counteract these irritating effects. Ascorbate is the buffered form of vitamin C and is much gentler on the stomach than pure ascorbic acid. Note: people who have been told to restrict their salt intake should avoid sodium ascorbate.

## Timed-Release Capsules

Timed-release supplements make good sense in theory, but in reality they do not appear to be any better, and may even be less effective, than the standard vitamin preparation. It was thought that if vitamins and minerals were to dissolve at a slower rate in the intestine, more of them would be absorbed and less lost in the urine. Unfortunately, timed-release tablets are not acting according to the theory and are often more poorly absorbed than the regular supplements. In one study with niacin, when both a timed-release and a standard supplement were given to patients with elevated blood cholesterol levels, the standard supplement proved more effective in lowering blood cholesterol than the timed-release one.

## The Values and What They Mean

Different values are attached to the macronutrients (protein, carbohydrates, and fats) and the micronutrients (vitamins and minerals) and can be confusing to the lay person. Since I am often asked what they mean, I will give you a short summary. The body needs vitamins and minerals in varying amounts, and the relative weights of the amounts needed are generally given in metric units.

| UNIT | | APPROXIMATE EQUIVALENT |
|---|---|---|
| kilogram (kg) | = 1,000 g | = 2.2 lb. |
| gram (g) | = 1,000 mg | = 0.04 oz. |
| milligram (mg) | = 1,000 mcg | = 0.00004 oz. |
| ounce (oz.) | | = 28.35 grams |
| pound (lb.) | | = 454 grams |

Sometimes you will see IU listed next to fat-soluble vitamins such as A, E, and D. International Units (IU) do not measure weight; rather, they standardize the biological activity or potency of the vitamin. However, since they can be converted to measurements of weight, you may see amounts of vitamin E, for example, given in milligrams or micrograms. Conversions are different depending on the vitamin.

| FAT-SOLUBLE VITAMIN | WEIGHT AND BIOLOGICAL ACTIVITY | |
|---|---|---|
| Synthetic vitamin E (dl-alpha tocopherol) | 1 mg | = 1.0 IU |
| Natural vitamin E (d-alpha tocopherol) | 1 mg | = 1.49 IU |
| Vitamin D | 1 mcg | = 40 IU |
| Vitamin A (retinol) | 1 mcg | = 3.44 IU |

To confuse you even more, vitamin A can also be measured in retinol equivalents (RE). Sometimes you may see the RDA for vitamin A written as 800 RE or 4,000 IU. The convenient conversion factor varies with vitamin A, depending on whether you are talking about retinol or beta-carotene, but for convenience we often use an average that comes to 1 RE for every 5 IU.

## Miscellaneous Concerns About Supplements

+ Check the expiration date. Vitamins and minerals are relatively stable; however, they will lose their potency if they have passed their listed date. Unfortunately, not all products carry expiration dates, so be wary.

+ Try to spot additional additives and avoid products that include them. Don't pick up vitamins that contain dyes, binders, fillers, or preservatives.

+ Buy products that are packaged in opaque containers that will not permit easy penetration by light. Supplements lose their potency when exposed to light and air, so store them in a cool, dark place and make sure the container is tightly sealed. Don't store them in the refrigerator, where the dampness will damage them.

+ Purchase oil-based vitamins like vitamin E in smaller quantities, because they turn rancid easily. This is also true of cooking oils.

✦ One way of determining the quality of a supplement is by checking for a "USP" designation. The U.S. Pharmacopoeia, an independent, nonprofit body of experts, has provided a standard to determine if a supplement dissolves in a laboratory setting. If a tablet does not dissolve, the body will not absorb it. Not all products have a USP designation, but those that include it are legally responsible to the FDA for quality control. The USP seal of approval does not apply to timed-release supplements.

✦ As a general rule, take nutrients together in one multivitamin/ mineral formula for proper balance. If you require greater quantities because your particular supplement is lacking in an individual nutrient, add as needed. Do not exceed doses suggested in this book unless you are under a doctor's care.

# 16

# HEALTHY BEHAVIORS FOR THE HEART

Whatsoever things are honest,
whatsoever things are just,
whatsoever things are pure,
whatsoever things are lovely . . .
think on these things.

—PHILIPPIANS 4:8

Illness is caused by any number of interrelated factors. For many, heart disease develops after years of destructive dietary practices. For others, the disease may reflect maladaptive emotional behavior and unconscious psychological issues. Your personality, how you feel about life, and the way in which you express your emotions and cope with stress are as critical in causing or preventing heart disease as are high blood pressure, obesity, inactivity, and poor nutrition.

The sad truth is that many of us do not recognize obvious signs that scream out for us to take action. When we are not coping with the multiple stresses of our lives, be they crises or everyday aggravations, our body lets us know in a number of ways. The necessity of heeding these clues is emphasized by cardiologist Dr. Robert Eliot in the title of his groundbreaking book on stress and heart disease, *Is It Worth Dying For?* Dr. Eliot encourages people to pay attention to the various ways stress manifests in their body and behavior. He divides symptoms of stress into three groups: physical, behavioral, and emotional. Consider the following as you examine your diet and lifestyle.

## Physical Signs of Stress

Headaches

Indigestion

Weight gain or loss

Frequent illness

Sexual problems

Insomnia

Nausea

Nervous diarrhea

Constipation

Reliance on self-medication

## Emotional Signals of Stress

Apathy or "the blahs"

Feelings of sadness

Anxiety

Agitation

Insecurity

Sense of worthlessness

Irritability

Denial of problems

Ignoring symptoms

Arrogance

Argumentative or angry nature

Mental fatigue

Difficulty concentrating

Overcompensation

Exaggerating your importance

Working too hard

Feeling suspicious

## Behavioral Patterns that Signal Stress

Avoiding things like work

Keeping to yourself

Neglecting responsibility

Continually being late to work

Poor personal hygiene

Being accident-prone

Finding yourself in debt

Excessive drinking

Overeating

Excessive gambling

Excessive shopping

Sexual promiscuity

## GETTING PROFESSIONAL HELP

If you find yourself mentally checking off several familiar habits as you scan the list of stress signals, and especially if you have been living with them for decades, it behooves you to think about seeking professional help. To continue to repeat unhealthful habits sets you up for disease—if not specifically heart disease, some other disease of the body, mind, or soul.

The first step in Alcoholics Anonymous (AA) and the treatment of all addictions is to admit that you cannot cure yourself. Maybe you have tried and failed many times already and feel that your "weakness" is just who you are, that you are a victim of your genes. Not true. You can change any situation. Many people from all walks of life have proven it over and over again. It takes courage to face some problems head-on, but in the long run it is easier than struggling to mask them or pretending they don't exist.

I understand that therapy is frightening to many people. Spilling your secrets and unraveling your soul can be embarrassing and downright painful. But if you need emotional, psychological, or spiritual guidance, the experience of facing the truth of who you really are can unveil a new life for you and open up a world you never dreamed existed.

Dr. Bruno Cortis, author of *Heart & Soul: A Psychological and Spiritual Guide to Preventing and Healing Heart Disease*, finds that cardiac patients often ignore their own needs and deny themselves the ability to relax, enjoy life, and celebrate their successes. Learning why you are angry, why you can't let people you love into your inner world, and why you replay the same mistakes over and over can be the best gift you ever gave yourself. I know it was for me. My counselor, Carole, once shared with me that the truly saddest people she ever met were the ones who on their deathbed discovered they had never lived an authentic life. No one really knew them, but even worse, they never knew themselves.

Scott Peck, psychiatrist and author of *The Road Less Traveled*, speaks of therapy as the high road to obtaining personal and mental knowledge as well as spiritual growth. It is not a sign of weakness or mental incompetence to seek professional help. We don't hesitate to call for assistance in other areas of our lives. We go to a doctor for medical advice, consult a financial advisor to help us manage our money, and probe spiritual uncertainties with our minister, priest, or rabbi. Likewise, when we suspect our life isn't working for some reason, when our friends haven't been able to solve our problems, and when all the self-help books we have pored over haven't brought about change, it is probably time to consider outside intervention.

It was Gloria Steinem, in her book *Revolution from Within*, who most influenced me at a time when I was searching for answers in my own life. It comforted me to know that a woman who was rated one of the ten most confident women in the world could admit that she really didn't know herself all that well and, in her words, lacked a sense of internal reality. She recognized she had been unconsciously repeating patterns from her early childhood, allowing her past to shape her present behavior. Ms. Steinem's epiphany resonated with me and gave me courage to take steps toward seeking professional advice.

I learned from her, and later on in my own counseling sessions, that each of us has a child from the past lurking under the surface of our consciousness who often directs our everyday adult activities and decisions. Often, the way that innocent being was treated during our early years translates into the way we view ourselves as adults. If there was something missing or dysfunctional taking place in childhood, an unmet need or gigantic hole, it can haunt us and dominate our grown-up behavior until we take action to stop it. The good news is that it is possible to go back and revamp these aberrant behaviors if they are not serving us well as adults. Some individuals can do it on their own by reading good books or through visualization, self-talk, and prayer. Many of us require in-depth guidance to unravel the layers behind our actions. But it can be done. You do not have to remain a victim of your early upbringing. You can change if you want to and have the right person to help you.

When looking for a therapist, ask friends and relatives for references. It isn't easy to find the right fit, so don't be shy about interviewing several until you feel you have found one whom you trust implicitly.

## TEMPERING YOUR TEMPER

Do you frequently explode over insignificant events? Scream at your partner for leaving the toilet seat up? Cut in front of cars on the freeway? Sizzle inside when the line at the market moves too slowly? Grit your teeth when someone at the movies crinkles their candy wrapper? Hyperventilate when your client is half an hour late for an appointment? If you cannot tolerate situations like these, you may be slowly eroding your heart as much as if you were smoking or eating a cube of butter every day.

Anger, whether it is suppressed or ignites into uncontrollable rage, is toxic to the body. Most of the studies on the health consequences of anger grow out of research linking negative emotional behaviors with an increased risk of developing heart disease. It is clear that chronic anger can drive up blood pressure, produce irregular heartbeats, and increase the risk of heart disease. The literature also shows that learning to manage anger halts this detrimental process, so that healing can occur. Cardiologists like Stephen Sinatra, M.D., who offer comprehensive heart-healing workshops, teach people to redirect their inappropriate anger.

Anger has its place in a healthy life and can be a very positive response to any number of situations. When we are being hurt or abused, when our rights are violated, when someone is hurting another or something morally and ethically is not appropriate, we should respond with indignation and speak up. As a rule, women let little things slip by rather than make waves, but when they do speak up, watch out. Clarissa Pinkola Estes, Ph.D., writes in *Women Who Run with the Wolves* that most of the time wolves avoid confrontation, but when they must defend their territory, when something or someone constantly hounds or corners them, they explode. It doesn't happen often, but the ability to express this anger is within their repertoire, and it should be in ours, too. I don't think this suggests that we should withhold our anger until we reach the boiling point, then explode. We all know that this behavior is not healthy for our body or soul. What I think it tells us is that there are instances when an explosive outburst of emotion is appropriate and the best way to handle a situation.

## Learning from Your Anger

The dark emotions that we fight so hard to suppress can teach us about things in ourselves that secretly hover beneath our consciousness. Harriet Lerner, Ph.D., psychotherapist at the Menninger Clinic, tells us that anger can signal that we are not addressing an important emotional issue in our lives, or that too much of our self—our beliefs, values, desires, or ambitions—is being compromised. In her book *The Dance of Anger,* she enlightens us about the subtleties of anger. In analyzing the nature of our feelings of rage, we may discover that we are doing or giving more than we are capable of. Conversely, our anger may warn us that others are doing too much for us, at the expense of our personal growth. Inappropriate anger may reveal a great deal about ourselves and the nature of our relationships with those closest to us. Acknowledging anger can be an important tool that can transform us and foster a stronger sense of self.

Every expert who has written about this subject starts by encouraging us to admit that anger is a problem. Denying that every little incident pushes you over the edge or that you control yourself at a low boil on a regular basis just doesn't work. Dr. Pinkola Estes advises us not to think it is like a kidney stone—if you wait long enough it will pass. It won't. I suspect you have an inkling if anger is infringing on your life and health. Whether you steam in silence or fly off the handle regularly, you must have felt the accelerated heartbeat, rush of blood to the brain, stomach tightening, and general agitation that accompanies such episodes. If you are nodding in agreement, that is a good sign and the first step in changing.

## Identifying Triggers for Anger

Once you have identified the problem, take action by examining the specific situations that trigger your anger. Redford Williams, M.D., psychiatrist and stress researcher at Duke University, advises maintaining a hostility log, a written record of your thoughts, feelings, and actions in relation to specific aggressive outbursts. Keeping a journal allows you to carefully observe the situation and to see the patterns, frequency, and intensity of your outbursts clearly and rationally. Once the information is collected, then you can write an updated conclusion.

## Tempering Techniques

There are many ways of dealing with unbridled anger. One common method used by mental health professionals, called *repetitious internal dialogue*, helps you prepare for recurring episodes. For example, you can write out phrases like "I am a calm person," "I am in control of my life," "I am at peace with the world," or something that you feel would fit your personality and belief system. Some people I know borrow lines and sections from books of poetry or religious writings. Use whatever speaks to you, original words or famous sayings. Write your words or phrases on a small card or in your Daytimer so you don't forget them, and start reciting them daily while you put on your makeup or drive to work. Don't wait until a volatile event presents itself. Prepare your mind in advance.

Another helpful tool is to visualize common situations that make you angry and replay them with an ideal outcome. Imagining yourself in a situation that has occurred before and acting out in your mind how you would like to respond can start the process for change. Biofeedback, meditation, relaxation techniques, and prayer can help to support and accelerate your progress.

Dr. Williams suggests we analyze each angry outburst after it has subsided and our thinking is clearer by asking ourselves if our anger was justified. Sometimes people upset us unintentionally; lashing out at an innocent victim is not appropriate and can also be harmful to a relationship. I remember a time when I was furious with my three-year-old son, Joey, because he watered the inside plants with the outside hose. Was my anger real? You bet! Was it justified? No, he wasn't being malevolent. He was behaving like a typical helpful toddler. Each and every time your anger surges, ask yourself if it is warranted. Recognizing that every incident that spurs your anger isn't a personal affront to you may help temper your reaction. This is tedious work and requires patience and tenacity, but it will pay off.

Many experts suggest that you delay your angry response—not deny it is there, just postpone a reaction. "Count to ten and then count again" is a saying as old as time, and according to an authority on women's stress, Dr. Georgia Witkin, it still works. When you are angry, time gives you a chance to decide on an active, not reactive, response. You can think more clearly once the adrenaline has dropped, and in waiting you can regain a sense of control, something we all need. Breathing deeply while you count is both relaxing and stress reducing, and you can do it any time you feel anxious or unnerved. Delaying a reaction further by writing down your complaint may help in situations where it is not convenient to respond or you are so overwhelmed that you fear a face-to-face confrontation.

## THE RELAXATION RESPONSE

The cure for balancing stress in our lives is (relatively) simple: all we need to do is relax. The problem isn't knowing the answer but implementing it. As much as we would like to work daily meditation or relaxation exercises into our schedules, what happens in the real world is that life, with its interrupting stressors, swallows up our time. Given the amount of stress and tension we experience daily from the minor irritations of life—leaving the sunroof open on the car during the heaviest rain of the season, waiting all day for the plumber when he said he would be at the house in the morning, or forgetting to save two hours of tedious work on the computer—not to mention the devastating, heart-wrenching stress of divorce, illness, and death—guess which one wins out, stress or relaxation?

One way to counter the cumulative effects of stress is to practice relaxation or meditation on a regular basis. Making a habit of relaxation is a great boost to your health. If you are physically ill, specific relaxation techniques have proven helpful. Relaxation has been an integral part of Dr. Dean Ornish's program for reversing heart disease. Joan Borysenko, Ph.D., has shown that many diabetics can cut down on their need for insulin through the use of relaxation techniques. Herbert Benson, the father of the "Relaxation Response" along with his colleagues at the Mind/Body Medical Institute, lists in his book *Timeless Healing* the tremendous diversity of medical conditions that the relaxation response (together with other self-care strategies such as nutrition, exercise, and stress management) can heal or cure. The following is a partial list of some medical conditions that have been alleviated by learning how to relax:

✦ Patients with high blood pressure experienced decreases in blood pressure and were able to discontinue or reduce their medication over a three-year period.

✦ Patients with cardiac arrhythmias experienced fewer of them.

✦ Patients with chronic pain experienced less severity of pain, more activity, less anxiety, less depression, and less anger.

✦ Women suffering from PMS experienced a 57 percent decrease in its severity.

✦ Working people had fewer medical symptoms, fewer days off from work due to illness, improved performance, and lower blood pressure.

The physical effects of relaxation are opposite to those of stress. Practically every reaction is nullified or reversed. Heart rate and blood pressure drop; respiration and oxygen consumption slow down; brain waves move from the alert beta rhythm to a relaxed alpha rhythm; blood flow to the muscles decreases; and more blood is sent to the brain and skin. You feel rested and energized.

To evoke the relaxation response is quite easy, and according to Dr. Benson, it can be achieved using a smorgasbord of techniques, including meditation, prayer, autogenic training, progressive muscular relaxation, jogging, swimming, breathing exercises, yoga, tai chi chuan, chi gong, and if you can believe it, knitting and crocheting. Only two basic steps need to be followed: (1) you need to repeat a word, sound, phrase, or action, and (2) you need to passively disregard everyday thoughts that come to mind (as they will), and return to your repetitive sound or action.

The choice of the focused word or phrase should fit the individual. If you are religious, you might choose a phrase like "The Lord is my shepherd," "Hail, Mary, full of grace," or "Shalom." If you don't have a religious background or leaning, you may select words like "love," "peace," "calm," or "relax." Say whatever seems appropriate and engenders a feeling of peace and wellness.

Relaxation or meditation involves a ten- to twenty-minute exercise of sitting quietly in a comfortable position, closing your eyes, relaxing your muscles, and breathing slowly and naturally as you silently repeat your word or phrase. When thoughts creep in, acknowledge they are there and then let them go. Continue the repetition for a minimum of ten minutes, then sit quietly for a moment before opening your eyes and returning to the real world. Practice this technique once or twice a day, depending on your need.

Most health professionals recommend sitting and closing your eyes, but Dr. Benson says that you can also do it with your eyes wide open and even while you're jogging. He taught runners to meditate as they jogged and found that their bodies actually became more efficient than if they exercised without "help." Before too long, he says, there were small groups of runners and walkers using "aerobic prayer," short prayers in cadence with their steps. I knew somewhere in my soul that jogging had benefits far beyond those of the aerobic variety. Especially when I am alone, I find that while jogging I can totally clear my mind of stress, figure out unresolved issues, and pray for guidance. How about that—I can exercise, pray, and elicit the relaxation response all at one time, a triple threat to stress.

## CRYING FOR TENSION RELEASE

Crying is a powerful healer. It is the most basic form of release the human body has available to disseminate tension resulting from pain or anger. Our first and most continuous sound after birth is a loud, piercing wail. In Dr. Sinatra's healing workshops, he finds that the women and men who cannot cry tend to be the ones with heart disease. Crying is a necessary tool when the heartaches of life put you at risk for heart trouble. Psychoanalyst Alexander Lowen, M.D., writes that crying is the only way for adults to relieve the tension that results from the loss of love, whether it comes from a hurt from long ago or from a present loss. The process of mourning is ineffective in discharging the pain of loss unless it includes sobbing deeply.

Crying is natural healing at its best. It promotes deep breathing, enhances oxygen delivery, and initiates production of the hormones that positively stimulate the immune system. It discharges sadness and anger from the body and frees the heart of muscular tension and rigidity.

Physician and author Christiane Northrup writes that crying is one of the ways in which we rid our bodies of toxins. When we fully release our emotions, our body, mind, and spirit feel cleansed. And, strangely, when we shed tears, insight comes. When we hold back and don't allow ourselves to fully experience our emotions and instead turn to addictive processes such as tranquilizers, alcohol, or even running to get our "high," we actually create hormones (enkephalins) that repress our tears.

Maybe women lag behind men in our incidence of heart attacks not because of hormones but because we allow ourselves to cry. It is possible that our immunity comes not from estrogen but from tears.

## LAUGHTER IS GOOD MEDICINE

Like crying, laughing heals the body by promoting deep breathing and encouraging the distribution of oxygen to all our tissues and cells. It enhances blood flow to the extremities, lowers blood pressure, and improves cardiac function. A good belly laugh releases endorphins, the mood-elevating and painkilling chemicals, as well as the antiaging hormone DHEA. It frees up tension and raises your spirits when you are down. It may be a contributing factor in preventing and treating a host of diseases, including heart disease.

Norman Cousins, adjunct professor at UCLA's School of Medicine, championed the idea that humor is restorative. In his classic book *Anatomy of an Illness As Perceived by the Patient*, he chronicled how a healthy dose of laughter and vitamin C saved him from a nearly fatal collagen disease. His self-prescription of *Candid Camera* videos, Marx Brothers films, and humorous books eased his pain and gave him the additional years of life to write of his discovery. It is largely because of Norman Cousins that researchers and clinicians started taking laughter seriously and began to study its health benefits.

In his book *Anger Kills*, psychiatrist Redford Williams, M.D., explains that learning to laugh is one of the techniques for combating a hostile personality. He and others have identified hostility as one of the toxic emotions that can erode the heart. Given that so much of anger is petty, unjustified, and futile (for instance, what good does it do to get angry in traffic?), hostile people miss out on countless opportunities to laugh. Laughter is the ultimate antidote to all those negative emotions like irritation, frustration, annoyance, and outrage.

One of Dr. Williams's strategies is to laugh at your own feelings of self-importance by "catastrophizing" any situation you have blown out of proportion. For example, when the line at the bank moves at a snail's pace, make up a story about the elderly woman at the head of the line who seems to be transacting a lifetime's worth of financial arrangements. She probably waited outside just for you to come in to make your quick deposit and managed to sneak in ahead of you before you reached the line. Maybe she even set her alarm to make sure she would be early enough so she wouldn't miss you. Don't hold back—embellish, and let your sense of persecution run wild. It will amuse you—and it will also make the time go more quickly.

## EXPRESSIONS OF LOVE

The heart is symbolic of love. All major religions teach that love is the most powerful and the most vital of human emotions. In the

Bible, Paul writes to the Corinthians that the three primary emotions are faith, hope, and love, but the greatest of these is love. It is essential to life, like oxygen; without it we cannot survive. To love others and ourselves unconditionally is the most powerful healing force in the universe.

Since the beginning of time, poets, musicians, and authors have written about the beauty and pain of love. We are very much aware that love is a feeling, but we may not realize that, as a deeply felt human emotion, it elicits a series of physiological reactions within the body whenever we experience or remember a loving moment. Our heart rate jumps, our face turns red, our hands turn clammy, and we often lose the ability to speak coherently and rationally. And this is good thing. It is one of the healthiest ways to get the blood pumping and the oxygen flowing. To feel and express love, whether it is for a friend, family member, or lover, makes us feel elated in the moment and can have lasting positive effects on our physical health.

## Making Friends a Priority

A sense of social support is crucial to the recovery of heart patients. The literature of psychoneuroimmunology is filled with scientific evidence of the direct benefit of social support to patients. Even as little as a hug, a held hand, a pat on the arm, or a warm smile elicits a physiological change in the body that strengthens multiple systems. When people have more social and community ties, they have a stronger immune system and are likely to live longer. Researchers found that elderly women and men who had two or more sources of emotional support lived measurably longer lives after a heart attack than those with no support.

Loneliness predisposes an individual to heart trouble. Dr. James Lynch, founder and director of the Holistic Health Force in New York, extensively studied the importance of social contact in relation to heart problems. After investigating various countries and groups within the United States in which eating habits were less than healthy but the incidence of heart disease fell under the national average, he came to the conclusion that the emotional support from a close-knit community may be the deciding factor. People who channel their energies into loving, caring relationships appear to enjoy *cultural protection* from heart disease.

It is important to the health of your total being to connect with others. Join a service club, church, hiking group, reading club, or any other organization of people who share your interests. Get to know your neighbors, spend time cultivating new friends, volunteer at a local school or hospital, and start connecting with the wonderful people in your community. You will feel better mentally, spiritually, and physically.

## Volunteering Your Time

If you want to experience love in your life, reach out and help someone else. It may sound corny, but it is true. Allan Luks, former executive director of the Institute for the Advancement of Health, analyzed health profiles of people who frequently donate their time helping others and found that they generally experience better health than those who don't involve themselves in working with other people. When analyzing the responses of three thousand volunteers, he also found that over 90 percent of respondents reported immediate, positive physical sensations linked to helping others: exhilaration, strength, and tranquillity. You don't have to wait for the long-term benefits—there are short-term rewards as well.

If you are feeling isolated and alienated from the world, reconnect with other people. If you have never considered enriching your life in this way, start small by offering a few hours of your time a week, and see how it goes. You might start by looking for a service that uses skills you already have (cooking, crafts, math, listening). Follow your heart to help individuals you are particularly drawn to— children, the elderly, the sick, or the homeless. Make sure your volunteer work includes personal contact with individuals who need your help and support.

## Sexual Expressions of Love

Sex, or the expression of sexual desire, is conducive to maintaining a healthy heart. The physical act itself is close to an aerobic activity and has been equated with walking up two long flights of stairs.

During sex, the blood pressure and heart rate rise, breathing acceler-ates, and blood rushes to the extremities, making the skin pink and tingly. Tension builds up until it is ultimately released during orgasm.

Some studies suggest that failing to reach orgasm may have a negative effect on a woman's heart. In one study that surveyed two hundred hospitalized women aged forty to sixty, half of them had had heart attacks and the other half suffered from a variety of other aliments. Among the cardiac patients, 65 percent complained of sexual frigidity and sexual dissatisfaction, compared to 24 percent of the control group. According to Alexander Lowen, M.D., author of *Love, Sex, and Your Heart*, these figures are statistically significant and indicate that a lack of sexual satisfaction should be considered a risk factor for heart disease in women.

If there is a relationship between sexual dysfunction and heart disease, it is difficult to determine whether or not it is a direct causal one. Making love is more than an exercise—it involves a confluence of feelings, passion, fantasy, connection, support, and caring. It is true that married partners have a lowered incidence of heart attacks than single or widowed people, but regular touching and continued intimacy and support could factor just as easily into that equation. This is not to undermine the importance of a healthy sex life, espe-cially considering that unsatisfying sexual relationships often result in feelings of failure and isolation.

For those of you who have had a heart attack or are at risk for heart disease and are afraid of having a heart attack during sex, not to worry. The risk is minimal and does not appear to apply to *legiti-mate* partners. The *Japanese Study of Legal Medicine* in 1963 found that deaths related to sex accounted for only 0.6 percent of sudden deaths in men, and that in most cases the men were with someone other than their wives. Additional circumstances surrounding the deaths: the men were on the average thirteen years older than their female partners, and one-third of them were intoxicated.

## Loving a Pet

Pets are easy to love and hilarious to watch. They force you to laugh even when you have a case of the grumpies. For the most part, they are thrilled by your presence. Dogs always are; cats, birds, and fish you just can't be sure. They listen attentively to your whining, but most important, they love you unconditionally. Aside from the complete and utter enjoyment they offer, pets play a role in preventing and treating heart disease. Throwing a ball for your dog, stroking your cat, or just watching an exotic fish swim through the reeds in an aquarium can take your mind off your problems, force you to relax, and even go beyond that to lower your blood pressure.

Once you have suffered a heart attack, a pet can help restore your health. One study indicated that during the first year after a heart attack, patients not owning pets died at five times the rate of pet owners. The kind of pet was unimportant—dog or cat, fish or bird—even an iguana was listed as a potential pet. The authors suggested that the protection conferred by this relationship did not have so much to do with the love offered by the pet but rather stemmed from the patient's act of showing love and affection to the animal. I'm not sure how they arrived at this conclusion, since the love and attention received from an animal can be as powerful a force for healing. As I understand it, love is best when it is reciprocal, and usually with pets this is the case.

## GETTING IN TOUCH WITH YOUR SPIRITUAL SIDE

One's spiritual life has a profound influence on physical and emotional health. In a comprehensive review of the scientific literature on the medical effects of spiritual experiences collected by Dr. Dale Matthews and colleagues and reported in *The Faith Factor*, the investigators found that religious factors were correlated with reduced blood pressure and improved quality of life for patients with heart disease and cancer. Spirituality also increased the patients' survival rate; reduced alcohol, cigarette, and drug use; and reduced anxiety, depression, and anger. The greater the person's commitment to some kind of god, religion, or higher power, the better their health profile. This is not to say that if you join a monastery or become a nun you will necessarily experience abundant health for the rest of your life. It merely suggests a link between believing in something higher than yourself and a generally improved physical health.

Although it is beyond the scope of this book to discuss this in detail, I want to introduce the very ancient concept that the body, mind, and spirit are intertwined and when one area is skewed, disease in all areas is probable. Dr. Bruno Cortis, in his book *Heart & Soul*, introduces his readers to the possibility that having a heart problem is a spiritual wound as well as a physical wound, and that you cannot heal the physical heart without first attending to the spiritual heart. As he so eloquently describes it, "clearing the channels of spirituality is equivalent to opening the heart's arteries."

Finding our spiritual part—our soul or God or Higher Power, or whatever you want to call it—is a journey we all face. It starts like anything else: being open to learning and receiving the wisdom that is available. If this concept is new to you, but you want to investigate what's out there, you can start reading books about various religions and denominations, visit local places of worship, look into religious texts, participate in weekend retreats, and talk to other people about their faith. There is a saying: "When the student is ready, the teacher will appear."

In the comments and examples about religions that follow I have drawn on my Christian background and beliefs. I considered providing references to other religions, but because I feel I don't have the necessary familiarity to do so, I have stayed with what I know. Please understand that I don't suggest the Christian way is the only way, and that I hope you will apply the spirit of the examples to your own faith, belief, or religion—whatever it may be.

## It Pays to Go to Religious Services

No matter what their age or their ethnic or religious affiliation, individuals who regularly attend some form of worship service tend to be healthier and live longer than folks who shun organized religion. Epidemiologist William Strawbridge and his colleagues at the Public Health Institute analyzed almost three decades' worth of data on about five thousand Californians, predominantly Christians, although not all professed to be practicing. Those who attended weekly church services regularly experienced lower death rates than people who went to church occasionally or not at all. The researchers noted that regular congregation members who admitted to having bad health habits were more likely to make changes like cutting back on alcohol, quitting smoking, exercising more, becoming socially active, and staying married than were the infrequent churchgoers. Health professionals are always looking for inventive ways to motivate people to change their habits. It looks like joining an organized religious group is one definite answer.

It has been suggested that the reason for lower blood pressure rates and generally healthier profiles among religious people is that they drop the vices that aggravate these conditions. As I have mentioned, this is often the case, but it isn't necessarily true. Church attendance can lower your blood pressure even if you smoke. David Larson, president of the National Institute for Healthcare Research, conducted a research study that showed that smokers who go to church at least once a week are four times less likely to have high blood pressure than smokers who rarely attend. Moreover, Larson's research team found that smokers who say that religion is integral to their lives are seven times less likely to display hypertension than smokers who do not consider religion important. Larson reports that "the influence of spirituality on blood pressure is large enough to lower one's risk of cardiovascular disease by as much as 10 to 20 percent, which is enough of a difference to affect whether or not someone is put on medication."

## Prayer

There is an expanding body of evidence that confirms that prayer can be included on the list of complementary approaches to healing. The world of science is now reporting that prayer positively affects high blood pressure, wounds, heart attacks, headaches, and anxiety. The science is so strong that Dr. Larry Dossey has concluded, "not to employ prayer with my patients was the equivalent of deliberately withholding a potent drug or surgical procedure."

I wonder why this comes as such a shock to many people. From the beginning of time, faith and healing have been considered interrelated. The Bible is rich with proverbs uniting the body, mind, and spirit. We read "A merry heart doeth good like medicine, but a broken spirit drieth the bones" (Proverbs 17:22). This is not a revolutionary thought, but it does seem to have shaken the medical community, which in our culture has traditionally adhered to the separation of science and spirituality.

Science is founded on an analytical process of watching what happens in a controlled situation, drawing conclusions, and then replicating those conclusions with additional studies. This doesn't sound like something that is amenable to prayer, but some renegade researchers in the land of white coats and lab rats must have thought otherwise, because there are innumerable papers describing the scientific aspects of the power of prayer. Larry Dossey, M.D., one of the first clinicians who probed the medical literature, found that over one hundred experiments had been conducted on the efficacy of prayer, many under stringent laboratory conditions that even scientists couldn't fault.

The landmark study that generated interest in prayer was conducted by cardiologist Randolph Byrd in 1984 and published four years later. This particular test was important because it used the classic methodology known as a randomized, double-blind, controlled setting for intervention and evaluation.

Byrd examined the effects of intercessory prayer on 393 patients admitted to a coronary care unit at San Francisco General Hospital. Over a ten-month period, some of the participants were prayed for by an at-home prayer group of five to seven individuals, and the others were not. Neither the doctors, nurses, nor subjects knew which group the patients were in. Prayer groups were given the first names of their patients as well as a brief description of each patient's condition and diagnosis. They were asked to pray each day but not offered details as to how they were to do it or what they were to say. By the end of the study, patients in the group that received prayers were five times less likely to require antibiotics; they were three times less likely to develop pulmonary edema (a condition in which the lungs fill with fluid as a consequence of the failure of the heart to pump properly); none of them required endotracheal intubation (an artificial airway made in the throat); and fewer of them died. Pretty impressive, if you are skeptical about prayer.

So, if we want to make use of this information and use prayer to heal our hearts, how exactly do we go about it? And how do we know if we are doing it right? After reading evaluations of the various studies, it appears it doesn't really matter. In the Byrd study, the praying participants were told only to pray, not given instructions and not asked about the methods they employed. Dr. Herbert Benson's extensive research with the relaxation response showed the versatility of the spoken technique. You can repeat a word, phrase, or prayer—whatever your suits your personality. To even suggest there is a single right way to pray, Dr. Benson felt, would disenfranchise people and result in prayer dropouts.

Most people who pray have learned in the context of a religion. Some use formal, soliloquylike prayers; others prefer repetitious words and phrases that help them clear their mind of everyday distractions. Some just talk to God as they would normally speak to their father, mother, or dear friend. Some people pray to a personal God or Supreme Being, some to Jesus, and others to saints. Prayer can be very private. Christ recommended going into your closet to pray (they must have had walk-ins in those days). Prayer may be offered publicly in churches and synagogues, at Thanksgiving dinners, and in homes each night before dinner. People form small groups to pray for each other's daily concerns, and they come together in prayer when a family member is precariously ill, as my family did when my daughter grew a lemon-sized tumor on her spinal cord.

Dr. Larry Dossey, who has studied the effects of prayer and also uses it in his practice, writes that both directed and nondirected prayer is effective in creating change. A directed prayer is stated with a specific outcome in mind. For example, "Please let my daughter's tumor be benign," or "Give my father strength to survive the surgery." A nondirected prayer carries a more general tone, like "Whatever is best" or "Thy will be done." I guess the bottom line is that it doesn't matter how you do it—it only matters that you do it.

## MAKING PEACE WITH YOUR WEIGHT

Most of us who fall into the menopausal category have dieted a good portion of our lives. Our weight has fluctuated up and down like a seesaw as we have attempted weird weight-loss schemes that have promised us unrealistic results. When will it end? When are we finally going to decide on a healthy weight range and stop obsessing about each and every pound? We are older now, and, one hopes, wiser, so why don't we make peace with our bodies? If we are creeping close to the obesity range, then we do need to take action, but what if we are just not where we were twenty years ago? Is that a good enough reason to go back to carrot sticks and cottage cheese? I don't think so. Actually, I don't think we should ever, ever go back in time to the ultra low fat, low-calorie diets. They weren't healthy then, and they are still healthy and doomed to fail.

The aging female body is faced with a set of hormonal changes that make weight loss even more of a challenge. Skimping on food for decades further aggravates the situation. The harder we try to whittle down portions, the more futile our efforts seem to be. The hormonal situation that we face can be dealt with, but not in the same way we did in our earlier years. Have you noticed, during the midlife years, that many aspects of our lives must be approached from a new perspective? If you are feeling frustrated about losing extra pounds, read *Outsmarting the Midlife Fat Cell* by Debra Waterhouse, M.P.H., R.D. Her explanation of what is going on with fat cells at menopause is very helpful and encouraging.

Not everyone agrees that a thin person is healthier than one with a little extra padding. Dr. Rueben Andres, clinical director of the National Institute on Aging, contends that adults who fatten up a bit as they age live longer than those who lose weight. We probably all have different definitions for "a bit." To me it means five, maybe ten pounds higher than what we considered our normal weight in our thirties, and this would also depend on where we were on the weight scale two decades ago and on our body type.

Fitness is a better indicator of longevity and radiant health than is thinness. Research coming out of the famous Cooper Institute for Aerobics in Texas has shown that thin people who are out of shape are three times more likely to die prematurely than heavier people who are in shape. So, just because someone looks sleek in tight jeans doesn't mean they are necessarily healthier than those who sport an elastic waistband.

Losing weight is tough any time, whether you do it to improve your health or to look better in slacks. Experts are continually coming up with new diets to make it easy, yet 98 percent of the people who lose weight regain it. Just so we don't keep making the same mistakes, let's take a look at a few individuals who have been successful and see what works for them. There is no one way to lose weight. Different programs work for different people. But what are some of the common denominators that we can start with in determining what will work best for us?

One prevalent practice that I absolutely do *not* recommend because of its potential for harm is diet pills. They may help temporarily, but they have been proven to be ineffective over time. Researchers compiling a National Weight Registry surveyed almost eight hundred people who had kept off a minimum of 30 pounds for at least one year and discovered that only 4 percent of them used pills. Registered dietician Anne Fletcher located more than two hundred people who had kept their weight off for at least three years and found out that, although some had tried weight-loss drugs, virtually none were helped in the long run by the pills. Please do not consider taking diet pills to lose weight.

Dr. Judith Stern, professor of nutrition at the University of California at Davis, studied women dieters and established common behaviors among those who were successful and those who were not. The women who could not maintain their lowered weight shared similar behaviors. They limited their approach to one aspect of weight loss—watching what they ate. Exercise did not factor into their plan, nor did they endeavor to develop new behavioral skills such as conquering cravings. Interestingly, the unsuccessful group shared other common traits. They struggled not only with overeating but also with overdoing. These women overloaded their days with tasks, had a difficult time delegating responsibilities, and found it impossible to relax. Sound familiar?

The women who enjoyed long-term success learned an entire array of new habits that extended beyond what they ate for breakfast, lunch, and dinner. As you might expect, both groups took in fewer calories (there is just no way to get around this one), but the difference lay in the fact that the successful women started and continued exercising regularly, and they also learned individual ways of handling stress and dealing with food cravings.

Focus on foods that encourage good health and establish a realistic diet for life. Figure out what you have been eating, and start to incorporate nutrient-rich foods into your eating plan as you slowly minimize the food that drains your energy and health. Move your body more in the course of your daily activities, and begin any type of regular exercise that sounds appealing and you know you will continue. If you need help with uncontrollable eating, admit it and seek counseling.

## MOVING YOUR BODY

Your body was designed to move. The less active you are, the greater your risk of heart disease. As activity levels increase, heart disease risk decreases. It is as simple as that. Your heart is a muscle, and like all muscles it needs exercise, so be good to your heart and move your body.

### A Little Exercise Extends Life

Researchers wholeheartedly agree that any physical activity is health promoting. The debates heat up around what type of exercise to engage in and how much time should be devoted to it to get results. For those of you who think that you have to sweat for hours to achieve any reward, rest easy; even a little exercise can lengthen your life. It's like putting money in the bank: whatever you deposit in terms of activity, you will earn interest in years added to your life.

A study conducted at the Cooper Institute for Aerobics Research in Dallas involving both women and men showed that brisk walking for thirty to sixty minutes a day is all it takes to reduce the risk of dying from heart disease. According to the study's director, Dr. Stephen Blair, the walk doesn't have to last a full hour. You can split the time into two shorter walks and still experience a significant benefit. Dr. Blair stresses that anything you do to increase your activity level will extend your life, from extra steps around the mall to light gardening to taking the stairs instead of the escalator.

### Aerobics Strengthen the Heart

Most experts agree that aerobic activities, defined as exercises that increase the heart rate and breathing (at a labored intensity, for a minimum of twenty minutes) and are practiced regularly (three to four times a week), go a step further to condition the heart. When you engage in activities that use the large muscles, such as brisk walking, hiking, jogging, bicycling, aerobic dance, or cross-country skiing, your body goes through a series of chemical changes that directly strengthen the heart as well as contribute to your overall health. An aerobic activity forces your entire circulatory system to work more efficiently and helps to maintain the elasticity of your arteries. After a few months, your resting heart rate drops (which is a sign of fitness), your blood pressure falls, and your blood cholesterol profile changes favorably.

Side effects from continuous aerobic exercise include more energy, greater self-confidence, restful sleep, and improved moods. It also builds muscle while chipping away at fat, protects our bones from osteoporosis, maintains blood sugar levels, and normalizes hormones during erratic months or, for some of us, years, as we go through menopausal changes. The way the entire body responds to exercise offers us a better quality of life on a daily basis, which I think far outweighs the additional years we are told we can expect with regular exercise. To live each day feeling more alive and alert is to me a greater advantage than extending the number of days I will live, especially if I am not healthy.

Moderate exercise protects your heart in several ways:

+ It improves circulation.

+ It reduces high blood pressure.

+ It raises HDL cholesterol levels.

+ It lowers LDL cholesterol as well as triglyceride levels.

+ It decreases the stickiness of blood platelets, making it harder for clots to build up.

+ It burns fat, which helps in controlling and maintaining weight.

+ It helps control diabetes and insulin sensitivity.

+ It helps provide an outlet for stress and relieves depression.

For optimum benefit, it is suggested that you spend about four hours a week doing some aerobic work for a minimum of fifteen to twenty minutes at a time. You also want to make sure you are doing it hard enough that your breathing is somewhat labored, but not so hard that you can't maintain a conversation. Many books will teach you how to determine your specific target range, or you can learn this if you join a gym. If you haven't participated in any aerobic exercise before, take it slowly and work up to the twenty minutes. Most people quit their programs prematurely because they push too hard too soon. Build up your endurance and tolerance. Don't scare your body by inflicting pain. It will scream at you and then you will drop out, vowing never to exercise again. Unfortunately, many of us make the same mistakes when we are trying to diet: we take extreme measures, get discouraged, and stop. Make small changes, slowly. That's what works.

## Strength Training

During the last few years, working out with free weights or machines has gained a glowing reputation as studies confirm that it builds bone, improves the cholesterol profile, controls weight, decreases the risk for diabetes, enhances flexibility and balance, and relieves arthritis symptoms. It is important to add that most of these studies were conducted not with young, supple, athletic bodies, but on individuals past their so-called prime. Bodybuilding has come a long way from Arnold Schwarzenegger torsos to include young and midlife women and little gray-haired ladies who just want to look and feel as good as they can.

Strength training is especially good for women. We need to prevent muscle atrophy, which occurs naturally with aging, and the only way to do it is to work all the muscles of the body. Strength training can include free weights or weight machines at the gym or body-strengthening classes. It is essential that you have qualified instruction before venturing out on your own. It is very easy to hold the weight wrong or execute the move incorrectly. Good instruction is a must. Two to three days a week for half an hour is adequate for weight training. It is also best if you take a day off in between. Since this particular type of exercise can cause your blood pressure to rise, if you have hypertension, check with your doctor before starting.

Stretching is imperative before and after aerobic exercises and working out with weights, and it is good to do all by itself. It is always included in the classes I attend, and I have done it for so long that I know to stretch before and after I jog or hike. The gentle stretches of yoga, tai chi, and other Eastern exercises are likewise good for the body and soul.

There are many ways to go with exercise. Obviously, one size does not fit all. The trick is to find something that you will do on a regular basis and to have fun doing it. Try different things before giving up. Just because you once went to a class that you hated doesn't mean you shouldn't give another teacher, gym, or club a chance. Be open to finding something that will work for you. If you have had a heart attack, talk to your doctor before starting any exercise program.

Maybe you are not ready yet to entertain the idea of a strict routine. If this is the case, remember that any physical activity that you enjoy is beneficial, including walking, taking the stairs, vigorous gardening, or cleaning the house. All of them help you keep fit.

## BEING GOOD TO YOURSELF

Life is too short to waste. It isn't always apparent that we are pilfering our precious moments as we go about the business of life. Oftentimes it takes a shock like an illness or accident, to jar us into reality. The threat of a heart attack can initiate a major growth in our lives. It may be a gift that allows us to make the lifetime changes that we have thought about for several years. Rachel Naomi Remen, M.D., one of the early pioneers in developing a psychological approach to people with life-threatening illnesses, tells us that times of crisis are times of discovery, periods during which we cannot maintain our old ways of doing things and enter into a steep learning curve. We may be forced to learn about something we don't care to learn about; nevertheless, it is an opportunity to reevaluate what we are doing in our daily activities that is fostering ill health.

If you have been jolted into reality by a heart attack, my guess is you are already in the throes of reevaluating your priorities. You are probably making blanket promises to change the way you eat, exercise, lose weight, stop smoking, and anything else you think could help your heart condition. This is great, but as you plunge into major life changes, I would also suggest that you look at the small things you do on a daily basis that give you pressure and try to do things that will add to your enjoyment, fun, and creativity.

This advice is not only for those who have faced death—it is for all of us who get so caught up in the business of work, family, and friends that we forget to take time for ourselves. I think we lose touch with who we are when we don't pull back from the craziness of the world and examine what it is that fills our soul.

One of my favorite books of all time is *Gift from the Sea* by Anne Morrow Lindbergh. Since my husband gave it to me twenty years ago, I make it an annual practice to reread it, and each time, something new strikes me. One thing that has hit home at many stages of my life is that women are traditionally taught that we are always available to give away our time when there is a need. Don't we all jump when someone asks for help, whether or not we have the energy or experience to provide it? Not that this isn't a admirable trait, but taken to the extreme, it can be destructive to our health.

The words of Anne Lindbergh ring as true today as they did when she penned them in 1955. She writes, "Eternally woman spills herself away in driblets to the thirsty, seldom being allowed the time, the quiet, the peace, to let the pitcher fill up to the brim." She continues, "we are hungry and not knowing what we are hungry for, we fill up the void with endless distractions always at hand—unnecessary errands, compulsive duties, social niceties. And for the most part, to little purpose."

How do we get off the merry-go-round of endless chores and find real meaning in life? Obviously, we have to make a conscious choice to do it. If we wait for the right time or think we will do it when life slows down, it may never happen. As busy as you are this week, carve out a chunk of uninterrupted time and think about what truly enriches your life—what adds meaning and purpose to your life and what activities, people, and practices enhance or detract from that purpose. It is much easier to uncover the harmful practices that destroy our physical body than those that erode our mental and spiritual health. But taking emotional and soulful inventory is as vital to our hearts as evaluating our diet and lifestyle habits.

"If you want your life to come together, you have to start treating yourself better"—so says Sarah Ban Breathnach in *Simple Abundance*. How are you treating yourself? What is missing from your hectic life that you have been neglecting or saving for the future when you have more time? Ms. Breathnach suggests making a list of ten nice things you could do for yourself, and then picking one and doing it. Do you need a nudge to spur your imagination? How about reading a new novel, taking dance lessons, learning to play the piano, cultivating house plants, starting a vegetable garden, cross-country skiing, soaking in a bubble bath, getting a facial or a massage? I could go on, but if you need more ideas, pick up Jennifer Louden's *The Woman's Comfort Book*. It is loaded with suggestions.

## CONSIDERING YOUR OPTIONS

Are you a bit dazed by all this information about maintaining or reconstructing a healthy heart? It may be a bit daunting, so take some time to digest what you have read before jumping into a program that might be overly ambitious. It is easy for many of us to read a new book and then attempt too many changes too soon. What ultimately follows is discouragement, failure, and a return to old habits. So I am asking that you not run out to the grocery store and stock up on foods that are unfamiliar to you, or buy a year's supply of expensive vitamins. Rather, take some time to analyze your risk factors, notice what and how you eat, and mull over other lifestyle habits that may not be serving you well.

If you have thumbed through this book looking for the menus and a list of foods that you are supposed to follow each and every day in order to maintain a healthy heart, hunt no further; they are not included. Writing out daily food plans is popular, but while a perfectly designed daily diet appears to be simple and certainly looks impressive on paper, I find that in the long run, it is not practical or appropriate. One solitary plan cannot take into account everyone's likes and dislikes, nor their specialized nutritional needs.

We are all so different. Some are vegetarians, while others love beef and would never consider eliminating it from their diet. Many of you are open to experimenting with tofu and tempeh, but there are also women who resent anything remotely healthy. A large percentage of people dine almost exclusively in restaurants, and most dietary plans do not make allowances for eating outside the home.

I have provided a structure, an outline of foods and servings, and now you can figure out how to rearrange your present eating routine to include as many of the health-giving foods as you possibly can. Throughout the book, I have offered a variety of suggestions for each food group. When it is clear to you that you are not going to realistically reach the ideal recommendation in a specific area, then go directly to plan B and supplement.

Some doctors advocate changing your entire way of eating to follow their "perfect" diet. Given the threat of death, many of us would try anything—for a while. And I must interject here that if you are that rare individual who has totally changed your diet overnight or feel sure you could do so, more power to you; it's just not the norm. The numbers of people who deny all their favorite foods forever remain tiny compared to those who are helped by slowly making a few alterations, getting used to them, and moving on to a few more. There are times in our lives when more stringent dietary plans may be indicated. If you have just suffered a heart attack or some other condition that calls for extreme therapeutic measures, then you must follow the advice of your doctor. When your body normalizes and you are allowed a greater variety of food options, you can then make you *life plan* for health.

How diligent you are about your heart-healthy diet depends a great deal on how many risk factors you have. Therefore, let us first take a look at where you are, before going on to your action plan.

## GAUGING YOUR RISKS

Look over the following list and see if your risks are few or multiple. It goes without saying that the more items you check, the more careful you need to be about your food intake.

## Examining My Own Risk Profile

(Place a check in the blank to indicate yes.)

# Physical Risk Factors

Are you menopausal or older than 50? ____

Have you given birth to more than five children? ____

Did you start menopause before age forty-five, either naturally or by hysterectomy? ____

Are you more than twenty pounds over your ideal weight? ____

Are you shaped more like an apple than a pear? ____

Are you under 4'11" tall? ____

Did your parents or siblings die prematurely from a heart attack? ____

Do you have any congenital defects or existing heart conditions? ____

Are you diabetic? ____

Are you insulin-resistant? ____

Do you have high blood pressure? ____

Do you have high total cholesterol? ____

Do you have high triglyceride levels? ____

Do you have high LDL levels? ____

Do you have low HDL levels? ____

Do you have periodontal disease? ____

Have you had any abnormal medical tests?

    Uric acid (high)? ____

    Fibrinogen levels (high)? ____

    Hematocrit level (high)? ____

    Homocysteine level (high)? ____

    Lipoprotein(a) (high)? ____

## Emotional Risks

Are you continually stressed? _____

Are you clinically depressed? _____

Do you find yourself feeling angry several times a week? _____

Do you keep to yourself and avoid social involvement? _____

Do you live alone? _____

During the past year, have you lost a significant person in your life? _____

Is your primary subject of conversation yourself and your problems? _____

Do you feel you have little control over your life? _____

Do you have unresolved hurts from your childhood that you are afraid to confront? _____

Are you sexually unfulfilled? _____

## Lifestyle and Dietary Risks

Do you smoke or live with someone who does? _____

Do you drink more than three glasses of alcohol a day or none at all? _____

Do you move your body as little as possible? _____

Does fat comprise more than 30 percent of your diet? _____

Do you eat a lot of fried foods, frozen dinners, or cream sauces? _____

Do you snack on cookies, chips, and gooey desserts? _____

Do you often eat fatty cuts of meat (like prime rib and steak)? _____

Do you eat fried chicken, chicken with skin, or chicken nuggets? _____

Do you frequently eat at fast-food restaurants? _____

Do you eat fewer than two fruits a day? _____

Do you eat fewer than four vegetables a day?          _____

Do you rarely eat anything that is green, orange, or
yellow?          _____

Do you go for white bread, pasta, and rice?          _____

Do you drink more than nine cups of caffeine a day?     _____

Do you rarely drink water?          _____

This is not a test, but if you have checked over a third of these
items, then you need to be concerned about what you might be
doing in your life that is harming your body. Maybe you feel fine.
That makes it all the more difficult to change, but your heart health
is at risk. Make the changes now, before your body starts sending
you physical signals.

## DIETARY GUIDELINES

The following is a summary guideline of the foods and the amounts
recommended for a healthy diet, based on the research mentioned
in the book. Please go through and compare your daily or weekly
average with the ideal.

### Dietary Guidelines

| TYPE OF FOOD | DAILY OR WEEKLY SERVINGS | 1 SERVING EQUALS | EXAMPLES |
|---|---|---|---|
| Lean meats, poultry | 2 or fewer/day | 3 oz. cooked | Lean cuts with visible fat and skin removed; broiled, roasted, or baked; beef round steak, flank steak, chicken and turkey breast |
| Fish | 2/week | 3 oz. cooked | Broiled, baked, grilled; cod, flounder, halibut, sole, salmon, tuna |
| Eggs | up to 4/week | 1 egg | Hard-boiled, poached, scrambled, omelet, frittata |
| Milk, yogurt, cheese | 2–3 servings/ day | 1 cup milk or yogurt; 1½ oz. cheese | Skim or 1% milk, skim or low-fat buttermilk; nonfat or low-fat yogurt; part-skim mozzarella cheese, nonfat cheese |
| Beans, peas, legumes | 4–5 servings/ week | ½ cup cooked legumes | Kidney, red, black, pinto, lima, garbanzo beans; lentils |

| Nuts, seeds | 2–3 servings/ week | ³/₄ oz. or ¹/₆ cup nuts 1 tbsp. seeds | Almonds, filberts, mixed nuts, peanuts, walnuts, pecans, sunflower seeds |
|---|---|---|---|
| Soy | 2–5 servings/ week | 1 cup soy milk ¹/₂ cup tofu/tempeh ¹/₂ fresh soybeans ¹/₂ cup soy flour | Miso soup, soy or tofu burger, texturized vegetable protein |
| Cereals, rice, pasta or grains | 7–8 servings/ day | ¹/₂ cup cooked cereals, rice, or pasta 1 slice bread | Whole-grain breads, pita, English muffin, bagel, grits, oatmeal, corn, barley, millet, buckwheat |
| Fruits | 4–5 servings/ day | 1 med., ³/₄ cup juice, ¹/₂ cup canned, ¹/₄ cup dried | Apples, bananas, grapes, oranges, grapefruit, mangoes, melons, peaches, pineapples, prunes, raisins, strawberries |
| Vegetables | 4–5 servings/ day | 1 cup raw, leafy, ¹/₂ cup cooked, ³/₄ cup juice | Tomatoes, potatoes, carrots, peas, squash broccoli, turnip greens, kale, collards spinach, artichokes, sweet potatoes |
| Added oils, fats | 2–3 servings/ day | 1 tsp. oil butter, soft margarine, or regular mayo; 1 tbsp. low-fat mayo, regular salad dressing, or flaxseed; 2 tbsp. light salad dressing | olive or canola oil, soft margarine, low-fat salad dressings |

## DESIGNING YOUR STRATEGY

Writing goals down is helpful in creating change. Carolyn Myss, Ph.D., author of *Why People Don't Heal and How They Can*, says that every positive choice you make is a good one and activates a new current of energy in your body. You don't have to turn your life upside-down to start on a spiral to good health. Small changes can be highly effective in and of themselves; moreover, one tiny alteration can provide the inspiration and strength to take another step.

I am going to outline guidelines for effecting change. Don't just read through the following questions; participate by jotting down the answers as you see them right now. The points that stand out or strike a chord are probably the areas most in need of attention.

## A Twelve-Step Question-and-Answer Guide for Rebuilding and Maintaining a Healthy Heart

Commit to health: The fact that you are reading a health book is proof of your intention, but good intentions are not enough—you need to act. What is one thing that you can do today to start on a healthier road?

◆ What in your diet needs attention?

Saturated fat      _____

Total fat      _____

Fiber      _____

Fruits      _____

Vegetables      _____

Protein      _____

Portion sizes      _____

◆ What are your major nutritional nightmares?

Do you need additional supplementation?

Multivitamin and mineral tablet      _____

Calcium/magnesium      _____

Others      _____

◆ What heart-healthy foods could you easily incorporate into your present diet?

Fish      _____

Whole grains      _____

Soy      _____

Fruits      _____

Vegetables      _____

Garlic      _____

Green tea      _____

Others      _____

✦ What foods most need to be minimized in your diet?

Excess red meats          _____

Sweets          _____

Salt          _____

High-fat snacks          _____

Fried foods          _____

High-fat cheese          _____

Others          _____

✦ How can you generally increase your activity level?

✦ What regular exercise are you willing to commit to?

✦ Are you generally happy with your life?

✦ Do you involve yourself with other people?

✦ Are you attending to your spiritual needs?

✦ Do you need additional help (reading material, support group, or professional counseling)?

## A VISUAL AID

On the next two pages is a visual aid that I created while working on this book. I have included it because you may find it useful as a reminder for your healthy heart program. You can photocopy it—use brightly-colored paper, so it catches your attention—and post it on your refrigerator or bulletin board. Add your own comments and emphasis, use the space around the hearts for questions and new ideas. Share it with a friend, or your spouse or partner.

# THE TROUBLED HEART

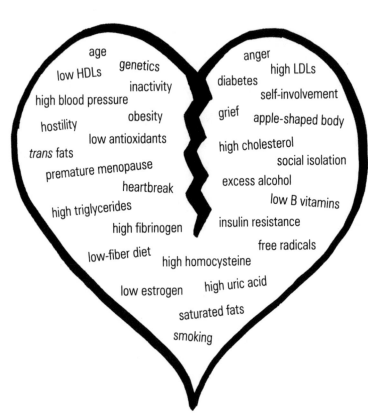

# THE HEALTHY HEART

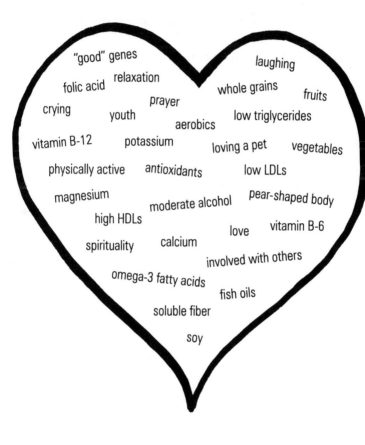

## FINAL THOUGHTS

Heart disease kills women, but with attention to and care for our body, emotions, and spirit, there is solid evidence that we can prevent or postpone it. The more life-preserving habits we follow, the more peace we will experience, knowing we have done what we can. Heart-healthy habits are not just about preventing a future catastrophe; they also help us to live more fully in the moment. And just maybe, that is enough.

*A votre santé* (to your health).

# Appendix A

# BODY MASS INDEX

| BMI | 19 | 20 | 21 | 22 | 23 | 24 | 25 |
|---|---|---|---|---|---|---|---|
| 4'10' | 91 | 96 | 100 | 105 | 110 | 115 | 119 |
| 4'11' | 94 | 99 | 104 | 109 | 114 | 119 | 124 |
| 5' | 97 | 102 | 107 | 112 | 118 | 123 | 128 |
| 5'1" | 100 | 106 | 111 | 116 | 122 | 127 | 132 |
| 5'2" | 104 | 109 | 115 | 120 | 126 | 131 | 136 |
| 5'3" | 107 | 113 | 118 | 124 | 130 | 135 | 141 |
| 5'4" | 110 | 116 | 122 | 128 | 134 | 140 | 145 |
| 5'5" | 114 | 120 | 126 | 132 | 138 | 144 | 150 |
| 5'6" | 118 | 124 | 130 | 136 | 142 | 148 | 155 |
| 5'7" | 121 | 127 | 134 | 140 | 146 | 153 | 159 |
| 5'8" | 125 | 131 | 138 | 144 | 151 | 158 | 164 |
| 5'9" | 128 | 135 | 142 | 149 | 155 | 162 | 169 |
| 5'10" | 132 | 139 | 146 | 153 | 160 | 167 | 174 |
| 5'11" | 136 | 143 | 150 | 157 | 165 | 172 | 179 |
| 6' | 140 | 147 | 154 | 162 | 169 | 177 | 184 |
| 6'1" | 144 | 151 | 159 | 166 | 174 | 182 | 189 |
| 6'2" | 148 | 155 | 163 | 171 | 179 | 186 | 194 |
| 6'3" | 152 | 160 | 168 | 176 | 184 | 192 | 200 |
| 6'4" | 156 | 164 | 172 | 180 | 189 | 197 | 205 |

Height (in feet and inches)

**Weight (in pounds)**

| BMI | 26 | 27 | 28 | 29 | 30 | 35 | 40 |
|---|---|---|---|---|---|---|---|
| 4'10' | 124 | 129 | 134 | 138 | 143 | 167 | 191 |
| 4'11' | 128 | 133 | 138 | 143 | 148 | 173 | 198 |
| 5' | 133 | 138 | 143 | 148 | 153 | 179 | 204 |
| 5'1" | 137 | 143 | 148 | 153 | 158 | 185 | 211 |
| 5'2" | 142 | 147 | 153 | 158 | 164 | 191 | 218 |
| 5'3" | 146 | 152 | 158 | 163 | 169 | 197 | 225 |
| 5'4" | 151 | 157 | 163 | 169 | 174 | 204 | 232 |
| 5'5" | 156 | 162 | 168 | 174 | 180 | 210 | 240 |
| 5'6" | 161 | 167 | 173 | 179 | 186 | 216 | 247 |
| 5'7" | 166 | 172 | 178 | 185 | 191 | 223 | 255 |
| 5'8" | 171 | 177 | 184 | 190 | 197 | 230 | 262 |
| 5'9" | 176 | 182 | 189 | 196 | 203 | 236 | 270 |
| 5'10" | 181 | 188 | 195 | 202 | 207 | 243 | 278 |
| 5'11" | 186 | 193 | 200 | 208 | 215 | 250 | 286 |
| 6' | 191 | 199 | 206 | 213 | 221 | 258 | 294 |
| 6'1" | 197 | 204 | 212 | 219 | 227 | 265 | 302 |
| 6'2" | 202 | 210 | 218 | 225 | 233 | 272 | 311 |
| 6'3" | 208 | 216 | 224 | 232 | 240 | 279 | 319 |
| 6'4" | 213 | 221 | 230 | 238 | 246 | 287 | 328 |

Height (in feet and inches)

**Weight (in pounds)**

# Appendix B

# RESOURCES

## ORGANIZATIONS

**American Heart Association**
National Center
7320 Greenville Avenue
Dallas, Texas 75231
(800) 242-8721
http://www.amhrt.org

**American Diabetes Association**
National Service Center
1006 Duke Street
Alexandria, Virginia 22314
(800) 342-2383
http://www.diabetes.org

**American Dietetic Association**
National Center for Nutrition and Dietetics
216 West Jackson Blvd., Suite 800
Chicago, Illinois 60606-6995
(800) 366-1655
http://www.eatright.org/

**National Heart, Lung, and Blood Institute**
Information Center
P.O. Box 30105
Bethesda, Maryland 20824-0105
(301) 951-3260

**Mind-Body Medical Institute**
Mercy Hospital and Medical Center
Stevenson Expressway at King Drive
Chicago, Illinois 60616-2477
(312) 567-6700

**DASH Diet**
(800) 575-WELL
http://www.dash.bwh.harvard.edu

# NEWSLETTERS

## General Health

*Harvard Health Letter*
P.O. Box 420300
Palm Coast, Florida 32142-0300
(800) 829-9045

*Tufts University Diet & Nutrition Letter*
P.O. Box 57857
Boulder, Colorado 80322-7857
(800) 274-7581

*U.C. Berkeley Wellness Letter*
P.O. Box 420148
Palm Coast, Florida 32142

*Nutrition Action Healthletter*
Center for Science in the Public Interest
1875 Connecticut Avenue, N.W., Suite 300
Washington, DC 20009-5728
http://www.cspinet.org

*Dr. Julian Whitaker's Health & Healing*
Phillips Publishing
7811 Montrose Road
Potomac, Maryland 20854
(800) 777-5005

## Women's Interest

*Dr. Christiane Northrup's Health Wisdom for Women*
7811 Montrose Road
Potomac, Maryland 20854

*Women's Health Advocate Newsletter*
P.O. Box 420235
Palm Coast, Florida 32142-0235
(800) 829-5876

*National Women's Health Network*
1325 G. Street, N.W.
Washington, DC 20005

*Harvard Women's Health Watch*
P.O. Box 420234
Palm Coast, Florida 32142-0234
(800) 829-5921

## Heart Specific

*HeartSense*
Phillips Publishing
7811 Montrose Road
Potomac, Maryland 20854-3394
(800) 211-7643

*Harvard Heart Letter*
P.O. Box 420289
Palm Coast, Florida 32142-9774

## INFORMATION ON NATURAL HORMONES

Women's International Pharmacy (800) 279-5708

Bajamar Women's Health Center (800) 255-8025

Madison Pharmacy Associates (800) 558-7046

## CATALOGUES FOR WOMEN

Transitions for Women (800) 888-6814

As We Change: Marketplace for Women (800) 203-5585

## SUPPLEMENTS FOR THE HEART

Optimum Health Line (800) 304-1708

Healthy Direction (800) 722-8008

## RECIPES FOR HEART AND HEALTH

*The American Heart Association Cookbook*, 5th edn. The American
Heart Association (New York: Ballantine Books, 1994).

*Dr. Dean Ornish's Program for Reversing Heart Disease*. Dean Ornish,
M.D. (New York: Ballantine Books, 1990).

*Estrogen the Natural Way.* Nina Shandler. (New York: Villard, 1997).

*Eat Well for a Healthy Menopause.* Elaine Moquette-Magee. (New York: John Wiley and Sons, 1996).

*Juicing For Life.* Cherie Calbom and Maureen Keane. (Garden City Park, NY: Avery Publishing Group,1992).

*The McDougall Program for a Healthy Heart.* John A. McDougall, M.D. and Mary McDougall. (New York: E. P. Dutton, 1996).

*The Natural Estrogen Diet.* Lana Liew, M.D., with Linda Ojeda, Ph.D. (Alameda, CA: Hunter House, 1998).

*Natural Kitchen: Soy: 75 Delicious Ways to Enjoy Nature's Miracle Food.* Dana Jacobi. (Rocklin, CA: Prima Publishing, 1996).

*Permanent Remissions.* Robert Haas, M.S. and Kristin Massey. (New York: Pocket Books, 1997).

*Recipes for Change.* Lissa DeAngelis and Molly Siple. (New York: Penguin USA, 1998).

*The Simple Soybean and Your Health.* Mark Messina, Ph.D. and Virginia Messina, R.D. with Ken Setchell (Garden City Park, NY: Avery Publishing Group, 1994).

*Super Soy: The Miracle Bean.* Ruth Winter, M.S. (New York: Crown, 1996).

*The 20-Day Rejuvenation Diet Program.* Jeffrey Bland, Ph.D. and Sara H. Benum. (New Canaan, CT: Keats Publishing, 1996).

# References

## Books

Benson, Herbert, M.D. *Timeless Healing: The Power and Biology of Belief.* New York: Simon & Schuster, 1997.

Bland, Jeffrey, Ph.D., with Sara H. Benum. *The 20-Day Rejuvenation Diet Program.* New Canaan, CT: Keats Publishing, 1997.

Bliznakov, Emile, M.D., and Gerald L. Hunt. *The Miracle Nutrient Coenzyme Q-10.* New York: Bantam Books, 1986.

Borysenko, Joan, Ph.D. *Minding the Body, Mending the Mind.* Reading, MA: Addison-Wesley Publishing Company, 1987.

Breathnach, Sarah Ban. *Simple Abundance: A Daybook of Comfort and Joy.* New York: Warner Books, 1995.

Brown, Judith E. *The Science of Human Nutrition.* New York: Harcourt Brace Jovanovich, 1990.

Calbom, Cherie, and Maureen Keane. *Juicing for Life.* Garden City Park, NY: Avery Publishing Group, 1992.

Carlson, Karen J., M.D., Stephanie A. Eisenstat, M.D., and Terra Ziporyn, Ph.D. *Harvard Guide to Women's Health.* Cambridge, MA: Harvard University Press, 1996.

Carper, Jean. *Food—Your Miracle Medicine.* New York: Harper Perennial, 1994.

———. *Miracle Cures.* New York: HarperCollins, 1997.

———. *Stop Aging Now.* New York: HarperCollins, 1995.

Cortis, Bruno, M.D. *Heart & Soul: A Psychological and Spiritual Guide to Preventing and Healing Heart Disease.* New York: Pocket Books, 1995.

Cousins, Norman. *Anatomy of an Illness As Perceived by the Patient.* New York: W. W. Norton, 1979.

Delany, Sarah L., and A. Elizabeth Delany, with Amy Hill Hearth. *Having Our Say.* New York: Bantam Doubleday Dell, 1993.

Dossey, Larry, M.D. *Healing Words: The Power of Prayer and the Practice of Medicine.* San Francisco: HarperCollins, 1997.

———. *Meaning and Medicine.* New York: Bantam Books, 1991.

Eades, Michael R., M.D., and Mary Dan Eades, M.D. *Protein Power.* New York: Bantam Books, 1996.

Eliot, Robert S., M.D., and Dennis L. Breo. *Is It Worth Dying For?* New York: Bantam Books, 1984.

Estes, Clarissa Pinkola, Ph.D. *Women Who Run with the Wolves.* New York: Ballantine Books, 1992.

Friedman, Meyer, M.D., and Ray H. Rosenman, M.D. *Type A Behavior and Your Heart*. New York: Alfred A. Knopf, 1974.

Friedman, Meyer, M.D., and Diane Ulmer, R.N. *Type A Behavior and Your Heart*. New York: Alfred A. Knopf, 1984.

Gittleman, Ann Louise, with J. Maxwell Desgrey. *Beyond Pritikin*. New York: Bantam Books, 1988.

Helfant, Richard H., MD. *Women Take Heart*. New York: G.P. Putnam's Sons, 1993.

Hendler, Sheldon Saul, M.D. *The Doctors' Vitamin and Mineral Encyclopedia*. New York: Simon & Schuster, 1990.

Keys, Ancel B. *Seven Countries: A Multivariate Analysis of Death and Coronary Heart Disease*. Cambridge, MA: Harvard University Press, 1980.

Klesges, Robert C., Ph.D., and Margaret DeBon, M.S. *How Women Can Finally Stop Smoking*. Alameda, CA: Hunter House, 1994.

Kushi, Michio, with Alex Jack. *Diet for a Strong Heart*. New York: St. Martin's Press, 1985.

Lee, John R., M.D. *What Your Doctor May Not Tell You About Menopause*. New York: Warner Books, 1996.

Legato, Marianne J., M.D., and Carol Colman. *The Female Heart: The Truth About Women and Heart Disease*. New York: Avon Books, 1991.

Lerner, Harriet, Ph.D. *The Dance of Anger*. New York: Harper & Row Publishers,1985.

Lindbergh, Anne Morrow. *Gift from the Sea*. New York: Pantheon, 1995.

Louden, Jennifer. *The Woman's Comfort Book: A Self-Nurturing Guide for Restoring Balance in Your Life*. San Francisco: HarperCollins Publishers, 1992.

Love, Susan M., M.D., with Karen Lindsey. *Dr. Susan Love's Hormone Book*. New York: Random House, 1997.

Lowen, Alexander. *Love, Sex and Your Heart*. New York: Macmillan Publishing Company, 1988.

Margen, Sheldon, M.D., and the Editors of the *University of California at Berkeley Wellness Letter*. *The Wellness Encyclopedia of Food and Nutrition*. New York: Rebus, 1992.

Matthews, D. A., et al. *The Faith Factor: An Annotated Bibliography of Clinical Research on Spiritual Subjects*. Vol. 1. John Temple Foundation, 1993.

Messina, Mark, Ph.D., and Virginia Messina, R.D., with Ken Setchell. *The Simple Soybean and Your Health*. Garden City Park, NY: Avery Publishing Group, 1994.

Murray, N.D., and Joseph Pizzorno, N.D. *Encyclopedia of Natural Medicine*. Rocklin, CA: Prima Publishing, 1991.

Myss, Caroline, Ph.D. *Why People Don't Heal and How They Can*. New York: Harmony Books, 1997.

National Women's Health Network. *Taking Hormones and Women's Health: Choices, Risks and Benefits*. Washington, DC: National Women's Health Network, 1995.

Nelson, Miriam E., Ph.D.. with Sarah Wernick, Ph.D. *Strong Women Stay Young*. New York: Bantam Books, 1997

Northrup, Christiane, M.D. *Women's Bodies, Women's Wisdom*. New York: Bantam Books, 1994.

Notelovitz, Morris, M.D., and Diana Tonnessen. *Essential Heart Book for Women*. New York: St. Martin's Press, 1996.

Ornish, Dean, M.D. *Dr. Dean Ornish's Program for Reversing Heart Disease*. New York: Ballantine Books, 1990.

Pashkow, Fredric J., M.D., and Charlotte Libov. *The Woman's Heart Book*. New York: Penguin Books, 1994.

Passwater, Richard A., Ph.D. *Chromium Picolinate*. New Canaan, CT: Keats Publishing, 1992.

Peck, M. Scott, M.D. *The Road Less Traveled*. New York: Simon & Schuster, 1978.

Remen, Rachel Naomi, M.D. *Kitchen Table Wisdom*. New York: Riverhead Books, 1996.

Sachs, Judith. *Natural Medicine for Heart Disease*. New York: Dell Publishing, 1997.

Siegel, Bernie S., M.D. *Peace, Love & Healing*. New York: Harper & Row, 1989.

Simon, Harvey B., M.D. *Conquering Heart Disease*. Boston: Little, Brown and Company, 1994.

Sinatra, Stephen, M.D. *Heartbreak and Heart Disease*. New Canaan, CT: Keats Publishing, 1996.

Steinem, Gloria. *Revolution from Within*. Boston, MA: Little, Brown and Company, 1992.

Tenney, Louise, M.H. *Today's Herbal Health: The Essential Reference Guide*. Pleasant Grove, UT: Woodland Publishing, 1997.

Waterhouse, Debra, M.P.H., R.D. *Outsmarting the Midlife Fat Cell*. New York: Hyperion, 1998.

Whitaker, Julian, M.D. *Is Heart Surgery Necessary?* Washington, DC: Regnery Publishing, 1995.

Whitten, David N., M.D., Ph.D., and Martin R. Lipp, M.D. *To Your Health! Two Physicians Explore the Health Benefits of Wine*. San Francisco: HarperCollins West, 1996.

Williams, Redford, M.D. *The Trusting Heart: Great News About Type A Behavior*. New York: Times Books, 1989.

Williams, Redford, M.D., and Virginia Williams, Ph.D. *Anger Kills*. New York: Harper Perennial, 1993.

Winter, Ruth, M.S. *Super Soy: The Miracle Bean.* New York: Crown Trade Paperbacks, 1996.

Witkin, Georgia, Ph.D. *It Must Be That Time of the Month and Other Lies That Drive Women Crazy.* New York: Penguin Books, 1997.

Wright, Jonathan V., M.D., and John Morgenthaler. *Natural Hormone Replacement.* Petaluma, CA: Smart Publications, 1997

## Selected Journals and Newsletters

## *Chapter 1: Heart Disease Kills Women Too*

Ayanian, John Z., et al. "Differences in the Use of Procedures Between Women and Men Hospitalized for Coronary Heart Disease." *The New England Journal of Medicine* 325 (4): 221–230 (1991).

Chernoff, Ronni. "Baby Boomers Come of Age: Nutrition in the 21st Century." *Journal of the American Dietetic Association* 95: 650–655 (1995).

Fieback, Nicholas H., et al. "Differences Between Women and Men in Survival After Myocardial Infarction: Biology or Methodology?" *The Journal of the American Medical Association* 263 (8): 1092–1096 (1990).

Healy, Bernardine. "The Yentl Syndrome." *The New England Journal of Medicine* 325 (4): 274–275 (1991).

Khan, S., et al. "Increased Mortality of Women in Coronary Artery Bypass Surgery: Evidence for Referral Bias." *Annals of Internal Medicine* 112: 561–567 (1990).

Luscher, T. F. "The Endothelium and Cardiovascular Disease—A Complex Relation." *The New England Journal of Medicine* 330 (15): 1081–1083 (1994).

Maynard, Charles, et al. "Gender Differences in the Treatment and Outcome of Acute Myocardial Infarction." *Archives of Internal Medicine* 152: 972–976 (1992).

Patlak, Margie. "Women and Heart Disease." *FDA Consumer* 28 (9): 7–10 (November 1994).

Prior, Jerilynn. "Correspondence." *The New England Journal of Medicine* 326: 705–706 (1992).

Rich-Edwards, et al. "The Primary Prevention of Coronary Heart Disease in Women." *The New England Journal of Medicine* 332: 1759–1766 (1995).

Steingart, Richard M., et al. "Sex Differences in the Management of Coronary Artery Disease." *The New England Journal of Medicine* 325: 226–230 (1991).

Tobin, N.J., et al. "Sex Bias in Considering Coronary Bypass Surgery." *Annals of Internal Medicine* 107: 19–25 (1987).

"Top Ten Medical Advances of 1995," *Harvard Health Letter* 21 (5): 6 (March 1996).

Wenger, Nanette K., et al. "Cardiovascular Health and Disease in Women." *The New England Journal of Medicine* 329 (4): 247–253 (1993).

"We're Talking Years." *University of California at Berkeley Wellness Letter* 13 (4): 8 (January 1997).

## Chapter 2: Risk Factors and Physical Traits

Dattilo, Anne M., and P. M. Kris-Etherton. "Effects of Weight Reduction on Blood Lipids and Lipoproteins: A Meta-analysis." *The American Journal of Clinical Nutrition* 56: 320–328 (1992).

"Healthy Gums, Healthy Heart?" *Women's Health Advocate Newsletter* 4 (3): 2 (May 1997).

Hubert, Helen B, et al. "Obesity as an Independent Risk Factor for Cardiovascular Disease: A 26-Year Follow-up of Participants in the Framingham Heart Study." *Circulation* 67 (5): 968–976 (1983).

Jeffrey, R.W., et al. "Weight Cycling and Cardiovascular Risk Factors in Obese Men and Women." *The American Journal of Clinical Nutrition* 55: 641–644 (1992).

Lee, I. M., and R. S. Paffengarger. "Change in Body Weight and Longevity." *The Journal of the American Medical Association* 268: 2045–2049 (1992).

Liebman, Bonnie, and Jayne Hurley. "The Heart of the Matter." *Nutrition Action Health Letter (Center for Science in the Public Interest)* 20 (8): 1–7 (October 1993).

Lissner, L., et al. "Variability of Body Weight and Health Outcomes in the Framingham Population." *The New England Journal of Medicine* 324: 1839–1844 (1991).

Manson, Joanne, et al. "A Prospective Study of Obesity and Risk of Coronary Heart Disease in Women." *The New England Journal of Medicine* 322 (13): 882–889 (1990).

Manson, Joanne, et al. "Body Weight and Mortality Among Women." *The New England Journal of Medicine* 333: 677–685 (1995).

Rodin, J., et al. "Weight Cycling and Fat Distribution." *Int. J Obes* 14: 303–310 (1990).

St. Jeor, Sachiko. "The Role of Weight Management in the Health of Women." *Journal of the American Dietetic Association* 93: 1007–1012 (1993).

Willett, W. C., et al. "Weight, Weight Change and Coronary Heart Disease in Women: Risk Within the 'Normal' Weight Range." *The Journal of the American Medical Association* 273 (6): 461–465 (1995).

## Chapter 3: Medical Profile

Anastos, Kathryn, et al. "Hypertension in Women: What Is Really Known?" *Annals of Internal Medicine* 115 (4): 287–293 (1993).

Appel, Lawrence J., et al. "A Clinical Trial of the Effects of Dietary Patterns on Blood Pressure." *The New England Journal of Medicine* 336: 1117–1124 (1997).

Barnard, James R., et al. "Role of Diet and Exercise in the Management of Hyperinsulinemia and Associated Atherosclerotic Risk Factors." *The American Journal of Cardiology* 69: 440–444 (1992).

Barrett-Connor, E., et al. "Why Is Diabetes Mellitus a Stronger Risk Factor for Fatal Ischemic Heart Disease in Women Than in Men? The Rancho Bernardo Study." *The Journal of the American Medical Association* 265 (5): 627–631 (1991).

"Calcium Supplements: Get the Lead Out." *Women's Health Advocate Newsletter* 4 (5): 5 (July 1997).

Castelli, William P., et al. "Incidence of Coronary Heart Disease and Lipoprotein Cholesterol Levels: The Framingham Study." *The Journal of the American Medical Association* 256 (20): 2835–2838 (1986).

Clarke, R., et al. "Variability and Determinants of Total Homocysteine Concentrations in Plasma in an Elderly Population." *Clinical Chemistry* 44 (1): 102–107 (1998).

Despres J. P., et al. "Hyperinsulinemia as an Independent Risk Factor for Ischemic Heart Disease." *The New England Journal of Medicine* 334: 952–957 (1996).

"Diabetes Prevention: The Test," *University of California at Berkeley Wellness Letter* 14 (1): 4–5 (October 1997).

Eckel, Robert H. "Insulin Resistance in Atherosclerosis." *The American Journal of Clinical Nutrition* 65: 164–165 (1997).

Elliot, W. J. "Earlobe Crease and Coronary Artery Disease." *American Journal of Medicine* 75: 1024–1032 (1983).

Foster, Daniel W. "Insulin Resistance—A Secret Killer?" *The New England Journal of Medicine* 320 (11): 733–734 (1989).

French, John K., et al. "Association of Angiographically Detected Coronary Artery Disease with Low Levels of High-Density Lipoprotein Cholesterol and Systemic Hypertension." *The American Journal of Cardiology* 71: 505–510 (1993).

Grossman E, and F. H. Messerli. "Diabetic and Hypertensive Heart Disease: Review." *Annals of Internal Medicine* 125: 304–310 (1996).

Helmrich, Susan, et al. "Physical Activity and Reduced Occurrence of Non-Insulin-Dependent Diabetes Mellitus." *The New England Journal of Medicine* 325 (3): 147–152 (1991).

Howell, Wanda H., et al. "Plasma Lipid and Lipoprotein Responses to Dietary Fat and Cholesterol: A Meta-Analysis." *The American Journal of Clinical Nutrition* 65: 1749–1759 (1997).

"The Latest on Hypertension." *University of California at Berkeley Wellness Letter* 12 (3): 4–5 (December 1995).

Lawn, Richard M. "Lipoprotein(a) in Heart Disease." *Scientific American* 266: 54–60 (June 1992).

Leaf, Alexander. "Management of Hypercholesterolemia: Are Preventive Interventions Advisable?" *The New England Journal of Medicine* 321: 680–684 (1989).

"*Mangia!* The Case for Pasta and Carbohydrates." *University of California at Berkeley Wellness Letter* 11 (8): 1–2 (May 1995).

Maseri, Attilio. "Inflammation, Atherosclerosis, and Ischemic Events— Exploring the Hidden Side of the Mood." *The New England Journal of Medicine* 336: 1014–1015 (1997).

Morgan, Peggy, with Susan C. Smith. "Do You Have Syndrome X?" *Prevention:* 111–186 (May 1997).

"New Definition for Diabetes." *Tufts University Health & Nutrition Letter* 15 (7): 1–6 (September 1997).

"New Guidelines: Broader Screening for Diabetes." *Harvard Health Letter* 22 (11): 6 (September 1997).

Northrup, Christiane. "New Dietary Guidelines for Preventing Diabetes." *Health Wisdom for Women* 2 (3): 6 (March 1995).

Persfghin, Gianluca, et al. "Increased Glucose Transport-Phosphorylation and Muscle Glycogen Synthesis After Exercise Training in Insulin-Resistant Subjects." *The New England Journal of Medicine* 335: 1357–1362 (1996).

Reaven, G. M. "Banting Lecture 1988: Role of Insulin Resistance in Human Disease." *Diabetes* 37: 1595–2607 (1988).

Ridker, Paul M., et al. "Inflammation, Aspirin, and the Risk of Cardiovascular Disease in Apparently Healthy Men." *The New England Journal of Medicine* 336: 973–979 (1997).

Salmeron, Jorge, et al. "Dietary Fiber, Glycemic Load, and Risk of Non-Insulin-Dependent Diabetes Mellitus in Women." *The Journal of the American Medical Association* 277: 474–477 (1997).

Savoroni I., et al., "Risk Factors for Coronary Disease in Persons with Hyperinsulinemia and Normal Glucose Tolerance." *The New England Journal of Medicine* 320: 702–707 (1989).

Schardt, David, and Stephen Schmidt. "How to Avoid Adult Onset Diabetes." *Nutrition Action Health Letter* 23 (7): 3–5 (September 1996).

Selhub, Jacob, et al. "Association Between Plasma Homocysteine Concentrations and Extracranial Carotid-Artery Stenosis." *The New England Journal of Medicine* 332: 286–291 (1995).

Sinatra, Stephen. "Are You Aware of the 'New' Risk Factors for Heart Disease?" *HeartSense* 3 (7): 2–3 (July 1997).

Stampfer, M. J., and M. R. Malinow. "Can Lowering Homocysteine Levels Reduce Cardiovascular Risk?" (Editorial) *The New England Journal of Medicine* 332: 328–329 (1995).

Steingart, Richard M., et al. "Sex Differences in the Management of Coronary Artery Disease." *The New England Journal of Medicine* 325: 226–230 (1991).

Whelton, Paul K., et al. "Effects of Oral Potassium on Blood Pressure." *The Journal of the American Medical Association* 277: 1624–1632 (1997).

Wilson, Peter W. F. "High-Density Dipoprotein, Low-Density Lipoprotein and Coronary Artery Disease." *The American Journal of Cardiology* 66: 7A–10A (1990).

Wilson, Peter, et al. "Cumulative Effects of High Cholesterol Levels, High Blood Pressure, and Cigarette Smoking on Carotid Stenosis." *The New England Journal of Medicine* 337: 516–522 (1997).

## Chapter 4: Risks Unique to Women

Bar, J., et al. "The Effect of Estrogen Replacement Therapy on Platelet Aggregation and Adenosine Triphosphate Release in Postmenopausal Women." *Obstetrics and Gynecology* 81: 261–264 (1993).

Barrett-Connor, Elizabeth, and Trudy L. Bush. "Estrogen and Coronary Heart Disease in Women." *The Journal of the American Medical Association* 265: 1861–1867 (1991).

Colditz, Graham A., et al. "The Use of Estrogens and Progestins and the Risk of Breast Cancer in Postmenopausal Women." *The New England Journal of Medicine* 332: 1589–1593 (1995).

———. "Menopause and the Risk of Coronary Heart Disease in Women." *The New England Journal of Medicine* 316: 1105–1110 (1987).

Matthews, Karen A., et al. "Menopause and Risk Factors for Coronary Heart Disease." *The New England Journal of Medicine* 321: 641–646 (1989).

"The Menopause and Hormone Therapy." *National Women's Health Report* 17 (4): 1–4 (July/August 1995).

Ness, R. A., et al. "Number of Pregnancies and the Subsequent Risk of Cardiovascular Disease." *The New England Journal of Medicine* 328: 1528–1533 (1993).

Notelovitz, Morris, M.D. "An Opposing View." *The Journal of Family Practice* 29 (4): 410–415 (1989).

Rosenberg, L., et al. "A Case-Control Study of Myocardial Infarction in Relation to Use of Estrogen Supplements." *American Journal of Epidemiology* 137: 54–63 (1993).

Stampfer, Meir, et al. "Postmenopausal Estrogen Therapy and Cardiovascular Disease: Ten-Year Follow-up from the Nurses' Health Study." *The New England Journal of Medicine* 325 (11): 756–762 (1991).

Stanford, J. L., et al. "Combined Estrogen and Progestin Hormone Replacement Therapy in Relation to Risk of Breast Cancer in Middle-aged Women." *The Journal of the American Medical Association* 274: 137–142 (1995).

Steinberg, Karen K., et al. "A Meta-analysis of the Effect of Estrogen Replacement Therapy on the Risk of Breast Cancer." *The Journal of the American Medical Association* 265 (15): 1985–1990 (1991).

The Writing Group for the PEPI Trial. "Effects of Estrogen or Estrogen/Progestin Regimens on Heart Disease Risk Factors in Postmenopausal Women: The Postmenopausal Estrogen/Progestin Intervention Trial." *The Journal of the American Medical Association* 85 (4): 529–537 (1995).

## Chapter 5: Risky Behaviors

"Alcohol and Health: Mixed Messages for Women." *Women's Health Advocate Newsletter* 2 (12): 4–8 (February 1996).

"Alcohol and HRT." *Women's Health Advocate Newsletter* 3 (12): 1–8 (February 1997).

Berkman, L., and S. Syme, "Social Networks, Host Resistance, and Mortality: A Nine-year Follow-up Study of Alameda County Residents." *American Journal of Epidemiology* 109: 186–204 (1982).

Blair, Stephen, et al. "Influences of Cardiorespiratory Fitness and Other Precursors on Cardiovascular Disease and All-Cause Mortality in Men and Women." *The Journal of the American Medical Association* 276: 205–210 (1996).

Blair, S. N., et al. "Physical Fitness and All-Cause Mortality: A Prospective Study of Healthy Men and Women." *The Journal of the American Medical Association* 262: 2395–2401 (1989).

"Benefits of Pumping Iron." *Tufts University Health & Nutrition Letter* 14 (12): 8 (February 1997).

Castelli, William P., et al. "Incidence of Coronary Heart Disease and Lipoprotein Cholesterol Levels: The Framingham Study." *The Journal of the American Medical Association* 256: 2835–2838 (1986).

Connor, William, et al. "Should a Low-Fat, High Carbohydrate Diet Be Recommended for Everyone? Clinical Debate." *The New England Journal of Medicine* 337: 562–567 (1997).

"Coronary Disease: Taking Emotions to Heart." *Harvard Health Letter* 21 (11): 1–3 (October 1996).

"Coronary Heart Disease Attributable to Sedentary Lifestyle—Selected States, 1988." *The Journal of the American Medical Association* 264 (11): 1390–1392 (1990).

Curfman, G. D. "The Health Benefits of Exercise." (Editorial) *The New England Journal of Medicine* 328: 574–576 (1993).

Denollet, Johan, et al. "Personality as Independent Predictor of Long-Term Mortality in Patients with Coronary Heart Disease." *The Lancet* 347: 417–421 (1996).

"Diet and Heart Disease: Unanswered Questions." *Harvard Women's Health Watch* IV (4): 6 (December 1996).

Dolnick, Edward. "Hotheads and Heart Attacks." *Health*: 58–64 (July/August 1995).

Duncan, John J., et al. "Women Walking for Health and Fitness: How Much Is Enough?" *The Journal of the American Medical Association* 266: 3295–3299 (1991).

Frankel, E. N., et al. "Inhibition of Oxidation of Human Low-Density Lipoprotein by Phenolic Substances in Red Wine." *The Lancet* 341: 454–456 (1993).

Fuchs, Charles S., et al. "Alcohol Consumption and Mortality Among Women." *The New England Journal of Medicine* 332: 1245–1250 (1995).

Gullett, Elizabeth, et al. "Effects of Mental Stress on Myocardial Ischemia During Daily Life." *The Journal of the American Medical Association* 277: 1521–1526 (1997).

Haertel, Ursula, et al. "Cross-Sectional and Longitudinal Associations Between High Density Lipoprotein Cholesterol and Women's Employment." *American Journal of Epidemiology* 135: 68–78 (1992).

Haynes, S. G., and M. Feinleib. "Women, Work and Coronary Heart Disease: Prospective Findings from the Framingham Heart Study." *American Journal of Public Health* 70 (2): 133–141 (1980).

Hertog, M.G.L., et al. "Dietary Antioxidant Flavenoids and Risk of Coronary Heart Disease: The Zutphen Elderly Study." *The Lancet* 342: 1007–1011 (1993).

House, James S., et al. "Social Relationships and Health." *Science* 241: 540–544 (1988).

Howard, G., et al. "Cigarette Smoking and Progression of Atherosclerosis Risk in Communities (ARIC) Study." *The Journal of the American Medical Association* 279 (2): 119–124 (1998).

Kilata, Gina. "Heart Attacks at 9:00 A.M." *Science* 233: 417–418 (July 25, 1986).

Kris-Etherton, P. M., and Debra Krummel. "Role of Nutrition in the Prevention and Treatment of Coronary Heart Disease in Women." *Journal of the American Dietetic Association* 93: 987–993 (1993).

Leaf, Alexander. "Preventive Medicine for Our Ailing Health Care System." *The Journal of the American Medical Association* 269 (5): 616–618 (1993).

Lesperance, F., and M. Frasure-Smith. "Negative Emotions and Coronary Heart Disease: Getting to the Heart of the Matter." *The Lancet* 347: 414–415 (1996).

Northrup, Christiane. "Should You Get off Premarin?" *Dr. Christiane Northrup's Health Wisdom for Women* 4 (2): 2–5 (February 1997).

Ornish, D., et al. "Can Lifestyle Changes Reverse Coronary Heart Disease? The Lifestyle Heart Trial." *The Lancet* 336: 129–133 (1990).

Paffenbarger, Ralph S. Jr., et al. "A Natural History of Athleticism and Cardiovascular Health." *The Journal of the American Medical Association* 252 (4): 491–495 (1984).

Powell, K. E., et al. "Physical Activity and the Incidence of Coronary Heart Disease." *Annals Review of Public Health* 8: 253–287 (1987).

Rabkin, S. W., et al. "Chronobiology of Cardiac Sudden Death in Men." *The Journal of the American Medical Association* 244 (12): 1357–1358 (1980).

Raymond, Chris. "Distrust, Rage May Be 'Toxic Core' That Puts 'Type A' Person at Risk. *The Journal of the American Medical Association* 261 (6): 813 (1989).

Renaud, S., and M. de Lorgeril. "Wine, Alcohol, Platelets and the French Paradox for Coronary Heart Disease." *The Lancet* 339: 1523–1526 (1992).

Scherwitz, L., et al. "Type A Behavior, Self-Involvement, and Coronary Atherosclerosis." *Psychosomatic Medicine* 45 (1): 45–57 (1983).

Schleifer, Stephen J., et al. "Suppression of Lymphocyte Stimulation Following Bereavement." *The Journal of the American Medical Association* 250 (3): 374–377 (1983).

Schnall, Peter, et al. "The Relationship Between 'Job Strain,' Workplace Diastolic Blood Pressure, and Left Ventricular Mass Index." *The Journal of the American Medical Association* 263: 1929–1935 (1990).

Schols, D., et al. "Current Cigarette Smoking and Risk of Acute Pelvic Inflammatory Disease." *American Journal of Public Health* 82: 1352–1355 (1992).

Siguel, Edward N., and Robert H. Lerman. "Role of Essential Fatty Acids: Dangers in the U.S. Department of Agriculture Dietary Recommendations ("Pyramid") and in Low-Fat Diets." *The American Journal of Clinical Nutrition* 60: 973–979 (1994).

"Taking Grief to Heart." *Harvard Health Letter* 21 (8): 8 (June 1996).

USDHHS. "The Health Benefits of Smoking Cessation: Report of the Surgeon General" (DHHS No. CDC 90–8416), Washington, DC: USGPO (1990) .

Willett, Walter C., et al. "Relative and Absolute Excess Risks of Coronary Heart Disease Among Women Who Smoke Cigarettes." *The New England Journal of Medicine* 317 (21): 1303–1309 (1987).

## Chapter 6: Cholesterol Confusion

Castelli, William P., et al. "Incidence of Coronary Heart Disease and Lipoprotein Cholesterol Levels: The Framingham Study." *The Journal of the American Medical Association* 256: 2835–2838 (1986).

French, John K., et al. "Association of Angiographically Detected Coronary Artery Disease with Low Levels of High-Density Lipoprotein Cholesterol and Systemic Hypertension." *The American Journal of Cardiology* 71: 505–510 (1993).

Hully, S. B., et al. "Health Policy on Blood Cholesterol." *Circulation* 56: 1026 (1992).

Johnson, Clifford, et al. "Declining Serum Total Cholesterol Levels Among U.S. Adults: The National Health and Nutrition Examination Surveys." *The Journal of the American Medical Association* 269: 3002–3007 (1993).

Leaf, Alexander. "Treating Hypercholesterolemia." *The New England Journal of Medicine* 321: 676–684 (1989).

"Management of Hypercholesterolemia: Are Preventive Interventions Advisable?" *The New England Journal of Medicine* 321: 680–683 (1989).

Retzlaff, Barbara, et al. "Effects of Two Eggs per Day Versus Placebo in Moderately Hypercholesterolemic and Combined Hyperlipidemic Subjects Consuming the NCEP Step-One Diet." *Circulation* 92: 1–350 (1995).

Stamler, Jeremiah, et al. "Is Relationship Between Serum Cholesterol and Risk of Premature Death from Coronary Heart Disease Continuous and Graded?" *The Journal of the American Medical Association* 256: 2823–2828 (1986).

"Triglycerides, HDL, and CAD." *Women's Health Watch* III (4): 7 (December 1995).

Wilson, Peter. "High-Density Lipoprotein, Low-Density Lipoprotein and Coronary Artery Disease." *The American Journal of Cardiology* 66: 7A–10A (1990).

## Chapter 7: Fat: Friend or Foe

Ascherio, Alberto, et al. "Dietary Fat and Risk of Coronary Heart Disease in Men: Cohort Follow-up Study in the United States." *British Medical Journal* 313: 84–90 (1996).

———. "Dietary Intake of Marine n-3 Fatty Acids, Fish Intake, and the Risk of Coronary Disease Among Men." *The New England Journal of Medicine* 332: 977–982 (1995).

Bang, H. O., et al. "The Composition of the Eskimo Food in North-Western Greenland." *The American Journal of Clinical Nutrition* 33: 2657–2661 (1980).

Blades, B., and A. Garg. "Mechanisms of Increase in Plasma Triacylglycerol Concentrations as a Result of High Carbohydrate Intakes in Patients with Non-Insulin-Dependent Diabetes Mellitus." *The American Journal of Clinical Nutrition* 62: 996–1002 (1995).

Blankenhorn, D. H., et al. "The Influence of Diet on the Appearance of New Lesions in Human Coronary Arteries." *The Journal of the American Medical Association* 263: 1646–1652 (1990).

Bonanome, Andrea, et al. "Effect of Dietary Monounsaturated and Polyunsaturated Fatty Acids on the Susceptibility of Plasma Low-Density Lipoproteins to Oxidative Modification." *Arteriosclerosis and Thrombosis* 12: 529–533 (1992).

Burr, M. L., et al. "Effects of Changes in Fat, Fish, and Fibre Intakes on Death and Myocardial Reinfarction: Diet and Reinfarction Trial (DART)." *The Lancet* II: 757–756 (September 1989).

Chen, Y. D., et al. "Why Do Low-Fat High-Carbohydrate Diets Accentuate Postprandial Lipemia in Patients with NIDDM?" *Diabetes Care* 18: 10–16 (1995).

Cobiac, Lynne, et al. "Lipid, Lipoprotein, and Hemostatic Effects of Fish vs. Fish-Oil n-Fatty Acids in Mildly Hyperlipidemic Males." *The American Journal of Clinical Nutrition* 53: 1210–1216 (1991).

Connor, William E., and Sonja L. Connor. "Should a Low-Fat, High Carbohydrate Diet Be Recommended for Everyone?" *The New England Journal of Medicine* 337: 562–563 (1997).

Daviglus, Martha L., et al. "Fish Consumption and the 30-Year Risk of Fatal Myocardial Infarction." *The New England Journal of Medicine* 336: 1046–1053 (1997).

"Dueling Food Pyramids: Which One Is Best for Women?" *Women's Health Advocate Newsletter* 1 (1): 4–6 (January 1995).

Gordon, D. J., and B. M. Rifkind. "High-Density Lipoprotein—The Clinical Implications of Recent Studies." *The New England Journal of Medicine* 321: 1311–1316 (1989).

Howell, Wanda, et al. "Plasma Lipid and Lipoprotein Responses to Dietary Fat and Cholesterol: A Meta-Analysis." *The American Journal of Clinical Nutrition* 65: 1747–1764 (1997).

"In Search of a Better Diet: A Mediterranean Odyssey." *Tufts University Diet & Nutrition Letter* 11 (6): 3–6 (August 1993).

Judd, Joseph R., et al. "Dietary *Trans* Fatty Acids: Effects on Plasma Lipids and Lipoproteins of Healthy Men and Women." *The American Journal of Clinical Nutrition* 59: 861–868 (1994).

Katan, Martijn, et al. "Beyond Low-Fat Diets." *The New England Journal of Medicine* 337: 563–567 (1997).

Kromhout, Daan, et al. "The Inverse Relation Between Fish Consumption and 20-Year Mortality from Coronary Heart Disease." *The New England Journal of Medicine* 312: 1205–1209 (1985).

Kushi, Lawrence H., et al. "Health Implications of Mediterranean Diets in Light of Contemporary Knowledge: Meat, Wine, Fats, and Oils." *The American Journal of Clinical Nutrition* 61 (suppl): 1416S–1427S (1995).

Leaf, A. "Cardiovascular Effects of Omega-3 Fatty Acids." *The New England Journal of Medicine* 318: 549–557 (1988).

Mann, George V. "Metabolic Consequences of Dietary *Trans* Fatty Acids," *The Lancet* 343: 1268–1271 (1994).

Marchmann, Peter, et al. "Low-Fat, High-Fiber Diet Favorably Affects Several Independent Risk Markers of Ischemic Heart Disease: Observations on

Blood Lipids, Coagulation, and Fibrinolysis from a Trial of Middle-Aged Danes." *The American Journal of Clinical Nutrition* 59: 935–939 (1994).

Mensink, Ronald P., and Martijn B. Katan. "Effect of Dietary *Trans* Fatty Acids on High-Density and Low-Density Lipoprotein Cholesterol Levels in Healthy Subjects." *The New England Journal of Medicine* 323: 439–445 (1990).

Milner, M. R. "Usefulness of Fish Oil Supplements in Preventing Clinical Evidence of Restenosis after Percutaneous Transluminal Coronary Angioplasty." *The American Journal of Cardiology* 64 (5): 294–299 (1989).

Ornish, Dean, et al. "Can Lifestyle Changes Reverse Coronary Heart Diseases? The Lifestyle Heart Trial." *The Lancet* 336: 129–133 (1990).

Sabate, Joan, et al. "Effects of Walnuts on Serum Lipid Levels and Blood Pressure in Normal Men." *The New England Journal of Medicine* 328: 603–607 (1993).

Sacks, Frank M., and Walter C. Willett. "More on Chewing the Fat." *The New England Journal of Medicine* 325 (24): 1740–1741(1991).

Schardt, David, et al. "Going Mediterranean." *Nutrition Action* 21 (10): 1–5 (December 1994).

Siguel, Edward N., and Robert H. Lerman. "Role of Essential Fatty Acids: Dangers in the U.S. Department of Agriculture Dietary Recommendations ("Pyramid") and in Low-Fat Diets." *The American Journal of Clinical Nutrition* 60: 973–979 (1994).

Simon, Joel, et al. "Serum Fatty Acids and the Risk of Stroke." *Stroke* 26: 778–782 (1995).

Simopoulos A., "Omega-3 Fatty Acids in Growth and Development and in Health and Disease." *Nutrition Today* 23 (3): 12–18 (May/June 1988).

"Varied Diet Lower Pressure." *Harvard Health Letter* 22 (4): 8 (February 1997).

Von Schacky, Clemens. "Prophylaxis of Artherosclerosis with Marine Omega-3 Fatty Acids." *Annals of Internal Medicine* 107: 890–899 (1987).

Willett, Walter C., et al. "Mediterranean Diet Pyramid: A Cultural Model for Healthy Eating." *The American Journal of Clinical Nutrition* 61 (suppl.): 1402S–1406S (1995).

Willett, Walter C., et al. "Intake of *Trans* Fatty Acids and Risk of Coronary Heart Disease Among Women." *The Lancet* 341: 581–585 (1993).

Wolk, Alicja, et al. "A Prospective Study of Association of Monounsaturated Fat and Other Types of Fat with Risk of Breast Cancer." *Archives of Internal Medicine* 158: 41–45 (1988).

Wootan, Margo, and Bonnie Liebman. "The Great Trans Wreck." *Nutrition Action Health Letter* 20 (9): 10–12 (November 1993).

Wootan, Margo, et al. "*Trans:* The Phantom Fat." *Nutrition Action Health Letter* 23 (7): 1–11 (September 1996).

## Chapter 8: Fabulous Fiber

Anderson, J. W., et al. "Serum Lipid Response of Hypercholesterolemic Men to Single and Divided Doses of Canned Beans." *The American Journal of Clinical Nutrition* 51: 1013–1019 (1990).

————. "Hypocholesterolemic Effects of Oat-Bran or Bean Intake for Hypercholesterolemic Men." *The American Journal of Clinical Nutrition* 40: 1146–1155 (1984).

Baig, Mirza Mansoor, and James John Cerda. "Pectin: Its Interaction with Serum Lipoproteins." *The American Journal of Clinical Nutrition* 34: 50–53 (1981).

Cerda, J. J., et al. "The Effects of Grapefruit Pectin on Patients at Risk for Coronary Heart Disease Without Altering Diet or Lifestyle." *Clinical Cardiology* 11: 589–594 (1988).

DeGroot, A. P., et al. "Cholesterol-Lowering Effect of Rolled Oats." *The Lancet* 2: 303–304 (1963).

Davidson, M. H., "The Hypocholesterolemic Effects of B-glucan in Oatmeal and Oat Bran." *The Journal of the American Medical Association* 285: 1833–1839 (1991).

"Dietary Fiber." *Harvard Women's Health Watch* 3 (1): 2–3 (September 1995).

Glore, Stephen, et al. "Soluble Fiber and Serum Lipids: A Literature Review." *Journal of the American Dietetic Association* 94: 425–436 (1994).

Haskell, William, et al. "Role of Water-Soluble Dietary Fiber in the Management of Elevated Plasma Cholesterol in Healthy Subjects." *The American Journal of Cardiology* 69: 433–439 (1992).

Hunninghake, Donald, et al. "Hypcholesterolemic Effects of a Dietary Fiber Supplement." *The American Journal of Clinical Nutrition* 59: 1050–1054 (1994).

"It's Back! Fiber Is Good for the Heart." *Harvard Health Letter* 21 10: 6–7 (August 1996).

Kushi, Lawrence, et al. "Health Implications of Mediterranean Diets in Light of Contemporary Knowledge: Plant Foods and Dairy Products." *The American Journal of Clinical Nutrition* 61 (suppl.): 1407S–1415S (1995).

Lanza, Elaine, et al. "Dietary Fiber Intake in the U.S. Population." *The American Journal of Clinical Nutrition* 46: 790–797 (1987).

Liebman, Bonnie. "Oat Bran: It's B-a-a-a-ck." *Nutrition Action Health Letter* 23 (4): 8–9 (May 1996).

————. "The Whole Grain Guide." *Nutrition Action Health Letter* 24 (2): 1–11 (March 1997).

Matson, Fred H., et al. "Optimizing the Effect of Plant Sterols on Cholesterol Absorption in Man." *The American Journal of Clinical Nutrition* 35: 697–700 (1982).

"Oats in the Offing." *Tufts University Health & Nutrition Letter* 15 (1): 7 (March 1997).

Pietinen, Pirjo, et al. "Intake of Dietary Fiber and Risk of Coronary Heart Disease in a Cohort of Finnish Men." *Circulation* 94: 2720–2727 (1996).

Ripsin, Cynthia, et al. "Oat Products and Lipid Lowering: A Meta-Analysis." *The Journal of the American Medical Association* 267: 3317–3325 (1992).

Robertson, J., et al. "The Effect of Raw Carrot on Serum Lipids and Colon Function." *The American Journal of Clinical Nutrition* 32: 1889–1892 (1979).

Topping, David L. "Soluble Fiber Polysaccharides: Effects on Plasma Cholesterol and Colonic Fermentation." *Nutrition Review* 49: 195–200 (1991).

Willett, Walter C., et al. "Dietary Fat and Fiber in Relation to Risk of Breast Cancer." *The Journal of the American Medical Association* 268: 2037–2044 (1992).

Wolever, Thomas, et al. "Method of Administration Influences the Serum Cholesterol-Lowering Effect of Psyllium." *The American Journal of Clinical Nutrition* 59: 1055–1059 (1994).

Wynder, Ernst L., et al. "High Fiber Intake: Indicator of a Healthy Lifestyle." *The Journal of the American Medical Association* 275 (6): 486–487 (1996).

## Chapter 9: Protein: Animal Versus Plant

Anderson, J. W., et al. "Dietary Fiber and Diabetes: A Comprehensive Review and Practical Application." *Journal of the American Dietetic Association* 87: 1189–1197 (1987).

———. "Meta-Analysis of the Effects of Soy Protein Intake on Serum Lipids." *The New England Journal of Medicine* 333: 276–82 (1995).

"As the Chicken Turns." *Tufts University Diet & Nutrition Letter* 11 (11): 1–2 (January 1994).

Brody, Jane E. "New Research on the Vegetarian Diet." *The New York Times,* Sciences Section, October 12, 1983.

Bergman, J. G., and P. T. Brown. "Nutritional Status of 'New Vegetarians.'" *Journal of the American Dietetic Association* 76: 151–155 (1980).

Cassidy, A., et al. "Biological Effects of a Diet of Soy Protein Rich in Isoflavones on the Menopausal Cycle of Premenopausal Women." *The American Journal of Clinical Nutrition* 60: 333–340 (1994).

Erdman, John Jr., and Elizabeth Fordyce. "Soy Products and the Human Diet." *The American Journal of Clinical Nutrition* 49: 725–737 (1989).

"Flocking to Chicken Wings." *Tufts University Diet & Nutrition Letter* 12 (12): 1 (February 1995).

Foster, Daniel W. "Insulin Resistance—A Secret Killer?" *The New England Journal of Medicine* 320 (11): 733–734 (1989).

Fraser, Gary. "Diet and Coronary Heart Disease: Beyond Dietary Fats and Low-Density-Lipoprotein Cholesterol." *The American Journal of Clinical Nutrition* 59 (suppl): 1117S–1123S (1994).

Gaddi, Antonia, et al. "Dietary Treatment for Familial Hypercholesterolemia—Differential Effects of Dietary Soy Protein According to the Apoliprotein E Phenotypes." *The American Journal of Clinical Nutrition* 53: 1191–1196 (1991).

Hurley, Jayne, and Stephen Schmidt. "Hard Artery Cafe?" *Nutrition Action Health Letter* 23 (8): 1–7 (October 1996).

"Is There Soy in Your Future?" *Tufts University Diet & Nutrition Letter* 12 (12): 4 (February 1995).

Kanazawa, et al. "Anti-Atherogenicity of Soybean Protein." *Annals New York Academy of Science* 676: 202–214 (1993).

Kato, H., et al. "Epidemiologic Studies of Coronary Heart Disease and Stroke in Japanese Men Living in Japan, Hawaii, and California: Serum Lipids and Diet." *American Journal of Epidemiology* 97: 372–385 (1973).

Kito, M. T., et al. "Changes in Plasma Lipids in Young Healthy Volunteers by Adding an Extruder Cooked Soy Protein to Conventional Meals." *Biosci Biotech Biochem* 57: 354–355 (1993).

Kushi, Lawrence H., et al. "Health Implications of Mediterranean Diets in Light of Contemporary Knowledge: Meat, Wine, Fats, and Oils." *The American Journal of Clinical Nutrition* 61 (suppl): 1416S–1427S (1995).

"The Latest Story on Soy." *Harvard Women's Health Watch* IV (9): 6 (May 1997).

"Lean Beef Shown to Be as Healthy as Chicken or Fish." *Food Chemical News* 32 (39): 6 (1990).

Liebman, Bonnie, and Jayne Hurley. "A Meat & Poultry Primer." *Nutrition Action Health Letter* 22 (9): 12–13 (November 1995).

Northrup, Christiane. "Have You Discovered Your Personal Dietary Truth?" *Dr. Christiane Northrup's Health Wisdom for Women* 4 (3): 3–5 (March 1997).

Phillips, R. L., et al. "Coronary Heart Disease Mortality Among Seventh–Day Adventists with Differing Dietary Habits: A Preliminary Report." *The American Journal of Clinical Nutrition* 31: S191–S194 (1978).

Potter S. M., et al. "Depression of Plasma Cholesterol in Men by Consumption of Baked Products Containing Soy Protein." *The American Journal of Clinical Nutrition* 58: 501–506 (1993).

Raines, E. W., and R. Ross. "Biology of Atherosclerotic Plaque Formation: Possible Role of Growth Factors in Lesion Development and the Potential Impact of Soy." *Journal of Nutrition* 125: 624S–630S (1995).

Reaven, G. M. "Banting Lecture 1988: Role of Insulin Resistance in Human Disease." *Diabetes* 37: 1595–1607 (1988).

Resnicow, Ken, et al. "Diet and Serum Lipids in Vegan Vegetarians: A Model for Risk Reduction." *Journal of the American Dietetic Association* 91: 447–453 (1991).

Sacks, F. M., et al. Effects of Ingestion of Meat on Plasma Cholesterol of Vegetarians." *The Journal of the American Medical Association* 246: 660–664 (1981).

———. "Blood Pressure in Vegetarians." *American Journal of Epidemiology* 100: 390–398 (1974).

Sirtori, C. R., et al. "Soybean-Protein Diet in the Treatment of Type II Hyperlipoproteinaemia" *The Lancet* 5: 275–277 (1977).

———. "Soybean Protein Diet and Plasma Cholesterol: From Therapy to Molecular Mechanisms." *Annals New York Academy of Sciences* 676: 188–201 (1993).

Slavin, Joanne. "Nutritional Benefits of Soy Protein and Soy Fiber." *The Journal of the American Dietetic Association* 91: 816–819 (1991).

Snowdon, D. A., et al. "Meat Consumption and Fatal Ischemic Heart Disease." *Preventive Medicine* 13: 490–500 (1984).

Tsai, A. C., et al. "Effects of Soy Polysaccharide on Postprandial Plasma Glucose, Insulin, Glucagon, Pancreatic Polypeptide, Somatostatin, and Triglyceride in Obese Diabetic Patients." *The American Journal of Clinical Nutrition* 45: 596–601 (1987).

Van Raaij, J. M., et al. "Effects of Casein Versus Soy Protein Diets on Serum Cholesterol and Lipoproteins in Young Healthy Volunteers." *The American Journal of Clinical Nutrition* 34: 1261–1265 (1981).

———. "Influence of Diets Containing Casein, Soy Isolate and Soy Concentrate on Serum Cholesterol and Lipoproteins in Middle-aged Volunteers." *The American Journal of Clinical Nutrition* 35: 925–934 (1982).

Verrillo, A., et al. "Soybean Protein Diets in the Management of Type II Hyperlipoproteinaemia." *Atherosclerosis* 54: 321–331 (1985).

Vesby, B., et al. "The Effects of Lipid and Carbohydrate Metabolism of Replacing Some Animal Protein by Soy-Protein in a Lipid-Lowering Diet for Hypercholesterolemic Patients." *Human Nutrition: Applied Nutrition* 36A: 179–189 (1982).

Wilcox, J. N., and B. F. Blumenthal. "Thrombotic Mechanisms in Atherosclerosis: Potential Impact of Soy Proteins." *Journal of Nutrition* 125: 631S–638S (1995).

Willett, Walter C., et al. "Mediterranean Diet Pyramid: A Cultural Model for Healthy Eating." *The American Journal of Clinical Nutrition* 61 (suppl); 1402S–1406S (1995).

## Chapter 10: Antioxidants

The Alpha Tocopherol, Beta Carotene Cancer Prevention Study Group. "The Effect of Vitamin E and Beta Carotene on the Incidence of Lung Cancer and Other Cancers in Male Smokers." *The New England Journal of Medicine* 330: 1029–1035 (1994).

Baggio, E., et al. "Italian Multicenter Study on the Safety and Efficacy of Coenzyme Q10 as Adjunctive Therapy in Heart Failure." *Molecular Aspects in Medicine* (suppl): S287–S294 (1994).

Bellizzi, M. C., et al. "Vitamin E and Coronary Heart Disease: The European Paradox." *European Journal of Clinical Nutrition* 48: 822–831 (1994).

"Beta Carotene Pills: Should You Take Them?" *University of California at Berkeley Wellness Letter* 12 (7): 1–2 (April 1996).

"Better Beta Carotene Advice." *University of California at Berkeley Wellness Letter* 13 (8): 4 (May 1997).

Brown, Katrina, et. al. "Vitamin E Supplementation Suppresses Indexes of Lipid Peroxidation and Platelet Counts in Blood of Smokers and Nonsmokers but Plasma Lipoprotein Concentrations Remain Unchanged." *The American Journal of Clinical Nutrition* 60: 383–383 (1994).

Di Mascio, Paolo, et al. "Antioxidant Defense Systems: The Role of Carotenoids, Tocopherols, and Thiols." *The American Journal of Clinical Nutrition* 53: 194S–299S (1991).

Fairley, Janet A. "Antioxidant Vitamins and Coronary Heart Disease." *The New England Journal of Medicine* 328: 1487 (1993).

Folkers, K., et al. "Biochemical Rationale and Myocardial Tissue Data on the Effective Therapy of Cardiomyopathy with Coenzyme Q10." *Procedures of the National Academy of Sciences* 82: 901–904 (1985).

Fuller, Cindy, and Ishwarlal Jialal. "Effects of Antioxidants and Fatty Acids on Low-Density-Lipoprotein Oxidation." *The American Journal of Clinical Nutrition* 60 (suppl): 1010S–1013S (1994).

Gatto, L. M. "Basic Research in Antioxidant Inhibition of Steps in Atherogenesis." *Journal of American College of Nutrition* 15: 154–158 (1996).

Gey, K. Fred, et al. "Increased Risk of Cardiovascular Disease at Suboptimal Plasma Concentrations of Essential Antioxidants: An Epidemiological Update with Special Attention to Carotene and Vitamin C." *The American Journal of Clinical Nutrition* 57 (suppl): 787S–797S (1993).

———. "Inverse Correlation Between Plasma Vitamin E and Mortality from Ischemic Heart Disease in Cross Cultural Epidemiology." *Acta Cardiologica* 44: 493–494 (1989).

Greenberg, E., et al. "A Clinical Trial of Antioxidant Vitamins to Prevent Colorectal Adenoma." *The New England Journal of Medicine* 331: 141–147 (1994).

Hankinson, Susan, and Meir Stampfer. "All That Glitters Is Not Beta Carotene." *The Journal of the American Medical Association* 272: 1455–1456 (1994).

Hallfrisch, Judith, et al. "High Plasma Vitamin C Associated with High Plasma HDL and HDL-2 Cholesterol." *The American Journal of Clinical Nutrition* 60: 100–105 (1994).

Hertog, Michael, et al. "Dietary Antioxidant Flavenoids and Risk of Coronary Heart Disease: The Zutphen Elderly Study." *The Lancet* 342: 1007–1011 (1993).

Hodis, Howard, et al. "Serial Coronary Angiographic Evidence That Antioxidant Vitamin Intake Reduces Progression of Coronary Artery Atherosclerosis." *The Journal of the American Medical Association* 273: 1849–1854 (1995).

Jandak, J., et al. "Alpha-Tocopherol, An Effective Inhibitor of Platelet Adhesion." *Blood* 72: 141–149 (1989).

Kagan, Valerian E., et al. "Recycling of Vitamin E in Human Low–Density Lipoproteins." *Journal of Lipid Research* 33: 385–390 (1992).

Kardinaal, A., et al. "Antioxidants in Adipose Tissue and Risk of Myocardial Infarction: The EURAMIC Study." *The Lancet* 342: 1379–1384 (1993).

Kok, Frans J., et al. "Decreased Selenium Levels in Acute Myocardial Infarction." *The Journal of the American Medical Association* 261: 1161–1164 (1989).

Kushi, Lawrence, et al. "Dietary Antioxidant Vitamins and Death from Coronary Heart Disease in Postmenopausal Women." *The New England Journal of Medicine* 334: 1156–1162 (1996).

Langsjoen, P. H., et al. "Long–Term Efficacy and Safety of Coenzyme Q10 Therapy for Idiopathic Dilated Cardiomopathy." *The American Journal of Cardiology* 65: 521–523 (1990).

Littarru, G. P., et al. "Deficiency of Coenzyme Q10 in Human Heart Disease Part II." *International Journal of Vitamin and Nutrition Research* 42: 413 (1972).

McKeown, L. A., "Vitamin E May Cut Heart Risk." *Medical Tribune* 33: 1 (1992).

Meydani, Simin, et al. "Vitamin E Supplementation and In Vivo Immune Response in Healthy Elderly Subjects." *The Journal of the American Medical Association* 277: 1380–1386 (1997).

Morris, D. L., et al. "Serum Carotenoids and Coronary Heart Disease: The Lipid Research Clinics Coronary Primary Prevention Trial and Follow-up Study." *The Journal of the American Medical Association* 272: 1439–1431 (1994).

Nakamura, Yoshiro, et al. "Protection of Ischemic Myocardium with Coenzyme Q10." *Cardiovascular Research* 16 (3): 132–137 (1982).

Natraj, C. V., et al. "Lipoic Acid and Diabetes: Effect of Dihydrolipoic Acid Administration in Diabetic Rats and Rabbits." *Journal of Bioscience* 6: 37–46 (1984).

Packer, Lester. "Protective Role of Vitamin E in Biological Systems." *The American Journal of Clinical Nutrition* 53: 1050S–1055S (1991).

Resnick, A. Z., et al. "Vitamin E Supplements in the Aged." *Journal of Optimum Nutrition* 1: 65–68 (1992).

Rimm, E. R., et al. "Vitamin E Consumption and the Risk of Coronary Heart Disease in Men." *The New England Journal of Medicine* 326: 1450–1456 (1993).

Sachse G., and B. Willms. "Efficiency of Thiotic Acid in the Therapy of Peripheral Diabetic Neuropathy." *Hormone and Metabolic Research* (Supplement) 9: 105 (1980).

Salonen, J. T. "Association Between Cardiovascular Death and Myocardial Infarction and Serum Selenium in a Matched-Pair Longitudinal Study." *The Lancet* 2: 175–179 (1982).

Schone, N.W., et al. "Effects of Selenium Deficiency on Aggregation and Thromboxane Formation in Rat Platelet." *Fed. Proc.* 43: 477 (1984).

Simon, Emmanuelle, et al. "Plasma and Erythrocyte Vitamin E Content in Asymptomatic Hypercholesterolemic Subjects." *Clinical Chemistry* 43 (2): 285–289 (1997).

Sinatra, Stephen, M.D. "Coenzyme Q10: Truly a Miracle in Our Midst." *HeartSense* 2 (7): 1–2 (July 1996).

———. "The Knights of the Roundtable: Alpha Lipoic Acid: The Lancelot." *HeartSense* 3 (9): 4–6 (September 1997).

Singh, Ram B., et al. "Effect of Antioxidant-Rich Foods on Plasma Ascorbic Acid, Cardiac Enzyme, and Lipid Peroxide Levels in Patients Hospitalized with Acute Myocardial Infarction." *Journal of the American Dietetic Association* 95: 775–780 (1995).

Stampfer, Meir J., et al. "Vitamin E Consumption and the Risk of Coronary Heart Disease in Women." *The New England Journal of Medicine* 326: 1444–1449 (1993).

Stephens, Nigel, et al. "Randomised Controlled Trial of Vitamin E in Patients with Coronary Disease: Cambridge Heart Antioxidant Study (CHAOS)." *The Lancet* 347: 781–786 (1996).

"To Take Antioxidant Pills or Not? The Debate Heats Up." *Tufts University Diet & Nutrition Letter* 2 (3): 3–6 (May 1994).

Varma, Shambhu. "Scientific Basis for Medical Therapy of Cataracts by Antioxidants." *The American Journal of Clinical Nutrition* 53: 335S–345S (1991).

"Vitamin E and Immune Function." *Harvard Health Letter* 22 (9): 8 (July 1997).

Wander, Rosemary, et al. "Effects of Interaction of RRR-Alpha-Tocopherol Acetate and Fish Oil on Low-Density-Lipoprotein Oxidation in Postmenopausal Women with and Without Hormone-Replacement Therapy." *The American Journal of Clinical Nutrition* 63: 184–193 (1996).

"When Food Falls Short." *Women's Health Advocate Newsletter* 2 (4): 5 (June 1995).

Whitaker, Julian, M.D. "Conventional Medicine Is Frozen. *Dr. Julian Whitaker's Health & Healing* 6 (12): 6–8 (December 1996).

———. "To Avoid Heart Attacks, Take Vitamin E." *Dr. Julian Whitaker's Health & Healing* 6 (9): 1–2 (September 1996).

## Chapter 11: Bolstering the B Vitamins

Boushey, C. J., et al. "A Quantitative Assessment of Plasma Homosycteine as a Risk Factor for Vascular Disease." *The Journal of the American Medical Association* 274: 1049–1057 (1995).

Bower, C. "Folate and Neural Tube Defects." *Nutrition Review* 53 (suppl.): S33–S38 (1995).

Brattstrom, Lars E., et al. "Postmenopausal Homocysteinemia." *Metabolism* 34 (11): 1073–1074 (1985).

Brevetti, G., et al. "Increases in Walking Distance in Patients with Peripheral Vascular Disease Treated with L–Carnitine: A Double-Blind, Cross-Over Study." *Circulation* 77: 767–773 (1988).

Brown, W. Virgil. "Clinical Trials Including an Update on the Helsinki Heart Study." *The American Journal of Cardiology* 66: 11A–15A (1990).

"The B Vitamins: Why Women Need Them." *Women's Health Advocate Newsletter* 2 (9): 4–5 (November 1995).

Driskell, J. A. "Vitamin B-6 Requirements of Humans." *Nutrition Research* 14: 293–324 (1994).

Ferrari, R., et al. "The Metabolic Effects of L-Carnitine in Angina Pectoris." *International Journal of Cardiology* 5: 213 (1984).

"For Your Heart's Sake, More B Vitamins." *Tufts University Diet & Nutrition Letter* 2 (12): 1–2 (February 1994).

Graham, Ian, et al. "Plasma Homocysteine as a Risk Factor for Vascular Disease: The European Concerted Action Project." *The Journal of the American Medical Association* 277: 1775–1781 (1997).

Goodman, DeWitt S., and Expert Panel. "Report of the National Cholesterol Education Program Expert Panel on Detection, Evaluation, and Treatment of High Blood Cholesterol in Adults." *Arch Internal Medicine* 148: 36–69 (1988).

Gorostiaga, E. M., et al. "Decrease in Respiratory Quotient During Exercise Following L-Carnitine Supplementation." *International Journal of Sports Medicine* 10: 169–174 (1989).

Herbert, Victor, and Jean Bigaouette. "Call for Endorsement of a Petition to the Food and Drug Administration to Always Add Vitamin B-12 to Any Folate Fortification or Supplement." *The American Journal of Clinical Nutrition* 65: 572–573 (1997).

Joosten, E, A., et al. "Metabolic Evidence That Deficiencies of Vitamin B-12 (Cobalamin), Folate, and Vitamin B-6 Occur Commonly in Elderly People." *The American Journal of Clinical Nutrition* 58: 468–476 (1993).

Kant, A. K., and G. Block. "Dietary Vitamin B-6 Intake and Food Sources in the U.S. Population: NHANES II, 1976–1980." *The American Journal of Clinical Nutrition* 52: 707–716 (1990).

Kelly, Patrick, et al. "Unmetabolized Folic Acid in Serum: Acute Studies in Subjects Consuming Fortified Food and Supplements." *The American Journal of Clinical Nutrition* 65: 1790–1795 (1997).

Landgren, F., et al. "Plasma Homocysteine in Acute Myocardial Infarction: Homocysteine-Lowering Effect of Folic Acid." *Journal of Internal Medicine* 237: 381–388 (1995).

Lindenbaum, J., et al. "Prevalence of Cobalamin Deficiency in the Framingham Elderly Population." *The American Journal of Clinical Nutrition* 60: 2–11 (1994).

Lowik, M. R., et al. "Long-Term Effects of a Vegetarian Diet on the Nutritional Status of Elderly People (Dutch Nutrition Surveillance System)." *Journal of the American College of Nutrition* 9: 600–609 (1990).

McCorkindale, C., et al. "Nutritional Status of HIV-Infected Patients During the Early Disease Stages." *Journal of the American Dietetic Association* 90: 1236–1241 (1990).

McCully, K. S. Vascular Pathology of Homocystemia: Implications for the Pathogenesis of Arteriosclerosis." *American Journal of Pathology* 56: 111–128 (1969).

Morrison, Howard, et al. "Serum Folate and Risk of Fatal Coronary Heart Disease." *The Journal of the American Medical Association* 275: 1893–1896 (1996).

Naurath, H. J., et al. "Effects of Vitamin B-12, Folate, and Vitamin B-6 Supplements in Elderly People with Normal Serum Vitamin Concentrations." *The Lancet* 346: 85–89 (1995).

"Niacin: Double-Edged Sword for Lowering Cholesterol." *Tufts University Diet & Nutrition Letter* 12 (6): 1 (August 1994).

Nygard, Ottar, et al. "Plasma Homocysteine Levels and Mortality in Patients with Coronary Artery Disease." *The New England Journal of Medicine* 337: 230–236 (1997).

Oakley, Godfrey. "Let's Increase Folic Acid Fortification and Include Vitamin B-12." *The American Journal of Clinical Nutrition* 65: 1889–1890 (1997).

Opie, L. H. "Role of Carnitine in Fatty Acid Metabolism of Normal and Ischemic Myocardium." *American Heart Journal* 97: 375–388 (1979).

Pancharuniti, Nonglak, et al. "Plasma Homocysteine, Folate, and Vitamin B-12 Concentrations and Risk for Early-Onset Coronary Artery Disease." *The American Journal of Clinical Nutrition* 59: 940–948 (1994).

"Preventing Heart Attacks: B Vitamins Could Be the Big Players." *University of California at Berkeley Wellness Letter* 14 (2): 1–2 (November 1997).

Rauma, A. L., et al. "Vitamin B-12 Status of Long-Term Adherents of a Strict Uncooked Vegan Diet ('Living Food Diet') Is Compromised." *Journal of Nutrition* 125: 2511–2515 (1995).

Robinson, K., et al. "Hyperhomocysteinemia and Low Pyridoxal Phasphate— Common and Independent Reversible Risk Factors for Coronary Artery Disease." *Circulation* 92: 2825–2830 (1995).

Selhub, Jacob, et al. "Association Between Plasma Homocysteine Concentrations and Extracranial Carotid-Artery Stenosis." *The New England Journal of Medicine* 332: 286–291 (1995).

———. "Vitamin Status and Intake as Primary Determinants of Homocysteinemia in an Elderly Population." *The Journal of the American Medical Association* 270: 2693–2698 (1993).

Stampfer, Meir , et al. "Folate and Cardiovascular Disease: Why We Need a Trial Now." *The Journal of the American Medical Association* 275: 1929–1930 (1996).

———. "A Prospective Study of Plasma Homocysteine and Risk of Myocardial Infarction in U.S. Physicians." *The Journal of the American Medical Association* 268: 877–881 (1992).

———. "Homocysteine and Marginal Vitamin Deficiency: The Importance of Adequate Vitamin Intake." *The Journal of the American Medical Association* 270: 2726–2727 (1993).

Subar, A. F., et al. "Folate Intake and Food Sources in the U.S. Population." *The American Journal of Clinical Nutrition* 50: 508–516 (1989).

Ubbink, J. B., et al. "Vitamin Requirements for the Treatment of Hyperhomocysteinemia in Humans." *Journal of Nutrition* 124: 1927–1933 (1994).

———. "Vitamin B-12, Vitamin B-6, and Folate Nutritional Status in Men with Hyperhomocysteinemia." *The American Journal of Clinical Nutrition* 57: 47–53 (1993).

Whitaker, Julian. "The Smoking Gun in Heart Disease and Stroke." *Dr. Julian Whitaker's Health & Healing* 7 (8): 1–3 (August 1997).

## Chapter 12: The Mighty Minerals

Abraham, Abraham S., et al. "The Effects of Chromium on Established Atherosclerotic Plaques in Rabbits." *The American Journal of Clinical Nutrition* 33: 2294–2298 (1980).

Ackley, Scott, et al. "Dairy Products, Calcium and Blood Pressure." *The American Journal of Clinical Nutrition* 38: 457–461 (1983).

Altura, Burton M., et al. "Magnesium Deficiency and Hypertension: Correlation Between Magnesium-Deficient Diets and Microcirculatory Changes in Situ." *Science* 223: 1315–1317 (1984).

Altura, B. M., and B. T. Altura. "New Perspectives on the Role of Magnesium in the Pathophysiology of the Cardiovascular System." *Magnesium* 4: 226–244 (1985).

Anderson, Richard A. "Chromium Metabolism and Its Role in Disease Processes in Man." *Clinical Physiology and Biochemistry* 4: 31–41 (1986).

Anderson, Richard A., and A. S. Kozlovsky. "Chromium Intake, Absorption and Excretion of Subjects Consuming Self-Selected Diets." *The American Journal of Clinical Nutrition* 41: 1177–1183 (1985).

Anderson, Richard, and Marilyn Polansky. "Chromium May Prevent Type II Diabetes Onset." *Science News* 137: 214 (1990).

Anderson, Richard A., et al. "Chromium Supplementation of Human Subjects: Effects of Glucose, Insulin and Lipid Parameters." *Metabolism* 32: 894–899 (1983).

———. "Effects of Supplemental Chromium on Patients with Symptoms of Reactive Hypoglycemia." *Metabolism* 36 (4): 351–355 (1987).

Belizan, Jose, et al. "Reduction of Blood Pressure with Calcium Supplementation in Young Adults." *The Journal of the American Medical Association* 249: 1161–1165 (1983).

Brattstrom, Lars, et al. "Folic Acid Responsive Postmenopausal Homocysteinemia." *Metabolism* 34 (11): 1073–1077 (1985).

Bucher, Heiner C., et al. "Effects of Dietary Calcium Supplementation on Blood Pressure: A Meta-Analysis of Randomized Controlled Trials." *The Journal of the American Medical Association* 275: 1016–1022 (1996).

Bunker, W., et al. "The Uptake and Excretion of Chromium by the Elderly." *The American Journal of Clinical Nutrition* 39: 797–802 (1984).

———"Calcium: Too Much of a Good Thing?" *Harvard Women's Health Watch* V (2): 7 (October 1997).

Campbell, Wayne, and Richard Anderson. "Effects of Aerobic Exercise and Training on the Trace Minerals Chromium, Zinc, and Copper." *Sports Medicine* 46: 1007 (1987).

Carlson, I. A., et al. "Effect of Oral Calcium upon Serum Cholesterol and Triglycerides in Patients with Hyperlipidemia." *Atherosclerosis* 14: 391 (1971).

Chipperfield, B., and J. R. Chipperfield. "Heart-Muscle Magnesium, Potassium and Zinc Concentrations After Sudden Death from Heart-Disease." *The Lancet* 2: 293 (1973).

Cohen, L., and R. Kitzes. "Magnesium Sulfate and Digitalis-Toxic Arrhythmias." *The Journal of the American Medical Association* 249: 2808–2810 (1983).

Crawford, T., and M. D. Crawford. "Prevalence and Pathological Changes of Ischemic Heart Disease in a Hard-Water and in a Soft-Water Area." *The Lancet* 1: 229 (1967).

Dyckner, T., and P. O. Wester. "Intracellular Potassium After Magnesium Infusion." *British Medical Journal* 286: 1847 (1983).

England, Michael R., et al. "Magnesium Administration and Dysrhythmias After Cardiac Surgery: A Placebo-Controlled, Double-Blind, Randomized Trial." *The Journal of the American Medical Association* 268: 2395–2402 (1992).

Evans, Gary W. "An Inexpensive, Convenient Adjunct for the Treatment of Diabetes." *Western Journal of Medicine* 155 (5): 549 (1991).

Garland, C., E. Barrett-Connor, A. Rossof, et al. "Dietary Vitamin D and Calcium and Risk of Colorectal Cancer: A 19-Year Prospective Study in Men." *The Lancet* 1: 307–309 (1985).

Gordon, Jeffrey. "An Easy and Inexpensive Way to Lower Cholesterol?" *Western Journal of Medicine* 154: 352 (1991).

Gruchow, H. W., et al. "Calcium Intake and the Relationship of Dietary Sodium and Potassium to Blood Pressure." *The American Journal of Clinical Nutrition* 48: 1463–1470 (1988).

"Guidelines Boost Calcium Requirements." *Harvard Health Letter* 22 (12): 7 (October 1997).

Hamet, P. "The Evaluation of the Scientific Evidence for a Relationship Between Calcium and Hypertension." Bethesda, MD: Life Sciences Research Office, *FASEB*, 1993.

Harvey, J. A., et al. "Calcium Citrate: Reduced Propensity for the Crystallization of Calcium Oxalate in Urine Resulting from Induced Hypercalciuria of Calcium Supplementation." *Journal of Clinical Endocrinology* 61: 391–393 (1985).

Heaney, R. P., et al. "Meal Effects on Calcium Absorption." *The American Journal of Clinical Nutrition* 49: 372–376 (1989).

Henderson, D. G., et al. "Effect of Magnesium Supplementation on Blood Pressure and Electrolyte Concentrations in Hypertensive Patients Receiving Long-Term Diuretic Treatment." *British Medical Journal* 293: 664 (1986).

Henry, H. J., et al. "Increasing Calcium Intake Lowers Blood Pressure: The Literature Reviewed." *Journal of the American Dietetic Association* 85: 182–185 (1985).

Holbrook, T. L., et al. "Dietary Calcium and Risk of Hip Fracture: 14-Year Prospective Study." *The Lancet* 2: 1046–1049 (1988).

"Is Chromium Essential for Humans?" *Nutrition Review* 46: 17–20 (1988).

Johansson, G., et al. "Effects of Magnesium Hydroxide in Renal Stone Disease." *Journal of the American College of Nutrition* 1: 179 (1982).

Johnson, N. E., et al. "Effects of Blood Pressure on Calcium Supplementation of Women." *The American Journal of Clinical Nutrition* 42: 12–17 (1985).

Kaplan, N. M. "Non-Drug Treatment of Hypertension." *Annals of Internal Medicine* 102: 359–373 (1985).

Karanja, N., et al. "Impact of Increasing Calcium in the Diet on Nutrient Consumption, Plasma Lipids, and Lipoproteins in Humans." *The American Journal of Clinical Nutrition* 59: 900–907 (1994).

Khaw, K-T., and E. Barrett-Connor. "Dietary Potassium and Stroke-Associated Mortality: A 12-Year Prospective Population Study." *The New England Journal of Medicine* 316: 235–240 (1987).

Khaw, K-T., and S. Thom. "Randomized Double-Blind Cross-Over Trial of Potassium on Blood Pressure in Normal Subjects." *The Lancet* 2: 1127–1129 (1982).

Kok, F. J., et al. "Dietary Sodium, Calcium, and Potassium and Blood Pressure." *American Journal of Epidemiology* 123: 1043–1048 (1986).

Kozlovsky, Adriene S., et al. "Effects of Diets High in Simple Sugars on Urinary Chromium Losses." *Metabolism* 35 (6): 515–518 (1986).

Krishna, G. G., et al. "Increased Blood Pressure During Potassium Depletion in Normotensive Men." *The New England Journal of Medicine* 320: 1177–1182 (1989).

Kurtz, T. W., et al. "'Salt-Sensitive' Essential Hypertension in Men: Is the Sodium Ion Alone Important?" *The New England Journal of Medicine* 317: 1043–1048 (1987).

Langford, H. G. "Dietary Potassium and Hypertension: Epidemiologic Data." *Annals of Internal Medicine* 98 (Part 2): 770–772 (1983).

Levenson, D. I., and R. S. Bockman. "A Review of Calcium Preparations." *Nutrition Review* 52: 221–232 (1994).

Lloyd, Tom, et al. "Dietary Caffeine Intake and Bone Status of Postmenopausal Women." *The American Journal of Clinical Nutrition* 65: 1826–1830 (1997).

MacGregor, Graham, et al. "Moderate Potassium Supplementation in Essential Hypertension. *The Lancet* 2: 567–570 (1982).

McCarron, David A. "Role of Adequate Dietary Calcium Intake in the Prevention and Management of Salt-Sensitive Hypertension." *The American Journal of Clinical Nutrition* 65 (suppl): 712S–716S (1997).

McCarron, D. A., et al. "Randomized Placebo-Controlled Trial of Oral Ca+2 in Human Hypertension." *Clinical Research* 32: 37A (1984).

———. "Dietary Calcium in Human Hypertension." *Science* 217: 267 (1982).

Meneely, G. R., and H. D. Battarbee. "High Sodium–Low Potassium Environment and Hypertension." *The American Journal of Cardiology* 38: 768–785 (1976).

Miller, J. Z., et al. "Calcium Absorption from Calcium Carbonate and a New Form of Calcium (CCM) in Healthy Male and Female Adolescents." *The American Journal of Clinical Nutrition* 48: 1291–1294 (1988).

New, Susan A., et al. "Nutritional Influences on Bone Mineral Density: A Cross-Sectional Study in Premenopausal Women." *The American Journal of Clinical Nutrition* 65: 1831–1839 (1997).

Nicar, M. J., and C.Y.C. Pak. "Calcium Bioavailability from Calcium Carbonate and Calcium Citrate." *Journal of Clinical Endocrinology* 61: 393 (1985).

NIH Consensus Development Panel on Optimal Calcium Intake. "Optimal Calcium Intake." *The Journal of the American Medical Association* 272: 1942–1948 (1994).

Ophir, O., et al. "Low Blood Pressure in Vegetarians: The Possible Role of Potassium." *The American Journal of Clinical Nutrition* 37: 755–762 (1983).

Parrot-Garcia, M., and D. A. McCarron. "Calcium and Hypertension." *Nutrition Review* 42: 205 (1984).

Peterson, D. R., et al. "Water Hardness, Arteriosclerotic Heart Disease, and Sudden Death." *American Journal of Epidemiology* 92: 90 (1970).

Press, Raymond, et al. "The Effect of Chromium Picolinate on Serum Cholesterol and Apolipoprotein Fractions in Human Subjects." *Western Journal of Medicine* 152: 41–45 (1990).

Rasmussen, H. S., et al. "Influence of Magnesium Substitution Therapy on Blood Lipid Composition in Patients with Ischemic Heart Disease." *Archives of Internal Medicine* 149: 1050–1053 (1989).

Recker, R. R., et al. "Calcium Absorption and Achlorhydria." *The New England Journal of Medicine* 313: 70–73 (1985).

Resnick, L. M. "Outpatient Therapy of Essential Hypertension with Dietary Calcium Supplementation." *Journal of the American College of Cardiology* 3: 616 (1984).

Riales, R., and M. Albrink. "Effect of Chromium Chloride Supplementation on Glucose Tolerance and Serum Lipids Including High-Density Lipoproteins of Adult Men." *The American Journal of Clinical Nutrition* 34: 2670–2678 (1981).

Ruddell, H., et al. "Effect of Magnesium Supplementation in Patients with Labile Hypertension." *Journal of the American College of Nutrition* 6: 445 (1987).

Saito, K. H., et al. "Effect of Oral Calcium on Blood Pressure Response in Salt-Loaded Borderline Hypertensive Patients." *Hypertension* 13: 219–226 (1989).

Seelig, M., and A. Heggtveit. "Magnesium Interrelationships in Ischemic Heart Disease: A Review." *The American Journal of Clinical Nutrition* 27: 59–79 (1974).

Simonoff, Monique. "Chromium Deficiency and Cardiovascular Risk." *Cardiovascular Research* 18: 591–596 (1984).

Staub, H., et al. "Serum Cholesterol Reduction by Chromium in Hypercholesterolemic Rats." *Science* 166: 746–747 (1969).

Turlapaty, P. D., and B. M. Altura. "Magnesium Deficiency Produces Spasms of Coronary Arteries: Relationship to Etiology of Sudden Death Ischemic Heart Disease." *Science* 208: 199–200 (1980).

Weinberger, M. H., et al. "The Blood Pressure Effects of Calcium
    Supplementation in Humans of Known Sodium Responsiveness."
    *American Journal of Hypertension* 6: 799–805 (1993).

Witterman, J.C.M., et al. "A Prospective Study of Nutritional Factors and
    Hypertension among U.S. Women." *Circulation* 80: 1320–1327 (1989).

"Yes, But Which Calcium Supplement?" *Tufts University Health & Nutrition
    Letter* 14 (12): 4–5 (February 1997).

## Chapter 13: Quasi-Supplements and Healing Foods and Herbs

Adler, Adam J., and Bruce Holub. "Effect of Garlic and Fish-Oil
    Supplementation on Serum Lipid and Lipoprotein Concentrations in
    Hypercholesterolemic Men." *The American Journal of Clinical Nutrition* 65:
    445–450 (1997).

Baghurst, K. I., et al. "Onions and Platelet Aggregation." *The Lancet* I: 101
    (1977).

Balieu, E. E., "Dehydroepiandrosterone (DHEA): A Fountain of Youth?"
    *Journal of Clinical Endocrinology and Metabolism* 81: 3147–3151 (1996).

Barrett-Connor, Elizabeth, et al. "A Prospective Study of
    Dehydroepiandrosterone Sulfate, Mortality, and Cardiovascular Disease."
    *The New England Journal of Medicine* 315: 1519–1524 (1986).

Block, E. "The Chemistry of Garlic and Onions." *Scientific American* 252:
    114–119 (March 1985).

"Can Green Tea Help Prevent Cancer?" *University of California at Berkeley
    Wellness Letter* 14 (3): 1–2 (December 1997).

"DHEA: The Next HRT." *Harvard Women's Health Watch* III (7): 6 (March
    1996).

"DHEA—The Promise of Youth and Health." *University of California at
    Berkeley Wellness Letter* 12 (4): 1–2 (January 1996).

Ebeling P., and V. A. Koivisto. "Physiological Importance of
    Dehydroepiandrosterone." *The Lancet* 343: 1479–1482 (1994).

Fulder, S. "Garlic and the Prevention of Cardiovascular Disease." *Cardiology in
    Practice* 7: 30–35 (1989).

Haffner, S. M., et al. "Relation of Sex Hormones and Dehydroepiandrosterone
    Sulfate (DHEA–SO4) to Cardiovascular Risk Factors in Postmenopausal
    Women." *American Journal of Epidemiology* 142: 925–934 (1995).

Ishikawa, T., et al. "Effect of Tea Flavenoid Supplementation on the
    Susceptibility of Low-Density Lipoprotein to Oxidative Modification." *The
    American Journal of Clinical Nutrition* 66 (2): 261–266 (1997).

Jain, Adesh K., et al. "Can Garlic Reduce Levels of Serum Lipids? A Controlled
    Clinical Study." *The American Journal of Medicine* 94: 632–635 (1993).

Kamer, Russell, et al. "Does Eating Garlic Lower Cholesterol?" *Annals of Internal Medicine* 120: 969 (1994).

Kendler, B. S. "Garlic *(Allium Sativum)* and Onion *(Allium Cepa)*: A Review of Their Relationship to Cardiovascular Disease." *Preventive Medicine* 16: 670–685 (1987).

Kono, S., et al. "Relation of Green Tea Consumption to Serum Lipids and Lipoproteins in Japanese Men." *Journal of Epidemiology* 6L: 128–133 (1996).

Kosolcharoen, P., et al. "Improved Exercise Tolerance after Administration of Carnitine." *Current Therapeutic Research* 30: 753–764 (1981).

Lau, B.H.S., et al. "*Allium Sativum* (Garlic) and Atherosclerosis: A Review." *Nutrition Research* 10: 137–144 (1987).

Louria, D. B., et al. "Onion Extract in Treatment of Hypertension and Hyperlipidemia: A Preliminary Communication." *Current Therapeutic Research* 37: 127–131 (1985).

Mitchell, L. E., et al. "Evidence for an Association Between Dehydroepiandrosterone Sulfate and Nonfatal, Premature Myocardial Infarction in Males." *Circulation* 89 (1): 89–93 (1994).

Morales, A. J., et al. "Effects of Replacement Dose of Dehydroepiandrosterone in Men and Women of Advancing Age." *Journal of Clinical Endocrinology and Metabolism* 78 (6): 1360–1367 (1994).

"Pressing Garlic for Possible Health Benefits." *Tufts University Diet & Nutrition Letter* 12 (7): 3–4 (September 1994).

"Reduced Salt Area (A Look at Salt Replacers)." *Tufts University Health & Nutrition Letter* 15 (3): 6 (May 1977).

Regelson, W., et al. "Dehydroepiandrosterone (DHEA)—The 'Mother Steroid.'" *Annals New York Academy of Sciences* 719: 543–552 (1994).

Schardt, David, and Bonnie Liebman. "Garlic: Clove at First Sight." *Nutrition Action Health Letter* 22 (6): 3–5 (July/August 1995).

Sinatra, Stephen. "DHEA: Should You or Shouldn't You?" *HeartSense* III (5): 2–5 (May 1997).

Vacha, Gian Maria, et al. "Favorable Effects of L-Carnitine Treatment on Hypertriglyceridemia in Hemodialysis Patients: Decisive Role of Low Levels of High-Density Lipoprotein-Cholesterol." *The American Journal of Clinical Nutrition* 38: 532–540 (1983).

Visudhiphan, S., et al. "The Relationship Between High Fibrinolytic Activity and Daily Capsicum Ingestion in Thais." *The American Journal of Clinical Nutrition* 35: 1452–1458 (1982).

Warshafsky, Stephen, et. al. "Effect of Garlic on Total Serum Cholesterol: A Meta-Analysis." *Annals of Internal Medicine* 119: 599–604 (1993).

Whitaker, Julian. "DHEA Can Prevent Heart Disease." *Dr. Julian Whitaker's Health & Healing* 4 (12): 7–8 (December 1994).

## Chapter 14: Eating and Drinking for Heart Health

"Dueling Food Pyramids: Which One Is Best for Women?" *Women's Health Advocate Newsletter* 1 (11): 4–6 (January 1995).

Heimendinger, Jerianne, and Mary Ann S. Van Duyn. "Dietary Behavior Change: The Challenge of Recasting the Role of Fruit and Vegetables in the American Diet." *The American Journal of Clinical Nutrition* 61 (suppl): 1397S–1401S (1995).

Hertog, M. "Dietary Antioxidant Flavonoids and Risk of Coronary Heart Disease: The Sutphen Elderly Study." *The Lancet* 342: 1007–1011 (1993).

Kawachi, I., et al. "A Prospective Study of Coffee Drinking and Suicide in Women." *Annals of Internal Medicine* 156 (5): 521 (1996).

Liebman, Bonnie. "DASH: A Diet for All Diseases." *Nutrition Action Health Letter* 24 (5): 10–13 (October 1997).

National Research Council. "Diet and Health: Implications for Reducing Chronic Disease Risk." Washington, DC: National Academy Press, 1989.

Palmer, J. R., et al. "Coffee Consumption and Myocardial Infarction in Women." *American Journal of Epidemiology* 141 (8): 724–731 (1995).

Patterson, B. H. "Fruits and Vegetables in the American Diet: Data from the NHANES II Survey." *American Journal of Public Health* 80: 1443–1449 (1990).

Schardt, David, Bonnie Liebman, and Stephen Schmidt. "Going Mediterranean." *Nutrition Action Health Letter* 21 (10): 1–9 (December 1994).

Serafini, M. "Red Wine, Tea and Antioxidants." *The Lancet* 344: 626 (1994).

"Should You Be Eating More Protein—or Less?" *University of California at Berkeley Wellness Letter* 12 (9): 4–5 (June 1996).

U.S. Department of Agriculture. "The Food Guide Pyramid." *Human Nutrition Information Service*, 1992 (publication HG249).

Weinmann, S., et al. "Caffeine Intake in Relation to the Risk of Primary Cardiac Arrest." *Epidemiology* 8 (5): 505–508 (1997).

Willet, W. C., et al. "Coffee Consumption and Coronary Heart Disease in Women: A Ten-Year Follow-up." *The Journal of the American Medical Association* 275 (6): 458–462 (1996).

## Chapter 15: Filling in the Blanks

"Is Your Supplement Dissolving?" *Tufts University Health & Nutrition Letter* 15 (9): 4–5 (November 1991).

Jenkins, D.J.A., et al. "Glycemic Index of Foods: A Physiological Basis for Carbohydrate Exchange." *The American Journal of Clinical Nutrition* 53: 1021S–1026S (1981).

Lachance, R., and L. Langseth. "The RDA Concept: Time for a Change?" *Nutrition Review* 52: 266–270 (1994).

Northrup, Christiane, M.D. "My Healthy Heart Action Plan For You." *Dr. Christiane Northrup's Health Wisdom for Women* 4 (12): 4–6 (December 1997).

Rosenberg, I. H. "Nutrient Requirements for Optimal Health: What Does That Mean?" *Journal of Nutrition* 124: 1777S–1780S (1994).

Sinatra, Stephen, M.D. "Heart Disease Prevention: Answers to Your Questions." *HeartSense* Supplement: 1–8 (1997).

## Chapter 16: Healthy Behaviors for the Heart

"The Angry Woman." *Women's Health Advocate Newsletter* 1 (5): 3–7 (July 1994).

Associated Press. "Road Rage Blamed for More Deaths on Highways." *Marin Independent Journal,* July 18, 1997: A9.

Byrd, Randolph C. "Positive Therapeutic Effects of Intercessory Prayer in a Coronary Care Unit Population." *Southern Medical Journal* 81: 7 (1988).

Mattox, William R. "Church-Going Smokers Reap a Stress Benefit." *The Orange County Register.* Metro 9 (April 9, 1997).

Strawbridge, William J., et al. "Frequent Attendance at Religious Services." *American Journal of Public Health* 86 (6).

# Index

# Index

# ORDER FORM

10% DISCOUNT on orders of $50 or more —
20% DISCOUNT on orders of $150 or more —
30% DISCOUNT on orders of $500 or more —
*On cost of books for fully prepaid orders*

NAME

ADDRESS

CITY/STATE                                    ZIP/POSTCODE

PHONE                                         COUNTRY (outside U.S.)

| TITLE | QTY | PRICE | TOTAL |
|---|---|---|---|
| *Her Healthy Heart* (paperback) | @ | $14.95 | |
| *Menopause Without Medicine* (paperback) | @ | $14.95 | |

*Prices subject to change without notice*

Please list other titles below:

| | | | |
|---|---|---|---|
| | @ | $ | |
| | @ | $ | |
| | @ | $ | |
| | @ | $ | |
| | @ | $ | |
| | @ | $ | |
| | @ | $ | |
| | @ | $ | |

**Shipping Costs:**
First book: $3.00 by book post ($4.50 by UPS or Priority Mail, or to ship outside the U.S.)
*Each additional book: $1.00*
For rush orders and bulk shipments call us at (800) 266-5592

TOTAL _____
Less discount @ _____ %     ( _____ )
TOTAL COST OF BOOKS _____
Calif. residents add sales tax _____
Shipping & handling _____
**TOTAL ENCLOSED** _____
*Please pay in U.S. funds only*

❏ Check    ❏ Money Order    ❏ Visa    ❏ Mastercard    ❏ Discover

Card # _____    Exp date _____

Signature _____

*Complete and send to:*
## Hunter House Inc., Publishers
PO Box 2914, Alameda CA 94501-0914
**Orders: 1-800-266-5592    email: ordering@hunterhouse.com**
Phone (510) 865-5282  Fax (510) 865-4295
❏ Check here to receive our book catalog

HHH 8/98